PHARMACOLOGY - RESEARCH, SAFETY TESTING AND REGULATION

STATINS

PHARMACOLOGY, CLINICAL IMPLICATIONS AND ADVERSE EFFECTS

PHARMACOLOGY - RESEARCH, SAFETY TESTING AND REGULATION

Additional books in this series can be found on Nova's website under the Series tab.

Additional e-books in this series can be found on Nova's website under the e-book tab.

BIOCHEMISTRY RESEARCH TRENDS

Additional books in this series can be found on Nova's website under the Series tab.

Additional e-books in this series can be found on Nova's website under the e-book tab.

PHARMACOLOGY - RESEARCH, SAFETY TESTING AND REGULATION

STATINS

PHARMACOLOGY, CLINICAL IMPLICATIONS AND ADVERSE EFFECTS

BENEDETTA LA GRUA
AND
ALESSANDRO MOLINELLI
EDITORS

Nova Science Publishers, Inc.
New York

For permission to use material from this book please contact us:
Telephone 631-231-7269; Fax 631-231-8175
Web Site: http://www.novapublishers.com

NOTICE TO THE READER

Library of Congress Cataloging-in-Publication Data

Library of Congress Control Number: 2012934334

ISBN: 978-1-62081-367-6

Published by Nova Science Publishers, Inc. † New York

Contents

Preface

Statins work by reducing cholesterol synthesis by inhibiting the enzyme HMG-CoA reductase. The decrease in cholesterol levels is associated with increased expression of receptors of hepatocytes, with a greater extraction of plasma LDL-C and a lower diffusion of it into the tissues. In this book, the authors present current research in the study of the pharmacology, clinical implications and adverse effects of statins. Topics include the pleiotropic effects of statins beyond cholesterol lowering; anti-inflammatory activity of statins in asthma and COPD; statins as anticancer agents; statin use in patients with carotid disease; and the Alzheimer's disease risk-lowering effect of lipophilic statins.

Chapter I - Background: 3-hydroxy-3-methylglutaryl coenzyme A reductase inhibitors (statins) have been increasingly shown among the most effective drugs in reducing the risk of stroke and major cardiovascular events in populations at high vascular risk. Carotid artery disease is an established risk marker for atherosclerosis complications and vascular morbidity and mortality. Advantages of statin therapy have been suggested by surrogate imaging results and by clinical data. The topic of this review is to analyze the effect of statins in patients with carotid stenosis.

Methods: Literature was systematically searched for studies evaluating the outcomes of statins use on carotid revascularization, carotid plaque and occurrence of cerebrovascular clinical events.

Results: Twelve meta-analyses, 27 randomized trials or mega-trials and 8 not-randomized clinical series addressing outcomes after the use of statins in patients with carotid disease, were reviewed. Statins use was various for type, duration and dosage of the drug. Nevertheless, there was consensus on advantages provided by statins in patients with carotid disease and detectable at both early subclinical and later clinical stages. Current evidence indicates that statins therapy significantly benefits patients undergoing carotid surgery or endovascular treatment for carotid stenosis reducing perioperative and long-term morbidity and mortality. Reasons for benefit in carotid revascularization are not only due to the lipid-lowering effect but other pleiotropic mechanisms statins-related are likely implied. Furthermore, statins may stop progression or induce regression of intima-media thickness and may also stop plaque growth by inducing plaque remodeling. Finally, statins appear to reduce the stroke risk and the hazard of all cardiovascular events in patients with carotid stenosis. It seems that with each 1.0 mmol/L reduction in LDL cholesterol by statins the annual rate of major vascular events (ischemic stroke, heart attach, revascularization) is safely reduced by over a fifth.

Conclusions: The benefits provided by statins in patients with carotid disease are confirmed by clinical and imaging data. Mounting evidence supports a link between statins exposure and improved outcomes in patients with carotid stenosis receiving or not a revascularization procedure, even though the mechanisms behind the statin effects are not totally defined. Ongoing research should better clarify this issue as well as how to optimize dosage and duration of statins treatment in these patients.

Chapter II - 3-hydroxy-3-methylglutaryl (HMG)-CoA reductase is a rate-limiting enzyme of the mevalonate pathway for cholesterol synthesis. Statins inhibit this enzyme, thus having functions for lowering cholesterol. There is also a growing body of evidence that statins have pleiotropic effects, independent of lowering cholesterol. These pleiotropic effects are partly exerted by inhibiting synthesis of isoprenoids, which are downstream molecules of the mevalonate pathway, involved in the activation of small GTPases that eventually modulate an intracellular signal cascade. These effects include: (i) anti-atherosclerosis and plaque stabilizating effects by inhibiting various steps of athelogenic and plaque formation cascades; (ii) inhibiting inflammation, which plays a pivotal role in the pathogenesis of atherosclerosis; (iii) neovascularizing or increasing blood flow in ischemic tissue, leading to cardio- and neuroprotective effects and subsequent improvements of vascular dementia; (iv) favorable effects on such neurodegenerative diseases as Alzheimer disease and Parkinson disease; (v) improving bone health through stimulation of bone formation and osteoclast inhibition ; (vi) improving renal dysfunction and preventing the progression of chronic kidney diseases; and finally (vii) negative or at least neutral effects on the development of some kinds of cancers. This chapter highlights current knowledge on the potential mechanisms for statin-mediated pleiotropic effects. Since these pleiotropic effects are significant on the aging-related or lifestyle-related diseases which have increasingly attracted global health concern, e.g. metabolic, neurological, and neoplastic diseases, this chapter will help researchers to develop new treatment strategies that incorporate statins as comprehensively effective agents, ultimately leading to prevent or regress such diseases.

Chapter III - Statins are conventionally known as 3-hydroxy-3-methylglutaryl coenzyme A (HMG-CoA) reductase inhibitors that deplete mevalonic acid. Statins possess pleiotropic effects on the inhibition of multiple inflammatory signals independent of their cholesterol-lowering capacity. Statins suppress mevalonic acid-induced smooth muscle proliferation. In animal studies, statins could inhibit eosinophilic and neutrophilic airway inflammation, a key pathology of asthma and COPD respectively, by modulating a variety of signal transductions. These include the inhibition of guanosine triphosphatase, nuclear factor-κB mediated activation of inflammatory / matrix remodelling pathways, and p38 MAPK mediated eosinophilic inflammation. In addition, statins attenuate airway remodeling, particularly the suppression of airway smooth muscle hyperplasia, and therefore improve airway hyperresponsiveness in asthma. Clinical studies suggested that statins enhance anti-inflammatory effects of corticosteroids on eosinophilic airway inflammation in asthma through the induction of the immunosuppressive indoleamine 2, 3-dioxygenase activity and the release of an anti-inflammatory cytokine, IL-10. Statins also mediate their effective anti-inflammatory effects through the suppression of the mevalonic acid cascade in alveolar macrophages that have emerged as critical modulators in the COPD pathophysiology. This chapter provides the proposed molecular mechanisms underlying the anti-inflammatory / anti-airway remodeling actions and the clinical effectiveness of statins in both asthma and COPD.

Chapter IV - Statins are potent inhibitors of 3-hydroxy-3-methylglutaryl-coenzyme A (HMGCoA) reductase, the rate limiting enzyme in the mevalonate biosynthetic pathway for cholesterol synthesis. The mevalonate pathway is extremely important because it is also involved in the synthesis of sterol and non-sterol intermediates that are essential for tumor cell survival and growth. Specifically, HMGCoA reductase catalyze the conversion of 3-hydroxy-3-methylglutaryl-coenzyme A to mevalonate, which subsequently produces isoprenoid intermediates such as farnesyl pyrophosphate and geranylgeranyl pyrophosphate that are required for posttranslational modification (isoprenylation) of various small GTP-binding proteins and heterotrimeric G-protein γ-subunit. Isoprenylation is needed for anchoring these signaling proteins to the cell membrane in close proximity to growth factor receptors so that these signaling proteins can be activated following receptor activation, and subsequently participate in turning on downstream mitogenic signaling pathways such as MAPK and Akt. HMGCoA reductase activity is characteristically elevated and/or unregulated in many forms of cancer and thereby, acts to promote cancer cell survival and proliferation by providing an abundance of non-sterol intermediates.

As a result, a great deal of attention has been focused on the development of agents that target and inhibit HMGCoA reductase activity for use in cancer chemotherapy. This review will focus on the growing body of research that demonstrates a role for statins as anticancer agents, starting with the origins of statin development as cholesterol lowering therapy and following the unique path they have taken towards anticancer agents. Finally, recent developments in the field will be discussed that indicate statins are poised to make the next step towards providing significant health benefits in the prevention and treatment of various forms of cancer.

Chapter V - Statins are the most potent lipid-lowering agents available today in the pharmaceutical market. They are currently the drugs of choice for the treatment of hypercholesterolemia, several clinical trials have shown that statins substantially reduce cardiovascular morbidity and mortality in patients with and without existing coronary heart disease.

Statins work by reducing cholesterol synthesis by inhibiting the enzyme HMG-CoA reductase. The decrease in cholesterol levels is associated with increased expression of receptors of hepatocytes, with a greater extraction of plasma LDL-C and a lower diffusion of it into the tissues. In addition to its activity on LDL-C, statins increase levels of HDL-C and lead to a decrease in triglycerides. These lipid-lowering activities must add a number of pleiotropic properties that together with the above make this group of drugs an important weapon for influencing the cardiovascular risk patient.

We are in a family of substances with a good safety profile, but its potential toxicity is a fact that should not be ignored. The HMG-CoA reductase inhibitors may be associated with hepatotoxicity and myopathy, which normally do not occur, but in certain circumstances such as interactions, liver failure or differences in gene expression may manifest.

Chapter VI - Statins, the most used lipid-lowering drugs, act classically like inhibitors of HMG-CoA reductase enzyme, blocking one of the most important cholesterol pathways. Reducing production of endogen cholesterol, statins determine an increased expression of LDL receptors that consent removal of "bad cholesterol" from blood by the liver; a reduction of VLDL hepatic production that induce an hipotrygliceridemic effect too; and at the same time an increased HDL production according to statin's different kind. Indeed, statins effectiveness is different and it is demonstrated that atorvastatin and rosuvastatina are more effective than simvastatin, pravastatin, lovastatin and fluvastatin. About their use in clinical practice, physicians exploit their classic effect and their pleiotropic effect too. Statins improve endothelial function, plaque stability and reduce inflammation and platelet aggregation. So today, statins are a very important weapon in the hand of physician. Specifically, importance of statins in secondary prevention of coronary heart disease (CHD) is established from a long time but their use in CHD primary prevention is still discussed because, if the protective effect is proven, on the other hand NNT and costs are so high. Statins find another important employment in prevention of periprocedural outcomes in patients that undergo PCI. For their capacity of plaque stabilization and inflammation lowering, and for an emerging direct effect on Central Nervous System (CNS), statins use is broadened to prevent ischemic stroke and, for the same reason, it is demonstrated their preventing role in CHF progression in particular in patients with metabolic syndrome. At least statins are helpful for management of patients with peripheral artery disease where symptoms reduction and progression are proved. Moreover it was tried to use them in subjects with aortic valve stenosis too, but it is unclear if there is an effective benefit in terms of progression of disease. On the other side, statins are burdened with important side effects that need accurate follow up, considering onset of symptoms, increased hepatic enzyme and attendant use of drugs that interact with P450 cytochrome or that increase myopathy possibility, like fibric acid derivates. Indeed, classical side effects of statins are hepatotoxicity and myopathy up to rhabdomyolysis. These side effects haven't an important incidence but they are more common in case of combination of statins and fibrates. It is also important underline like today research involves itself in study of correlation between statins and cancer and like this dispute is still open. The twelve years follow-up of the 4S studies showed not an increase but a decrease of new cases of cancer using simvastatin.

Chapter VII - Alzheimer's Disease (AD) is considered to be a multifactorial neurodegenerative disorder with a strong genetic component and the role of cholesterol in this pathology is attracting increasing attention. The association of genetic alterations of proteins involved in cholesterol production, distribution and removal from the central nervous system (CNS) and an higher risk of AD point an important link between this lipid and neurodegenerative disease.

Cholesterol has well-known neuroprotective effects, influences synaptic function and its disturbed homeostasis is involved in the pathogenesis of AD.

The use of pharmacological methods to reduce plasma cholesterol levels may have little effect on brain cholesterol if the drugs cannot cross the Blood-Brain-Barrier (BBB) but the most prescribed Statins for AD theraphies are lipophilic ones and long-term treatments could have adverse effects; in fact, a recent study shows an impaired synaptic vesicle release when neuronal cholesterol biosynthesis is inhibited with Lovastatin.

Probably Statins anti-atherosclerotic pleiotropic properties have influenced the outcome of many studies on AD patients because their anti-oxidant and anti-inflammatory effects improve oxygenation of the brain and they be responsible for the apparent reduction in AD risk.

Further studies are required, especially trials able to compare side effects on neuronal cholesterol of hydrophilic statins versus lipophilic ones and design of new drugs in neuropathology field must focus on the importance of brain lipidic pool, avoiding any alteration of it.

In: Statins
Editors: Benedetta La Grua and Alessandro Molinelli
ISBN: 978-1-62081-367-6

Chapter I

Statins Use: Clinical Implications in Patients with Carotid Disease

Paola De Rango, Enrico Cieri, Luca Farchioni, Alessandra Manzone, Paolo Bonanno and Fabio Verzini
Vascular and Endovascular Surgery, Hospital S. M. Misericordia, Perugia, Italy

Abstract

Background: 3-hydroxy-3-methylglutaryl coenzyme A reductase inhibitors (statins) have been increasingly shown among the most effective drugs in reducing the risk of stroke and major cardiovascular events in populations at high vascular risk. Carotid artery disease is an established risk marker for atherosclerosis complications and vascular morbidity and mortality. Advantages of statin therapy have been suggested by surrogate imaging results and by clinical data. The topic of this review is to analyze the effect of statins in patients with carotid stenosis.

Methods: Literature was systematically searched for studies evaluating the outcomes of statins use on carotid revascularization, carotid plaque and occurrence of cerebrovascular clinical events.

Results: Twelve meta-analyses, 27 randomized trials or mega-trials and 8 not-randomized clinical series addressing outcomes after the use of statins in patients with carotid disease, were reviewed. Statins use was various for type, duration and dosage of the drug. Nevertheless, there was consensus on advantages provided by statins in patients with carotid disease and detectable at both early subclinical and later clinical stages. Current evidence indicates that statins therapy significantly benefits patients undergoing carotid surgery or endovascular treatment for carotid stenosis reducing perioperative and long-term morbidity and mortality. Reasons for benefit in carotid revascularization are not only due to the lipid-lowering effect but other pleiotropic mechanisms statins-related are likely implied. Furthermore, statins may stop progression or induce regression of intima-media thickness and may also stop plaque growth by inducing plaque remodeling. Finally, statins appear to reduce the stroke risk and the hazard of all cardiovascular events in patients with carotid stenosis. It seems that with each 1.0 mmol/L reduction in LDL cholesterol by statins the annual rate of major vascular events (ischemic stroke, heart attach, revascularization) is safely reduced by over a fifth.

Conclusions: The benefits provided by statins in patients with carotid disease are confirmed by clinical and imaging data. Mounting evidence supports a link between statins exposure and improved outcomes in patients with carotid stenosis receiving or not a revascularization procedure, even though the mechanisms behind the statin effects are not totally defined. Ongoing research should better clarify this issue as well as how to optimize dosage and duration of statins treatment in these patients.

Introduction

Increasing evidence supports the benefit of lipid lowering in patients with cardiovascular diseases (CVD). However, the effects of use of 3-hydroxy-3-methylglutaryl coenzyme A reductase inhibitors (statins) in patients with carotid stenosis and at higher stroke risk are less evident. In the last years there has been a notable evolution of research also in this field and today there are reasonable data to support the benefit of the use of statins in patients with carotid stenosis disease. Particularly, published data showed benefits from statins in improving

1. stroke prevention.
2. operative outcomes in patients with carotid stenosis.
3. subclinical carotid disease (intimal-media thickness [IMT], carotid plaque regression /endothelial dysfunction).

Literature was systematically searched for studies evaluating the outcomes of statins use on occurrence of cerebrovascular clinical events, carotid revascularization and carotid plaque. Twelve meta-analyses, 27 randomized trials or mega-trials (8 primary prevention, 6 high-risk subgroups, 13 secondary prevention) and 8 not-randomized clinical series addressing outcomes after the use of statins in patients with carotid disease, were identified. Statins use was various for type, duration and dosage of the drug. The current literature reporting on these three major issues is summarized as following.

1. Statins Use and Stroke Prevention

The majority of studies analyzing the effect of statins and carotid disease were focused on clinical outcome reporting on the benefit of statins and stroke prevention. However, the relationship between cholesterol level and stroke risk still remains less clear than that of statins and cardiovascular risks. Abnormal levels of serum lipids, including Low Density Lipoprotein (LDL) and High Density Lipoprotein (HDL) cholesterol (LDL-C, HDL-C), are today well regarded as greater risk factors for coronary artery disease (CAD) according to a number of randomized clinical trials (RCT). The association between hypercholesterolemia and stroke has indeed become more apparent from data of prospective cohort studies (non randomized) that showed higher risks of ischemic stroke with increasing levels of total cholesterol in both men and women.[1,2] Accordingly, elevated levels of total cholesterol confers approximately twofold relative increase in the stroke risk. However, the risk of stroke has been investigated as an endpoint in several RCTs even if these studies were mainly focused on coronary patients or high-risk vascular patients and not specifically analyzed stroke patients. Here, the current evidence from meta-analyses and RCTs reporting on stroke incidence and statins use is summarized.

Meta-Analyses

Several published meta-analyses have provided cumulative data on stroke risk according to pooled results from statins studies.

Comprehensive Meta-Analyses on Stroke Risk of RCTs and Non Randomized Statin Trials

Amarenco et al, *Meta*-Analysis[3,4]

Amarenco et al, performed a systematic review of all RCTs testing statins drugs updated to 2008. The objective of this meta-analysis was to investigate the effect of statins and LDL-C on stroke incidence and stroke mortality, the specific effect of statins on the incidence of hemorrhagic stroke, the relationship between the magnitude of LDL-C reduction and the effect of statins treatment on stroke incidence and, as an ancillary analysis, the relationship between LDL-C reduction and carotid artery IMT change, expressed as percentage increase or decrease per year in IMT studies.

Twenty-four randomized statin trials that included 165,792 individuals at high risk of stroke were identified. Incidence of all strokes was reduced by 18% (95% Confidence Interval [CI] 13–23%, P<0.0001), incidence of fatal stroke was reduced by 13% (95%CI –3 to 27, P=0.10), although this did not reach statistical significance, and incidence of hemorrhagic stroke did not increase (Relative Risk [RR] 1.03, 95%CI, 0.75–1.41, P=0.88), without evidence of heterogeneity across the trials. In a meta-regression analysis of all major statin trials, each 1 mmol/L (39 mg/dL) decrease in concentration of LDL cholesterol equated to a relative risk reduction for stroke of 21.1% (95%CI 63–33.5, P=0.009).

In secondary prevention of non-cardioembolic stroke, intense reduction of LDL cholesterol by statins also significantly reduced the risk of recurrent stroke (RR 0.84, 95%CI 0.71–0.99, P=0.03) and major cardiovascular events (RR 0.80, 95%CI 0.69–0.92, P=0.002).

The combined analysis of all the 6 randomized trials assessing the effect of intensive lipid lowering therapy (including 42,054 patients) showed that, compared with standard statins therapy, intensive statins decreased the risk of any stroke (fatal and nonfatal) by 13% (RR 0.87; 95%CI 4-22%). For major cardiovascular events, including stroke, myocardial infarction (MI) and vascular death, the same meta-analysis found a relative risk reduction of 16% (RR 0.84; 95%CI 8-24%) in the intensive arm compared to the conventional arm.

Moreover, from an ancillary analysis, each 10% reduction in LDL-C was estimated to reduce the carotid IMT by 0.73% per year (95% CI 0.27 to 1.19), in accordance with the 9 trials that met the criteria of this meta-analysis.

In conclusion, from this meta-analysis of RCTs statins use showed a consistent 18% reduction in all strokes compared with control individuals without any increase in hemorrhagic strokes. This effect seemed to be associated with the extent of LDL cholesterol reduction: each LDL cholesterol reduction by 1mmol/L [39mg/dL] decreased the risk of stroke by 21.1%. Statins use also strongly decreased other cardiovascular events in patients with non-cardioembolic stroke regardless of ischemic stroke subtypes. Authors suggested further research to assess the effectiveness and safety of further LDL cholesterol reduction after a stroke.

O'Regan et al, *Meta*-Analysis[5]

O'Regan et al, conducted a comprehensive review of all randomized trials to determine the therapeutic potential of statins for all strokes.

The meta-analysis included any RCTs of any duration, on atorvastatin, fluvastatin, lovastatin, pravastatin, rosuvastatin, and simvastatin assessing statins therapy for all-stroke prevention. RCTs were included if comparing a statin to placebo or no treatment, and reporting on any of the following clinical cardiovascular outcomes: all-cause mortality, all-stroke, fatal stroke, hemorrhagic stroke, or ischemic stroke. Data were pooled using a random-effect model and analyzed with meta regression. Using these criteria, the literature search identified 42 trials for a total of 121,285 patients. Eight studies assessed atorvastatin (total n= 23,724), 6 studies assessed simvastatin (total n=26,146), 5 studies fluvastatin (total n=5,191), 18 pravastatin (total n=57,573), one of which stopped early, 4 studies assessed lovastatin (total n=8,102), and one evaluated any statin. No rosuvastatin trials met the inclusion criteria.

The pooled relative risk (RR) of statins therapy for all-cause mortality on 116,080 individuals was 0.88 (95% CI 0.83-0.93). Each unit increase in LDL resulted in a 0.3% increased RR of death (P =0 .02). Seventeen trials evaluated statins on cardiovascular death (in 57,599 individuals, RR 0.81, 95% CI 0.74-0.90), and 11 evaluated non-hemorrhagic cerebrovascular events (in 58,604 individuals, RR 0.81, 95% CI 0.69-0.94) showing significant decreases. Eleven trials reported hemorrhagic stroke incidence (in a total 54,334 patients, RR 0.94, 95% CI 0.68-1.30) and 21 trials reported on fatal strokes (in a total of 82,278 patients, RR 0.99, 95% CI, 0.80-1.21) without significant difference in rates among statins and controls. Only one trial reported on statins therapy for secondary prevention of stroke (RR 0.85, 95% CI 0.73-0.99, P = 0.04).

The meta-regression technique aimed to evaluate the effects of *a priori* identified covariates on outcomes. These included: specific statin within-class effects, underlying conditions and patient characteristics, dosage, lipid changes, and follow-up. Only absolute LDL changes predicted marked effects: every unit increase in LDL increased mortality risk by 0.3% (RR 1.003, 95% CI, 1.0005-1.006, P=0.02). With the exception of absolute LDL changes, the influence of any covariate using multivariate regression was unpredictable.

Despite the efficacy shown between LDL cholesterol decrease and decreasing mortality, authors were unable to display that cholesterol lowering effects of statins had a protective role in strokes, and suggested that the pleiotropic effect of statins could be more protective in ischemic stroke than LDL reduction alone.

In conclusion, according to this meta-analysis statins therapy seems to provide high levels of protection for all-cause mortality and non-hemorrhagic strokes. This reinforced the need to consider prolonged statins treatment in patients at high risk of major vascular events, but caution remained for patients at risk of bleeds. Authors suggested that other known effects of statins might be more important than LDL reduction in protecting against ischemic stroke. Furthermore, most clinical trials evaluating statins effectiveness occurred as primary prevention trials and few data were available for secondary prevention in stroke patients. Despite the compelling evidence of primary therapeutic protection for strokes, additional statins secondary prevention trials on stroke are needed.

Cholesterol Treatment Trialists' (CTT) Collaboration Meta-Analysis[6]

Cholesterol Treatment Trialists' (CTT) Collaboration meta-analysis was one of the largest and more comprehensive and updated meta-analysis to assess the safety and efficacy of more intensive LDL cholesterol with statins therapy in randomized trials.

Only individual participant data from randomized trials with at least 2 years' statins treatment duration were included. Both more versus less intensive statin regimens and statins versus control treatment trials were included. For each type of trial, the meta-analysis calculated not only the average risk reduction, but also the average risk reduction per 1.0 mmol/L LDL cholesterol reduction at 1 year after randomization. Pre-specified outcomes were cause-specific mortality, major coronary event (death or nonfatal myocardial infarction), stroke and coronary revascularization.

Overall, 26 RCTs were identified, 5 comparing more vs less intensive statin regimens and 21 comparing statins versus control treatment.

Taking all 26 trials together, the risk reduction in major vascular events was 22% ($P<0.0001$) per 1.0 mmol/L reduction in LDL cholesterol at 1 year, with a significant 12% reduction during the first year after randomization ($P<0.0001$) and highly significant reductions of about a quarter during each subsequent year ($P<0.0001$). The risk reduction of first strokes of any type was 16% (95% CI; $P<0.0001$) per 1.0 mmol/L LDL cholesterol reduction, with a highly significant reduction in ischemic stroke (1,427 vs 1,751; RR 0.79, 95% CI 0.74–0.85; $P<0.0001$) and a non-significant excess of hemorrhagic stroke (257 vs 220; RR 1.12, 95% CI 0.93–1.35; $P=0.2$).

In the five trials of more versus less intensive statins therapy (39,612 individuals; median follow-up 5.1 years), the weighted mean reduction in LDL cholesterol at 1 year was 0.51 mmol/L. First major vascular events were recorded in 3837 (4.5% per annum) of 19,829 participants allocated to more intensive versus 4,416 (5.3% per annum) of 19,783 allocated to less intensive therapy, corresponding to a highly significant proportional risk reduction of 15% (95% CI 11–18; $P<0{\cdot}0001$) further reduction in major vascular events, consisting of separately significant reductions in coronary death or nonfatal myocardial infarction of 13% (95% CI 7–19; $P<0.0001$), and in ischemic stroke of 16% (95% CI 5–26; $P=0.005$). Per 1.0 mmol/L reduction in LDL cholesterol, these further reductions in risk were similar to the proportional reductions in the trials of statins versus control. First strokes of any type were recorded in the five trials of more versus less intensive statins therapy in 572 (0.6% per annum) participants allocated to more intensive versus 663 (0.7% per annum) allocated to less intensive therapy. This significant risk reduction of 14% ($P=0.009$) represented a 16% reduction in the risk of ischemic stroke (440 vs 526; RR 0.84, 99% CI 0.71–0.99; $P=0.005$) and a non-significant excess of hemorrhagic stroke (69 vs 57; RR 1.21, 99% CI 0.76–1.91; $P=0.3$).

In the meta-analysis of 21 trials of statins versus control (129,526 individuals; median follow-up 4.8 years), 7,136 (2.8% per annum) of 64,744 participants allocated to statins therapy had first major vascular events versus 8934 (3.6% per annum) of 64,782 allocated to control, corresponding to a highly significant 22% ($P<0{\cdot}0001$) risk reduction with a 1.07

mmol/L LDL cholesterol reduction. In comparisons among these 21 trials, larger absolute reductions in LDL cholesterol were associated with larger proportional reductions in risk (trend P<0·0001). Overall, the weighted average reduction in major vascular events was 21% (P<0·0001) per 1·0 mmol/L reduction in LDL cholesterol. The proportional reduction in the incidence of stroke per 1.0 mmol/L LDL cholesterol reduction was non-significantly larger in the trials of more versus less intensive statins therapy (26% reduction) than in those of statins versus control (15% reduction).

Across all 26 trials, all-cause mortality was reduced by 10% per 1.0 mmol/L LDL reduction (RR 0.90, 95% CI 0·87–0·93; P<0.0001), largely reflecting significant reductions in deaths due to coronary heart disease (RR 0.80, 99% CI 0.74–0.87; P<0·0001) and other cardiac causes (RR 0.89, 99% CI 0.81–0.98; P=0.002), with non-significant effect on deaths due to stroke (RR 0.96, 95% CI 0.84–1.09; P=0.5) or other vascular causes (RR 0.98, 99% CI 0.81–1.18; P=0.8). No significant effects were observed on deaths due to cancer or other non-vascular causes (RR 0.97, 95% CI 0.92–1.03; P=0.3) or on cancer incidence (RR 1.00, 95% CI 0.96–1.04; P=0.9) even at low LDL cholesterol concentrations.

Deaths were recorded for 3,593 participants in the five trials of more versus less intensive statins therapy and for 12,376 in the 21 trials of statins versus control. For each category of deaths, the proportional reductions in risk per 1.0mmmol/L LDL cholesterol reduction did not differ between the two types of trial comparison.

This meta-analysis concluded that reduction in LDL cholesterol may safely produce further reductions in the incidence of ischemic stroke and cardiac complications with each 1.0mmmol/L reduction reducing the annual rate of these major vascular events by just over a fifth.

Meta-Analyses on Stroke Risk Focused on Primary Prevention Statin Trials

Cochrane Meta-Analysis[7]

The Cochrane Collaboration group undertook and recently published a systematic review to assess the effects, both harms and benefits, of statins in people with no history of Cardiovascular disease (CVD). RCTs of statins with minimum duration of one year and follow-up of six months, in adults with no restrictions on their total low LDL or HDL cholesterol levels, and where 10% or less had a history of CVD, were included. Outcomes included all cause mortality, fatal and nonfatal Cardiac Heart Disease (CHD), CVD and stroke events, combined endpoints (fatal and nonfatal CHD, CVD and stroke events), change in blood total cholesterol concentration, revascularization, adverse events, quality of life and costs.

Fourteen randomized control trials (16 trial arms; 34,272 participants) were included. Eleven trials recruited patients with specific conditions (raised lipids, diabetes, hypertension, microalbuminuria). Authors found that all-cause mortality was significantly reduced by statins (RR 0.84, 95% CI 0.73 to 0.96) as was combined fatal and nonfatal CVD endpoints (RR 0.70, 95% CI 0.61 to 0.79). Benefits were also seen in the reduction of revascularization rates (RR 0.66, 95% CI 0.53 to 0.83). Total cholesterol and LDL cholesterol were reduced in all trials but there was evidence of heterogeneity of effects. There was no clear evidence of any significant harm caused by statins prescription or of effects on patient quality of life.

Seven trials with 21,556 participants reported on combined fatal and nonfatal stroke events. Only one trial was stopped prematurely was able to demonstrate a significant reduction in this combined outcome with the use of statins. The significant reduction was maintained in the pooled analysis using a fixed effects model: 2.1% events; RR 0.78 (95% CI 0.65-0.94). Only one trial with 6,595 participants reported on fatal stroke events and another one with 255 participants on nonfatal stroke events. No significant risk reduction was seen for these endpoints: fatal stroke events, 0.2%; RR 1.50 (95% CI 0.42-5.30) and nonfatal stroke events, 0.4%; RR 2.98 (95%CI 0.12-72.39).

Only three trials with 17,452 participants reported a composite of fatal and nonfatal events for CHD, CVD and stroke. All three of the trials showed a significant reduction in this composite outcome with the treatment of statins which was maintained in the pooled analysis and using a fixed model: 5.4% events; RR 0.70 (95% CI 0.61-0.79).

The findings of this meta-analysis confirmed that reductions in all-cause mortality, major vascular events and revascularizations can be found with no excess of cancers or muscle pain among people without evidence of cardiovascular disease treated with statins. However, authors raised concerns that there was evidence of selective reporting of outcomes and failure to report adverse events. Only limited evidence showed that primary prevention with statins could be cost effective and could improve patient quality of life and authors concluded suggesting caution in prescribing statins for primary prevention among people at low cardiovascular risk.

Thavendiranathan et al, Meta-Analysis[8]

This meta-analysis included published RCTs with use of statins and 80% or more of the population without cardiovascular (CV) disease. Seven trials with 42,848 patients were included. Ninety percent had no history of CV disease. Mean follow-up was 4.3 years. According to this meta-analysis statins therapy reduced the relative risk (RR) of major coronary events, major cerebrovascular events, and revascularizations by 29.2% (95% CI 16.7%-39.8%; P<0.001), 14.4% (95%CI 2.8%-24.6%; P=0.02), and 33.8% (95% CI 19.6%-45.5%; P<0.001), respectively. Statins produced a non-significant 22.6% RR reduction in coronary heart disease mortality (95% CI 0.56-1.08; P=0.13). Non-significant reduction in overall mortality (RR, 0.92;95%CI, 0.84-1.01; P=0.09) was observed.

Thereby this pooled analysis of primary prevention trials on statins suggested that in patients without CV disease, statins therapy may decrease the incidence of major coronary and cerebrovascular events and revascularizations but not coronary heart disease or overall mortality.

Brugts et al, Meta-Analysis[9,10]

The meta-analysis of Brugts et al. examined the effectiveness of statins in reducing all cause mortality and major coronary and cerebrovascular events in people without established cardiovascular disease but with cardiovascular risk factors, and whether these effects were similar in men and women, in young and older (>65 years) people, and in people with diabetes mellitus.

Ten randomized trials for a total of 70,388 people, of whom 23,681 (34%) were women and 16,078 (23%) had diabetes mellitus, were included. Mean follow-up was 4.1 years.

Statins therapy was associated with a significant risk reduction in all cause mortality of 12%, in major coronary events of 30%, and in major cerebrovascular events of 19%. Specifically, Authors found that treatment with statins significantly reduced the risk of all cause mortality (odds ratio [OR] 0.88, 95% CI, 0.81 to 0.96), major coronary events (OR 0.70, 95%CI, 0.61 to 0.81), and major cerebrovascular events (OR 0.81, 95%CI 0.71 to 0.93). Overall, 2.3% (767/33793) of participants in the control group had a major cerebrovascular event compared with 1.9% (627/33683) in the statins group (19% risk reduction; OR 0.81, 95%CI 90.71 to 0.93). The annual rate for major cerebrovascular events with placebo was 0.6%. No heterogeneity in treatment effect was observed for endpoints in men and women and for age (≤65 and >65 years) or diabetic status. Furthermore, no evidence of an increased risk of cancer was observed with statins use. According to this meta-analysis in patients without established cardiovascular disease but with cardiovascular risk factors, statins use was associated with significantly improved survival and large reductions in the risk of major cerebrovascular and cardiovascular events. These results were in line with those previously published on the effects of statins in secondary prevention.

Meta-Analysis on Stroke Risk Focused on Secondary Prevention Statin Trials

Spector et al, Meta-Analysis[11]

Spector et al, recently published a meta-analysis on statin trials reporting on secondary prevention. To answer questions about the optimal statins dose in coronary artery disease patients, Authors performed simple and meta-analyses of 3 large long-term (approximately 5 years) dose-clinical response randomized trials and compared the results with older randomized trial including long-term safety data. Results of active comparator trials (trials comparing two different strategies of statins use) vs trials comparing statins vs placebo were also analyzed. A total of 15,488 patients under low statins dosage compared to 15,465 under high statins dosage and 2,221 under statins dosage compared to 2,223 under placebo were analyzed. The results showed that raising the dose of simvastatin or atorvastatin to 80mg conferred no mortality advantage, an increase in adverse reactions and only a slight decrease in myocardial infarctions and stroke versus a lower dose. Regarding stroke, in the combined analysis of active comparators trials stroke occurred in 608 (3.9%) of patients randomized to higher dosage vs 525 (3.4%) of those randomized to lower dosage resulting in 0.5% (95% CI 0.1 to 0.9) significant reduction in incidence. In trials with conventional comparison of statins vs placebo, the relative risk of stroke in statins group was 1.1% (95% CI 0.2 to 2.0). These results suggested a cost-effective approach of a single safe dose (40mg of inexpensive generic simvastatin or atorvastatin) for almost all CAD patients and might make treatment-to-goal and cholesterol monitoring unnecessary; moreover, simplifying statins dosage it was likely to improve the weakness in statins use (medication compliance).

Meta-Analysis on Hemorrhagic Stroke and Statins Use

Hackam et al, Meta-Analysis[12]

Hackam et al, undertook a systematic review to specifically assess the risk of intracerebral hemorrhage with the use of statins. Authors included published and unpublished data from 23 randomized trials (48% in primary prevention and 52% in secondary prevention settings) and 19 observational studies (including cohort studies and case-control series) for a total of 248,391 patients and 14,784 intracerebral hemorrhages. Authors did not find statistically increased risk of cerebral hemorrhage with the use of statins in each type of publication group. From the 23 randomized trials the median LDL cholesterol reduction achieved was 1.03 mmol/L [interquartile range (IQR) 0.93–1.36 mmol/L]. The summary random-effects Risk ratio (RR) for intracerebral hemorrhage was 1.10 (95% CI, 0.86–1.41) and the equivalent absolute risk increase was 0.027% (95% CI, -0.042 to 0.096). Authors also found reductions in total stroke (RR, 0.85; 95% CI, 0.78–0.93) and ischemic stroke (RR, 0.83; 95% CI, 0.75– 0.92) with statins use.

Furthermore, in meta-regression, among the randomized trials, no association between intracerebral hemorrhage and the degree of LDL lowering achieved (P=0.91), on-treatment LDL (P=0.90), or the type of statins used (P=0.53) was found.

From the 19 observational studies (117,948 patients) included, statins use was not associated with increased risk of intracerebral hemorrhage: in cohort studies, RR, 0.94; 95% CI,0.81–1.10; in or case-control studies, RR, 0.60; 95% CI, 0.41– 0.88.

This systematic review suggested that even if a risk of intracerebral hemorrhage from statins was been supposed, there was no enough evidence to support this risk. The absolute magnitude of intracerebral hemorrhagic risk from statins is likely to be small and outweighed by the other cardiovascular benefits of these drugs.

Meta-Analysis Focused on Complications in Statins Use (Diabetes)

Preiss et al, Meta-Analysis[13]

High dosage of statins may be associated with increased adverse event and lower tolerability. This meta-analysis aimed to investigate whether intensive-dose statins therapy was associated with increased risk of new-onset diabetes compared with moderate-dose statins therapy from published randomized trials on statins. Authors included randomized controlled endpoint trials that compared intensive-dose statins therapy with moderate-dose statins therapy and included more than 1,000 participants who were followed up for more than 1 year. Five statin trials were included. Authors found that from these trials with 32,752 participants without diabetes at baseline, 2,749 developed diabetes (1,449 assigned intensive-dose therapy, 1300 assigned moderate-dose therapy, representing 2.0 additional cases in the intensive-dose group per 1,000 patient years) and 6,684 experienced cardiovascular events (3,134 and 3,550, respectively, representing 6.5 fewer cases in the intensive-dose group per 1,000 patient-years) over a weighted mean follow-up of 4.9 years. Odds ratios were 1.12 (95% CI, 1.04-1.22) for new-onset diabetes and 0.84 (95%CI, 0.75-0.94) for cardiovascular events for participants receiving intensive therapy compared with moderate-dose therapy. As compared with moderate-dose statins therapy, the number needed to harm per year for intensive-dose statins therapy was 498 for new-onset diabetes while the number needed to treat per year for intensive-dose statins therapy was 155 for cardiovascular events. Odds ratios for specific components of the composite cardiovascular endpoint showed similar associations between intensive statins therapy and each cardiovascular endpoint component. Intensive-dose therapy was not associated with lower rates of nonfatal stroke as compared with moderate-dose statins therapy (OR, 0.90; 95% CI, 0.78-1.03; 4.75% in patients receiving intensive therapy vs 5.39% in patients receiving moderate doses) or with lower all-cause mortality compared with moderate- dose statins therapy.

Therefore, authors raised concerns that, according to the pooled analysis of data from 5 statin trials, intensive-dose statins therapy was associated with an increased risk of new-onset diabetes compared with moderate dose statins therapy.

Meta-Analyses Focused on Surrogate Endpoints (Lipid Levels) and Stroke Outcomes with Statins Use

Prospective Studies Collaboration. Meta-Analysis[14]

The Prospective Studies Collaboration group performed a meta-analysis to analyze the relationship between cholesterol levels and vascular events in primary prevention settings. This meta-analysis combined prospective studies of vascular mortality that recorded both blood pressure and total cholesterol at baseline, to determine the joint relevance of these two risk factors. Information was obtained from 61 prospective observational studies mostly in western Europe or North America, consisting of almost 900,000 adults without previous disease and with baseline measurements of total cholesterol and blood pressure. During nearly 12 million person years at risk between the ages of 40 and 89 years, there were more than 55,000 vascular deaths (34,000 ischemic heart disease [IHD], 12,000 stroke, 10,000 other). Information about HDL cholesterol was available for 150,000 participants, among whom there were 5000 vascular deaths (3000 IHD, 1000 stroke, 1000 other).

Authors found that 1 mmol/L lower total cholesterol was associated with about a half (hazard ratio [HR] 0.44 [95% CI 0.42–0.48]), a third (HR 0.66 [95% CI 0.65–068]), and a sixth (HR 0.83 [95% CI 0.81–0.85]) lower IHD mortality in both sexes at ages 40–49, 50–69, and 70–89 years, respectively. The proportional risk reduction decreased with increasing blood pressure, since the absolute effects of cholesterol and blood pressure were approximately additive. Of various simple indices involving cholesterol, the ratio total/HDL cholesterol was the strongest predictor of IHD mortality (40% more informative than non-HDL cholesterol and more than twice as informative as total cholesterol). Total cholesterol was weakly positively related to ischemic and total stroke mortality in early middle age (40–59 years), but this finding could be largely or wholly accounted for by the association of cholesterol with blood pressure. Moreover, a positive relation was seen only in middle ages and only in patients with below-average blood pressure; at older ages (70–89 years) and, particularly, for those with systolic blood pressure over about 145mmHg, total cholesterol was negatively related to hemorrhagic and total stroke mortality. Lower total cholesterol was weakly positively related to lower ischemic and total stroke mortality in early middle age (40-59 years, total stroke, HR 0.90 [95%CI 0.84-0.97], ischemic stroke n=225 HR 0.73 [95%CI 0.61-0.87]), but this finding could be largely or wholly accounted for by the association of cholesterol with blood pressure <145mmHg (total stroke HR 0.94[95%CI 0.90-0.99];ischemic stroke HR 0.92[95%CI 0.82-1.03]). The results for other vascular mortality were intermediate between those for IHD and stroke.

From this meta-analysis total cholesterol was positively associated with IHD mortality in both middle and old age and at all blood pressure levels. There was conclusive evidence from randomized trials that statins substantially reduced not only coronary event rates but also total stroke rates in patients with a wide range of ages and blood pressures. However, the absence of an independent positive association of cholesterol with stroke mortality, especially at older ages or higher blood pressures, remained unexplained requiring further research.

Kizer et al, Meta-Analysis[15]

The benefits from statins are often framed in terms of percent reductions in LDL-C from baseline or percent reduction between control and treatment groups, even though epidemiological data suggest that absolute inter-group difference in LDL-C (ΔLDLControl-Rx) is the more informative measure. The Kizer et al, meta-analysis aimed to evaluate the efficacy of statins for prevention of cardiovascular disease based on assessment of cholesterol levels. This meta-analysis underlined the relevance of absolute reductions in LDL-C to the design and interpretation of trials analyzing lipid- lowering therapies.

The Authors conducted a systematic review of large-scale trials of statins versus placebo, usual care or active (lower-dose statins) control to calculate updated summary estimates of risk reduction in coronary heart disease and all-cause mortality. Meta-regression analysis was used to ascertain the relations of different LDL-C metrics to outcome. Absolute inter-group difference in LDL-C (Δ LDL in Control vs treatment= Δ LDLContro-Rx) was analyzed.

Twenty large scale trials were included, for a total of 155,255 participants. Three trials were active comparators using in the control group a statin different from the treatment group. The remaining 17 trials focused on use of statins versus placebo or usual care.

In 20 included RCTs, there were significant overall reductions for CHD (OR=0.72, 95% CI=0.67–0.78) and mortality (OR=0.89, 95% CI=0.84–0.94), but with substantial variability in trial results. ΔLDLControl-Rx was the strongest determinant of CHD risk reduction, particularly after excluding active-comparator studies, and was independent of baseline LDL-C. By contrast, baseline LDL-C approached ΔLDLControl-Rx as the strongest determinant of mortality, but neither was significant after exclusion of the 3 active-comparator studies. The exclusion of 3 active comparators RCTs, however, rendered ΔLDLControl-Rx the predominant determinant of mortality reduction.

The findings of this meta-analysis underscored the relevance of absolute reductions in LDL-C to the design and interpretation of RCTs of lipid- lowering therapies.

Meta-Analysis Focused on Subclinical Carotid Stenosis (Plaque Progression) and Statins Use

Kang et al, Meta-Analysis[16]

Authors performed a systematic review to evaluate the efficacy and safety of statins therapy on the rate of carotid atherosclerosis progression through RCTs. Literature was searched from 1980–to 2003. Studies were included when reporting on symptomatic or asymptomatic early stage carotid atherosclerosis patients with hypercholesterolemia or familial hypercholesterolemia. Both studies using conventional dosage of statins (atorvastatin, simvastatin, pravastatin, lovastatin, fluvastatin, 20–40 mg/d) and aggressive dosage of statins (atorvastatin, simvastatin, pravastatin, lovastatin, fluvastatin, 80mg/d) were analyzed. Outcome was the progression of carotid atherosclerosis and plaque evaluated through measurement of B-mode ultrasound stratified by the use of statins: aggressive dosage or conventional dosage were compared with control group (placebo or conventional statins therapy).

Ten studies were selected, including 3,443 individuals, age range from 30 to 70 years old and follow-up for 1-4 years. Five studies used 40mg daily dosage of pravastatin, two studies lovastatin 20–40 and 80mg daily, respectively, another study fluvastatin 40mg daily, and another atorvastatin 80mg and simvastatin 40mg daily. In addition, a trial with atorvastatin 80mg and pravastatin 40mg daily was included. Duration of treatment was 4 years in two studies, 3 years in five studies, 2 years in two other studies, and 1 year in one study. In 8 studies treatment group with statins was compared to control group with placebo, in two trials treatment group with aggressive dosage of statins was compared to control group with conventional therapy (aggressive dosage of statins indicated atrovastatin 80mg/d, conventional therapy indicates simvastatin 20–40 mg/d or provastatin 40mg/d). All the 10 selected trials demonstrated that statins significantly improved hypercholesterolemia.

Eight studies showed that mean IMT was consistently significantly different between statins and placebo, the Z score for overall effect of IMT was 10.41 ($P < 0.00001$), total 95%CI of weighted mean difference (WMD) between two groups was −0.02235 [−0.02656, −0.01614] (mm/y). However the $\chi 2$ test for heterogeneity of IMT among eight studies showed significant differences ($P < 0.00001$). Although the heterogeneity was significant, studies indicated that conventional statins therapy was efficient in prevention of carotid atherosclerosis progression in the long-term.

Two reports between aggressive statins and conventional therapy demonstrated that the Z score for overall effect of IMT was 15.85 ($P < 0.00001$), total 95%CI of WMD between two groups was −0.06326 [−0.07108, −0.05544] (mm/y) with borderline $\chi 2$ -test for heterogeneity between different studies ($P = 0.050$).

The overall findings of this systematic review suggested that conventional statins therapy was efficient and safe to decrease the rate of carotid atherosclerosis progression in the long-term, and aggressive statins might provide superior efficacy for carotid atherosclerosis regression.

RCTs Reporting on Stroke Risk with Statins Use

Randomized trials to analyze the stroke risk with statins have been conducted in different settings of patients at stroke risk and with different dosage and strategies of statins use. Main findings by type of statins are shown in Tables I and II.

RCTs Reporting on Stroke Risk with Statins Use for Primary Prevention

West of Scotland Coronary Prevention Study (WOSCOPS)[17,18]

The West of Scotland Coronary Prevention Study (WOSCOPS) was the first trial to assess primary prevention of stroke with statins. The trial was performed in Scotland and demonstrated the effectiveness of pravastatin (40mg/d) in reducing morbidity and mortality from CHD in moderately hypercholesterolemic men. The trial was designed to test the hypothesis that reduction of serum cholesterol with pravastatin reduced the incidence of fatal and nonfatal myocardial infarction. The principal endpoints were: death due to coronary artery disease plus nonfatal myocardial infarction; death due to CAD; and nonfatal myocardial infarction.

Table I.

Trial Name	Primary or secondary prevention	Regimens	Pts.	Follow-up years	Inclusion criteria	Total Cholesterol level	RRR for Stroke	P value
Atorvastatin								
ASCOT [22,23]	primary	10mg/day vs placebo	10297	5.0	hypertension with at least other 3 risk factors	<252mg/dL	27%	0.024
CARDS [24]	primary	10mg/day vs placebo	2838	3.9	at least one of: retinopathy, albuminuria, smoking or hypertension	LDL<160mg/dL Triglyc<262mg/dL	48%	<0.05
ASPEN [28]	mixed	10mg/day vs placebo	2410	4.0	type 2 diabetes, LDL below guideline targets	LDL<140mg Triglyc<600mg/dL	n.s.	n.r.
4D[33]	mixed	20mg/day vs placebo	1255	4.0	type 2 diabetes, hemodialysis	LDL<121mg/dL	2.3%	0.04
ALLIANCE [45]	secondary	10-80 mg/day vs usual care	2443	4.3	CHD	LDL 130-250 mg/day without lipid-lowering therapy or 110-200 with lipid-lowering therapy	13%	n.s.
GREACE [46]	secondary	10-80mg/day vs usual care	1600	3.0	CHD	LDL>100mg/dL	47%	0.0017
MIRACL [48]	secondary	80mg vs placebo	3086	16 weeks	acute MI or unstable angina	<270 mg/dL	50%	0.04
Simvastatin								
HPS [29,30,31]	mixed	40mg/day versus placebo	20536 (3280 with previous stroke)	5.0	CHD, diabetes or other vascular disease (e.g. stroke)	>135mg/dL	25% ; 20% vascular events in pts. with stroke	0.0001
SHARP [35]	mixed	20mg/day+ ezetimibe 10 mg/day vs placebo	9270	4.9	chronic kidney disease (with no myocardial infarction or coronary revascularization)	-	25%	0.01

Table I. (Continued)

Trial Name	Primary or secondary prevention	Regimens	Pts.	Follow-up years	Inclusion criteria	Total Cholesterol level	RRR for Stroke	P value
4S [36,37]	secondary	10-40mg/day vs placebo	4444	5.4	MI, unstable angina	>270mg/dL	30%	0.024
Pravastatin								
WOSCOP [17,18]	primary	40mg/day vs placebo	6596	4.9	Hypercholesterolemia	LDL>270mg/dL	11%	n.s.
ALLHAT-LLT[20,21]	primary	40mg/day vs usual care	10355	4.8	Hypertension	LDL 120-198mg/dL or 100-129 with CHD and triglycerides <350mg/dL	9%	n.s.
KLIS [26]	primary	10-20mg/day vs placebo	5640	5.0	-	>220mg/dL	22%	n.s.
MEGA [27]	primary	10-20mg/day vs usual care	8114	5.3	hypercholesterolemia bodyweight of 40kg or more	220-270mg/dL	n.s.	0.33
PROSPER [32]	mixed	40mg/day vs placebo	5804 (3280 with previous stroke/TIA)	3.2	risk factors (hypertension, diabetes, smoke) or vascular disease (CHD, stroke)	150-350mg/dL	3%	n.s.
CARE [38]	secondary	40mg/day vs placebo	4159	4.8	MI	>249mg/dL and LDL 115-174 mg/dL	31%	0.03
LIPID [39]	secondary	40mg/day vs placebo	9014	6.1	MI, unstable angina	155-271mg/dL	19%	0.048
GISSI [40]	secondary	20mg/day vs no treatment	4271	1.9	acute MI	>200mg/dL	-9%	n.s.
SPARCL [41,42,43]	secondary	80mg/day vs placebo	4731	4.9	Cerebrovascular disease	LDL>100 and <190 mg/dL	33% in pts with carotid stenosis	0.02

Trial Name	Primary or secondary prevention	Regimens	Pts.	Follow-up years	Inclusion criteria	Total Cholesterol level	RRR for Stroke	P value
Lovastatin								
AFCAPS/ TexCAPS [19]	primary	20-40mg/day vs placebo	6605	5.2	no atherosclerotic cardiovascular disease, average or below average cholesterol levels	LDL 130–190mg/dL and HDL ≤45mg/dL for men and ≤47mg/dL for women	n.r.	n.r.
Rosuvastatin								
JUPITER [25]	primary	20mg/day vs placebo	17802	1.9	no history of cardiovascular disease	LDL<130mg/dL, hsCRP>2.0mg/L	48%	0.002
AURORA [34]	mixed	10mg/day vs placebo	2773	4.6	end stage renal disease and hemodialysis	LDL>100mg/dL	n.r.	0.42

Pts: Patients; RRR: Relative Risk Reduction; LDL: low density lipoprotein; Triglyc: Triglyceride; MI : Myocardial Infarction; CHD: Coronary Heart Disease; TIA: Transient Ischemic Attack; HDL: High density lipoprotein; hsCRP:high-sensitivity C-reactive protein; n.r.:not reported; n.s. :non-significant.

Table II. Active comparators

Trial Name	Primary or secondary prevention	Regimens	Pts.	Follow-up years	Inclusion criteria	Total Cholesterol level	RRR for Stroke	P value
A-to-Z trial[44]	secondary	simvastatin: 40mg/day (1 month) then 80mg/day; placebo (1 month then simvastatin 20mg/day)	4497	6-24 months	acute CHD	<250mg/dL	30%	n.s.
IDEAL[47]	secondary	atorvastatin 80mg/day vs simvastatin 20mg/day	8888	4.8	MI	-	13%	n.s.
SEARCH[49]	secondary	simvastatin 80mg/die vs 20mg/die	12064	6.7	MI	135mg/dL if already on a statin or 174mg/dL if not	9%	0.30
TIMI 22[50]	secondary	pravastatin 40mg/day versus atorvastatin 80mg/day	4162	2.0	acute CHD	<240mg/dL	-9%	n.s.
TNT[51,52]	secondary	atorvastatin 10mg/day vs 80mg/day	10001	4.9	CHD	LDL<130mg/dL	25% in favor of 80mg/day	0.02

Pts: patients; RRR: Relative Risk Reduction; MI: Myocardial Infarction; CHD: Coronary Heart Disease; LDL: low density lipoprotein; n.s.: non-significant.

In addition to the main endpoints, the effect of treatment on fatal and nonfatal strokes, death from cardiovascular causes, death from any cause, and the frequency of coronary revascularization procedures were analyzed.

6595 men aged 45-64 years were randomized to treatment with either pravastatin (40 mg/day) or placebo.

Pravastatin lowered plasma cholesterol levels by 20% and LDL-C levels by 26%, whereas there was no change with placebo. There were 248 definite coronary events (specified as nonfatal myocardial infarction or death from coronary heart disease) in the placebo group, and 174 in the pravastatin group (relative reduction in risk with pravastatin, 31%; 95 %CI, 17 to 43; P< 0.001). There were similar reductions in the risk of definite nonfatal myocardial infarctions, death from coronary heart disease and death from all cardiovascular causes. However, there was not relevant difference between treatment groups in the numbers of strokes that were only reduced by a non-significant 11% (95%CI -30 to 60; p=0.57) in the pravastatin group. Similarly, a non-significant 22% reduction in the risk of death from any cause in the pravastatin group (95 %CI, 0 to 40%; P=0.051) was found. There was no excess of deaths from non-cardiovascular causes in the pravastatin group.

From this primary prevention trial, treatment with pravastatin significantly reduced the incidence of myocardial infarction and death from cardiovascular causes but not of stroke in men with moderate hypercholesterolemia and no history of myocardial infarction.

Air Force/Texas Coronary Atherosclerosis Prevention Study (AFCAPS/TexCAPS)[19]

The Air Force/Texas Coronary Atherosclerosis Prevention Study (AFCAPS/TexCAPS) was the second trial analyzing effect of statins on primary prevention in a low-to-moderate risk cohort. The trial was a randomized, double-blind, placebo-controlled trial conducted at 2 sites in Texas that included healthy man and women with no evidence of atherosclerotic cardiovascular disease and average or below average cholesterol levels. At study entry, LDL-C had to be 130–190 mg/dL and HDL-C ≤45 mg/dL for men and≤47 mg/dL for women. Participants were randomized to either lovastatin 20–40 mg/day (n = 3304) or placebo (n = 3301) for a mean follow-up period of 5.2 years.

At 1 year, in the lovastatin group TC, LDL-C, and triglyceride (TG) were reduced by 18.4%, 25.0%, and 15%, respectively. HDL-C increased by 6.0%.

At 5 years, there was a significant 37% decrease in the relative risk for having a first acute coronary event (P=0.00008) and a significant 39% reduction in major coronary events (OR, 0.61; 95%CI 0.45-0.83) in the lovastatin versus placebo group. Women showed similar relative risk reduction as men. Older individuals benefited as much as younger ones from lovastatin. Subjects with ≥2 risk factors benefited more from statins than those with <2 risk factors. However, regarding the effect on cerebrovascular events, the use of lovastatin did not allow significant reduction of risks: 14 events occurred in the 3304 patients in lovastatin group vs 17 in the 3301 patients with placebo resulting in a non-significant reduction (OR 0.82 ,95%CI 0.40 to 1.67).

These first two trials on primary prevention confirmed that it was possible to reduce the risk of cardiovascular events in healthy individuals with the use of statins. However, the effect of the use of statins for primary prevention of cerebrovascular disease remained uncertain.

Antihypertensive and Lipid-Lowering Treatment to Prevent Heart Attack Trial (ALLHAT-LLT)[20,21]

The lipid-lowering trial (LLT) component of the Antihypertensive and Lipid-Lowering Treatment to Prevent Heart Attack Trial (ALLHAT) (ALLHAT-LLT) was originally intended as a double-blind trial to evaluate the effects of cholesterol lowering with a statin drug in a population that was hypertensive and moderately hypercholesterolemic but without evident vascular disease. The principal objectives of the ALLHAT-LLT were to evaluate the impact of large sustained cholesterol reductions on all-cause mortality in a hypertensive cohort with at least 1 other CHD risk factor and to assess CHD reduction and other benefits (including incidence of stroke and heart failure) in populations that had been excluded or underrepresented in previous trials, particularly older persons, women, racial and ethnic minority groups, and persons with diabetes.

Ambulatory persons (n=10,355), aged 55 years or older, with LDL-C of 120 to 189 mg/dL (100 to 129 mg/dL if known CHD) and triglycerides lower than 350 mg/dL, were randomized to pravastatin 40mg/d (n=5,170) or to usual care (n=5,185) in a ratio of 1:1.

Pravastatin did non-significantly reduce all-cause mortality or the incidence of coronary events or stroke, when compared with usual care. However, in the course of the study, nearly one-third of those allocated to usual care were treated with lipid-lowering drugs, which resulted in a smaller differential in total cholesterol reduction between the two groups.

After 2 years of follow-up, the total cholesterol level declined in both the pravastatin group and in the usual care group. The resultant absolute difference in the percentage change from baseline in total cholesterol between the pravastatin and usual care group was thus just 11% .

At year 4, total cholesterol levels continued to decline in both groups, with the total cholesterol differences between the pravastatin and usual care group narrowing slightly to about 10%: reduction by 17% with pravastatin vs 8% with usual care.

All-cause mortality was similar for the 2 groups (RR, 0.99; 95% CI, 0.89-1.11; P=0.88), with 6-year mortality rates of 14.9% for pravastatin vs 15.3% with usual care.

Rates of stroke were somewhat lower in the pravastatin than in the usual care group, but without statistical relevance. There were 209 total strokes in the pravastatin group and 231 in usual care (RR, 0.91; 95% CI, 0.75-1.09; P=0.31). Heart failure rates were similar in the 2 groups. Similarly CHD event rates were non-significantly different between the groups (RR, 0.91; 95% CI, 0.79-1.04; P=0.16), with 6-year CHD event rates of 9.3% for pravastatin and 10.4% for usual care.

A sub-analysis of ALLHAT, showed that non-blacks had higher benefit from pravastatin on stroke risk reduction when compared with usual care while blacks had a significantly lower benefit: RR 1.12 vs 0.74; P=0.03. At opposite, pravastatin showed a significant more favorable effect on CHD events in blacks than in non-blacks: RR 0.73 vs 1.02; P=0.03.

Unlike most other statin trials, ALLHAT-LLT did not show a significant lowering of CHD, stroke, or total mortality with statins use. This has been attributed to the modest difference in cholesterol lowering between the intervention and usual care groups (10%), which was less than half of the average for other long-term statin trials. In addition the trial results suggested that pravastatin was effective in preventing CHD in blacks.

Anglo-Scandinavian Cardiac Outcomes Trial—Lipid Lowering Arm (ASCOT-LLA)[22,23]

The Anglo-Scandinavian Cardiac Outcomes Trial—Lipid Lowering Arm (ASCOT-LLA), was a placebo-controlled randomized trial of the effects of atorvastatin 10 mg daily in the primary prevention of CHD in hypertensive subjects who had a total cholesterol level <6.5 mmol/L. ASCOT-LLA was part of a factorially designed trial in which hypertensive patients with no prior history of CHD were initially randomized to one of two antihypertensive treatment strategies [a beta-blocker adding a thiazide diuretic as required or a dihydropyridine calcium channel blocker (CCB), adding an angiotensin converting enzyme inhibitor as required (ASCOT-BPLA)].

Of the total 19,342 hypertensive patients enrolled in ASCOT-BPLA, 10,305 were further assigned to either atorvastatin, 10 mg/d, or placebo in the ASCOT-LLA trial. The primary outcome of ASCOT-LLA was combined CHD or nonfatal myocardial infarction. Secondary outcomes included fatal and nonfatal stroke, all coronary events, all cardiovascular events and procedures, cardiovascular mortality, all cause mortality, development of chronic stable angina, heart failure, and peripheral arterial disease. ASCOT-LLA was stopped prematurely after a median 3.3 years follow-up due to substantial benefits of atorvastatin on the primary endpoint of nonfatal myocardial infarction and fatal CHD, together with significant reductions in several other cardiovascular endpoints.

Despite the trial termination, Trial physicians were invited to offer atorvastatin to all ASCOT-LLA patients until the end of ASCOT-BPLA and the cardiovascular outcomes of those subjects originally assigned either atorvastatin or placebo in the LLA were followed-up to 5.5 years.

By the end of ASCOT-LLA, there was a 36% relative risk reduction in primary events (n =254) in favor of atorvastatin The occurrence of primary events was significantly reduced in the atorvastatin group in comparison with the placebo group (100 vs 154 events, HR 0.64; 95%CI 0.50-0.83; P=0.0005). Fatal and nonfatal strokes were also significantly reduced in the atorvastatin group compared with the placebo group (89 v 121 events; HR 0.73; 95%CI 0.56-0.86; P=0.024).

At the end of ASCOT-BPLA, 2.2 years later, despite extensive crossovers from and to statins usage, the relative risk reduction in primary events (n = 412) among those originally assigned atorvastatin remained at 36% (HR 0.64, 95% CI: 0.53–0.78, P = 0.0001). There were also significant reductions in a number of secondary endpoints at the end of LLA which were sustained until the end of BPLA, including fatal and nonfatal strokes (21% vs 23%), total cardiovascular events and procedure (23% vs 19%), total coronary events (29% vs 27%) and all cause mortality (13% vs 15%). The risk reduction in all stroke associated with assignment to atorvastatin (3.2% vs 4.1%, HR 0.77 , 95%CI 0.63-0.95; p=0.013) and the risk of reduction in all cause mortality (7.5% vs 8.7% , HR 0.85; 95%CI 0.74-0.98;p=0.022) achieved significance. For almost all other endpoints, risk reductions also remained essentially unchanged.

In conclusion, benefits in the extended follow-up with atorvastatin, albeit with substantial numbers of fatal and nonfatal events reported, accounted for unchanged relative risk reductions in most cardiovascular endpoints observed more than 2 years after ASCOT-LLA closed.

Collaborative Atorvastatin Diabetes Study (CARDS)[24]

The Collaborative Atorvastatin Diabetes Study (CARDS) was a double-blinded, randomized, placebo-controlled multicenter trial of atorvastatin (10mg/d) for the primary prevention of CVD in type 2 diabetes.

The trial hypothesis was that since LDL can vary considerably in its cholesterol content, lowering LDL-C as a goal of statins treatment implied the existence of considerable variation in the extent to which statins treatment removed circulating LDL particles. This consideration was particularly applicable in diabetes mellitus, in which LDL was frequently depleted of cholesterol.

In the CARDS study 2,838 Type 2 diabetes (68% men between 40 and 75years of age) from 132 centres in the UK and Ireland were randomly allocated to 10mg/day atorvastatin (n=1,154) or to placebo (n=1,196) for 1 year. The two arms of the trial were analyzed to compare spontaneous and statins-induced apolipoprotein B (apo B) concentrations (a measure of LDL particle concentration) at LDLC and non-HDL cholesterol (non-HDL-C) concentrations proposed as statins targets in type 2 diabetes.

The primary endpoint was first acute coronary heart disease event, stroke or coronary revascularization procedure. In addition information on all cause of deaths was collected.

To enter to the trial patients had to be free of macrovascular disease, to have serum LDL-C concentration <4.14mmmol/L (< 160mg/dL) and to have fasting serum triglyceride concentration <6.78mmol/l (<600mg/dL). In addition, study participants were required to have at least one cardiovascular risk factors including hypertension, retinopathy, proteinuria, or current smoking.

The trial was stopped 2 years earlier than planned at the request of the Safety Committee because of the clear benefit of statins treatment. The median time of patients participation in the trial was 3.9 years.

Patients allocated to atorvastatin had a significantly lower rate of cardiovascular events than those who received placebo (relative rate reduction 37% [95% CI –52 to –17], P=0.001). Treatment would be expected to prevent at least 37 major vascular events per 1000 such people treated for 4 years. Assessed separately, acute coronary heart disease events were reduced by 36%, coronary revascularizations by 31%, and rate of stroke by 48%. Atorvastatin reduced the death rate by 27% (P=0·059). No excess of adverse events was noted in the atorvastatin group.

Patients treated with atorvastatin produced lower serum apo B concentrations at any given LDL-C concentration than patients on placebo. An LDL-C concentration of 1.8 mmol/L (70 mg/dL) during atorvastatin treatment was equivalent to a non-HDLC concentration of 2.59 mmol/L (100 mg/dL) or an apo B concentration of 0.8 g/L.

At the more conservative LDL-C targets of 2.59 mmol/L (100 mg/dL) and 3.37 mmol/L (130 mg/dL) for non-HDLC, however, the apo B concentration exceeded the 0.9-g/L value anticipated in the Consensus Statement from the American Diabetes Association and the American College of Cardiology. The apo B concentration provided a more consistent goal for statins treatment than the LDLC or non-HDLC concentration.

From this primary prevention trial, atorvastatin 10mg daily was safe and efficacious in reducing the risk of first cardiovascular disease events, including stroke, in patients with type 2 diabetes and without high LDL-cholesterol levels.

Justification for the Use of Statins in Prevention: An Intervention Trial Evaluating Rosuvastatin (JUPITER)[25]

The Justification for the Use of statins in Prevention: an Intervention Trial Evaluating Rosuvastatin (JUPITER) was a randomized, double-blind, placebo controlled, multicenter trial to assess whether healthy patients (elevated high sensitivity C reactive protein levels but without hyperlipidemia) might benefit from statins treatment (rosuvastatin). The study was conducted at 1,315 sites in 26 countries. The tested hypothesis was whether rosuvastatin could decrease cardiovascular morbidity and mortality as compared with placebo in non-hyperlipidemic healthy subjects. JUPITER participants did not have to be qualified for statins therapy according to the existing guidelines for the management of dyslipidemia.

Men 50 years of age or older and women 60 years of age or older were eligible for the trial if they did not have a history of cardiovascular disease and if, at the initial screening visit, they had an LDL cholesterol level of less than 130 mg per deciliter (3.4 mmol per liter) and a high-sensitivity C-reactive protein (hs-CRP) level of 2.0 mg per liter or more. These apparently healthy men and women were randomly allocated in a 1:1 ratio to receive rosuvastatin 20mg daily or placebo and followed for all cause mortality, major cardiovascular events and adverse events including stroke.

The primary outcome was the occurrence of a first major cardiovascular event, defined as nonfatal myocardial infarction, nonfatal stroke, hospitalization for unstable angina, an arterial revascularization procedure, or confirmed death from cardiovascular causes. Secondary endpoints included the components of the primary endpoint considered individually — arterial revascularization or hospitalization for unstable angina, myocardial infarction, stroke, or death from cardiovascular causes — and death from any cause.

The trial was stopped after a median follow-up of 1.9 years (maximum, 5.0 years). JUPITER revealed that rosuvastatin 20 mg/d decreased LDL-C levels by 50% and hs-CRP levels by 37%. Also, rosuvastatin was associated with a significant decrease in the combined primary endpoint of myocardial infarction, stroke, arterial revascularization, hospitalization for unstable angina, or death from cardiovascular causes by 44% compared with placebo. Apart from this benefit in the primary endpoint, impressive reductions in the incidence of separate cardiovascular outcomes, including myocardial infarction (by 54%), stroke (by 48%) and revascularization for unstable angina (by 47%) compared with placebo were noted in the rosuvastatin-treated arm. A reduction by 47% was also observed in the secondary combined endpoint of myocardial infarction, stroke, or death from cardiovascular causes.

At the time of study termination the rates of the primary endpoint were 0.77 and 1.36 per 100 person years of follow-up in the rosuvastatin and placebo groups, respectively (HR for rosuvastatin, 0.56; 95% CI, 0.46 to 0.69; $P<0.00001$), with corresponding rates of 0.17 and 0.37 for myocardial infarction (HR, 0.46; 95% CI, 0.30 to 0.70; $P = 0.0002$), 0.18 and 0.34 for stroke (HR, 0.52; 95% CI, 0.34 to 0.79; $P = 0.002$), 0.41 and 0.77 for revascularization or unstable angina (HR, 0.53; 95% CI, 0.40 to 0.70; $P<0.00001$), 0.45 and 0.85 for the combined endpoint of myocardial infarction, stroke, or death from cardiovascular causes (HR , 0.53; 95% CI, 0.40 to 0.69; $P<0.00001$), and 1.00 and 1.25 for death from any cause (HR, 0.80; 95% CI, 0.67 to 0.97; $P = 0.02$).

The rosuvastatin group did not have a significant increase in myopathy or cancer but did have a higher incidence of physician-reported diabetes (270 reports of diabetes, vs. 216 in the placebo group; $P = 0.01$).

Since the first release of JUPITER, many secondary analyses of this study have come to the light with regard to the results of the study into separate subgroups of the study population. Also, JUPITER authors performed secondary analysis to assess the role of rosuvavstatin in subgroups and specifically analyzed in a separate analysis the effect on stroke.

Rosuvastatin was associated with a decrease in the risk of stroke by 48% compared with placebo, a rate which was similar also for nonfatal strokes. A decrease by 51% associated with rosuvastatin treatment was noted for ischemic strokes, which accounted for the majority of all strokes. Nevertheless, no effect of rosuvastatin treatment was noted with regard to the risk of hemorrhagic stroke or transient ischemic attacks.

Rosuvastatin-related benefits in the risk of stroke were similar in different groups according to age, sex, ethnicity, the presence of traditional risk factors for stroke, including age > 70 years, smoking, hypertension and a family history of premature stroke or a Framingham risk score > 10%. As with other vascular outcomes, the greatest reduction in stroke risk was noted among patients who achieved LDL-C levels < 70 mg/dL and hs-CRP < 2 mg/L.

In conclusion, in this trial of apparently healthy persons without hyperlipidemia but with elevated high-sensitivity C-reactive protein levels, rosuvastatin significantly reduced the incidence of major cardiovascular events and strokes without a systematic increase in reported adverse events. Nevertheless, physician-reported diabetes was more frequent in the rosuvastatin group.

The effect of statins use on stroke incidence for primary prevention was investigated by two Japanese trials,[26,27] suggesting the efficacy of pravastatin in lipid lowering and decreasing stroke risks in Asian populations. The efficacy was provided also with low drug dose:

Kyushu Lipid Intervention (KLIS)[26]

The Kyushu Lipid Intervention Study (KLIS), was the first large-scale primary prevention intervention study for hypercholesterolemia in Japan. A total of 5,640 male patients aged 45–74 years with a serum Total Cholesterol (TC) of 220 mg/dL (5.69 mmol/L) or greater were recruited by 902 physicians in the Kyushu District during the period from May 1990 to September 1993. Excluded from enrollment were those with a history of myocardial infarction, coronary bypass surgery, coronary angioplasty, cerebral hemorrhage, or Cerebral Infarction (CI); those with HDL-C concentration of 80 mg/dl (2.07 mmol/L) or greater; and those who had other specified life-limiting conditions.

In the protocol, pravastatin was prescribed at a dosage of 10–20 mg/day, and the conventional treatment included dietary and/or exercise therapy and medication with hypolipidemic drugs such as fibrates and nicotinic acid, excluding probucol, bezafibrate, and statins. The primary endpoint was CHD events such as fatal and nonfatal myocardial infarction, coronary artery surgery, coronary angioplasty, cardiac death, and sudden and unexpected death. CI was a secondary endpoint diagnosed as when typical symptoms and signs were accompanied with diagnostic findings on brain imaging or cerebral angiography; diagnosis based only on clinical signs and symptoms was regarded as a suspected case.

Pravastatin use was associated with statistically non-significant decreases in the risks of CHD events and CI in men with moderately elevated concentrations of serum TC. However, a greater reduction in serum TC was associated with a progressive decrease in the risk of CHD events as well as of CI. The decreased risk was more evident for CI. Men with a 15% or greater reduction in serum TC showed a statistically significant 61% decrease in the risk of CI, as compared with those with the least reduction in serum TC. As compared with those having an achieved concentration of TC 240 mg/dL (6.20 mmol/L) or higher, those with an attained concentration of less than 240 mg/dL (6.20 mmol/L) showed an approximately 50% lower risk of CHD events. The risk of CI was approximately 70% lower in the categories below 220 mg/dL (5.68 mmol/L).

From this Japanese trial it seemed that lowering serum total cholesterol below 220 mg/dL (5.68 mmol/L) was desirable with regard to the prevention of CI.

Management of Elevated Cholesterol in the Primary Prevention Group of Adult (MEGA)[27]

The Management of Elevated cholesterol in the primary prevention Group of Adult Japanese (MEGA) study, was a large-scale clinical study conducted in Japanese patients with mild or moderate hyperlipidemia to evaluate the primary preventive effect of pravastatin in daily clinical practice in Japan. In this prospective, randomized, open-labelled, blinded study, patients with hypercholesterolemia (total cholesterol 5.69–6.98 mmol/L) and no history of coronary heart disease or stroke were randomly assigned diet or diet plus 10–20 mg pravastatin daily. The primary endpoint was the first occurrence of coronary heart disease. Secondary endpoints included stroke, coronary heart disease plus cerebral infarction, all cardiovascular events, and total mortality.

Eligible patients were randomly assigned to either diet or diet plus pravastatin by computerized randomization by the permuted-block method. Treatment in the diet plus pravastatin group was started at 10mg per day pravastatin. During follow-up, the dose of pravastatin could be adjusted by the treating physician, with up-titration to 20mg per day if the total cholesterol concentration did not decrease to 5.69 mmol/L or less. This dose of pravastatin contrasted with the higher dose (20–40 mg) recommended in Europe and the USA. The follow-up period was initially scheduled for 5 years; however, on the basis of recommendations from the data and safety monitoring committee, the study was continued for an additional 5 years to increase the number of events.

3,966 patients were randomly assigned to the diet group and 3,866 to the diet plus pravastatin group. Mean follow-up was 5.3 years. At the end of study, mean total cholesterol was reduced by 2.1% (from 6.27 mmol/L to 6.13 mmol/L) and 11.5% (from 6.27 mmol/L to 5.55 mmol/L) and mean LDL cholesterol by 3.2% (from 4.05 mmol/L to 3.90 mmol/L) and 18.0% (from 4.05 mmol/L to 3.31 mmol/L) in the diet and the diet plus pravastatin groups, respectively.

Treatment with pravastatin was associated with a lower incidence of stroke than diet alone, although this difference was non-significant (HR 0.83, 95% CI 0.57–1.21; P=0.33). However, the incidence of coronary heart disease and cerebral infarction was significantly lower with pravastatin than with diet alone (HR 0.70, 95% CI 0.54–0.90; P=0.005). In addition, the rates of all cardiovascular events were significantly lower in the diet plus pravastatin group than in the diet group (HR 0.74, 0.59–0.94; P=0.01).

The incidence of coronary heart disease was significantly lower in the diet plus pravastatin group than in the diet group (HR 0.67, 95% CI 0.49–0.91; P=0.01). The number needed to treat (NNT) to prevent one coronary heart disease event with diet plus pravastatin was 119 during the average 5.3 years follow-up. The frequency of myocardial infarction was also significantly lower in the diet plus pravastatin group than in the diet group (HR 0.52, 95%CI 0.29–0.94; P=0.03; NNT 255). Although treatment with pravastatin was associated with lower total mortality than with diet alone, this result was non-significant (HR 0.72, 95%CI 0.51–1.01; P=0.055).

Authors also investigated the major endpoints at 5 years to assess the effect of extending the trial in those patients who consented to continue. Differently from early results, at 5 years, significant reductions were noted for stroke (P=0.03) and total mortality (P=0.048), although these data were from much smaller numbers of patients.

This study showed that in low-risk Japanese populations—eg, hypercholesterolemic patients with high HDL cholesterol— less aggressive cholesterol-lowering therapy (low doses of pravastatin) might be sufficient to produce a substantial and beneficial risk reduction for the primary prevention of coronary heart disease and stroke in the long term.

RCTs Reporting on Stroke Risk with Statins Use in High-Risk Populations and Mixed (Primary and Secondary) Prevention Settings

Atorvastatin Study for Prevention of Coronary Heart Disease Endpoints in Non-Insulin-Dependent Diabetes Mellitus (ASPEN)[28]

The purpose of Atorvastatin Study for Prevention of Coronary Heart Disease Endpoints in Non-Insulin-Dependent Diabetes Mellitus (ASPEN) was to assess the effect of 10mg of atorvastatin versus placebo on primary CVD prevention in subjects with type 2 diabetes and LDL cholesterol levels below contemporary guideline targets.

Subjects were randomly assigned to receive 10 mg of atorvastatin or placebo in a 4-year, double-blind, parallel-group study. The composite primary endpoint comprised cardiovascular death, nonfatal myocardial infarction, nonfatal stroke, recanalization, coronary artery bypass surgery, resuscitated cardiac arrest, and worsening or unstable angina requiring hospitalization.

A total of 2,410 subjects with type-2 diabetes were randomized. Mean LDL cholesterol reduction in the atorvastatin group over 4 years was 29% versus placebo ($P < 0.0001$). When comparing atorvastatin versus placebo, composite endpoint reductions were not statistically significant: composite primary endpoint rates 13.7% and 15.0%, respectively (HR 0.90; 95% CI 0.73-1.12).

Major cerebrovascular events occurred in similar rates among the two trial arms: in 27 of 959 patients under atorvastatin and in 29 of the 946 patents in the placebo group; OR 0.92 (95% CI 0.54 to 1.56).

For these reasons, the results of the ASPEN did not confirm the benefit of statins therapy but do not detract from the imperative that the majority of diabetic patients are at risk of coronary heart disease and deserve LDL cholesterol lowering to the recommended targets.

Heart Protection Study (HPS)[29,30,31]

The Medical Research Council and British Heart Foundation (MRC/BHF) Heart Protection Study (HPS), was established to assess the long-term efficacy and safety of lowering LDL cholesterol concentrations with statins treatment for stroke and cardiovascular disease prevention. This mega-trial included large numbers of people at substantial risk of death from both vascular and other causes including coronary disease, other occlusive arterial disease, or diabetes.

According to the original protocol, data were reported at 5 year follow-up. However, at the final follow-up, participants were encouraged to continue their allocated study treatment (unless it was contraindicated).The aim of the extended 11-year follow-up of the HPS was to assess long-term efficacy and safety of lowering LDL cholesterol with statins, and report cause-specific mortality and major morbidity in the in-trial and post-trial periods.

In this study, 20,536 men and women aged about 40–80 years, who were at increased risk of vascular events (with coronary disease, other occlusive arterial disease, diabetes or treated hypertension), were randomly allocated to receive 40 mg simvastatin daily or matching placebo. Previous myocardial infarction was reported by 8,510 (41%), other history of coronary disease by 4,876 (24%), and no history of coronary disease by 7150 (35%). Among the 7,150 participants without diagnosed coronary disease, 1,820 had cerebrovascular disease, 2,701 had peripheral arterial disease, and 3,982 had diabetes mellitus (with some having more than one of these three conditions), whereas among the 13,386 with known coronary disease, 1,460, 4,047, and 1,981, respectively, had these conditions. The large size of the study produced good balance between the treatment groups for the main pre-randomization prognostic features that were measured.

The primary outcome for analyses was the first post-randomization major vascular event (defined as nonfatal myocardial infarction or coronary death, fatal or nonfatal stroke, coronary or non-coronary revascularization). Secondary outcomes were: major vascular events during each year of follow-up and in various subcategories of patients; major coronary events (ie, nonfatal myocardial infarction or coronary death), strokes, and revascularizations separately; deaths from vascular and non-vascular causes separately; and cancers at all sites.

Mean follow-up during the in-trial period for all randomized participants was 5.3 years, and the mean total follow-up for participants who survived to the end of the post-trial period was 11.0 years. Of 20,536 participants, 17,519 were still alive at the start of the post-trial follow-up period: 8,863 allocated to simvastatin versus 8,656 to placebo. Overall, 96,784 person-years of follow-up were available for those originally allocated simvastatin and 95,084 for those allocated placebo.

During the in-trial period, allocation to simvastatin yielded an average reduction in LDL cholesterol of 1.0 mmol/L and a proportional decrease in major vascular events of 23% (95% CI 19–28; P<0.0001), with significant divergence each year after the first. During the post-trial period (when statins use and lipid concentrations were similar in both groups), no further significant reductions were noted in either major vascular events (risk ratio [RR] 0.95; 95%CI 0.89–1.02) or vascular mortality (RR 0.98, 95%CI 0.90–1.07).

During the in-trial period, all cause mortality was reduced among patients receiving simvastatin in comparison with those receiving placebo (12.9% vs 14.7%; P=0.0003) and similarly was reduced the rate of nonfatal myocardial infarction or coronary deaths. Fewer patients receiving simvastatin had a nonfatal stroke than patients receiving placebo: 444 (4.3%) vs 585 (5.7%), P<0.0001.

In a subgroup analysis of the 3,280 individuals with previous cerebrovascular disease, there was no apparent reduction in the stroke rate, which challenged the efficacy of statins in the secondary prevention of stroke. In HPS however, there was a 20% reduction in the rate of any major vascular event among cerebrovascular disease patients receiving statins therapy rather than placebo: 406 (24.7%) vs 488 (29.8%); P=0.001. The risk of stroke was reduced by about 25% in many other subgroups, including those with diabetes or coronary disease, those younger or older than 70 years of age and those presenting with various levels of blood pressure or lipids. The reduction in stroke incidence was non-significant during the first year, but was significant (P=0.0004) by the end of the second year.

During the combined in-trial and post-trial periods, non-significant differences were recorded in cancer incidence at all sites (RR 0.98, 95%CI 0·92–1.05) or any particular site, or in mortality attributed to cancer (RR 1.01, 95%CI 0.92–1.11) or to non-vascular causes (RR 0.96, 95%CI 0.89–1.03).

Collectively, findings of HPS provided compelling evidence that lowering LDL cholesterol by about 1 mmol/L reduced vascular mortality and morbidity including stroke by about a quarter in a wide range of patients (including elderly people and those with low cholesterol concentrations), without increasing the risk of non-vascular mortality or morbidity (apart from a small myopathy excess) during about 5 years of treatment.

More prolonged LDL-lowering statins treatment produced larger absolute reductions in vascular events. Moreover, even after study treatment stopped in HPS, benefits persisted for at least 5 years without any evidence of emerging hazards from statins use.

Prospective Study of Pravastatin in the Elderly at Risk (PROSPER)[32]

The aim of the PROspective Study of Pravastatin in the Elderly at Risk (PROSPER) study was to test the benefits of pravastatin treatment in an elderly cohort of men and women with, or at high-risk of developing, cardiovascular disease and stroke.

The study was a RCT in which 5,804 (2,520 from Scotland, 2,184 from Ireland, and 1,100 from the Netherlands) men (n=2,804) and women (n=3,000) aged 70—82 years with a history of, or risk factors for, vascular disease were assigned to pravastatin (40mg per day; n=2,891) or placebo (n=2,913). Baseline cholesterol concentrations ranged from 4.0 mmol/L to 9.0 mmol/L. Follow-up was 3.2 years on average and the primary endpoint was a composite of fatal or nonfatal stroke, coronary death, and nonfatal myocardial infarction.

Pravastatin lowered LDL cholesterol concentrations by 34% and significantly reduced the incidence of the primary endpoint to 408 events compared with 473 on placebo (HR 0.85, 95% Cl 0.74—0.97, P=0.014). Coronary heart disease death and nonfatal myocardial infarction risk was also reduced (292 events in treated patients vs 356 placebo, HR 0.81, 95% CI 0.69—0.94, P=0.006). Stroke risk was non-significantly changed between the two groups: 4.5% vs 4.7% events in placebo vs pravastatin group; HR 1,03, 95% CI 0.81—1.31, P=0.8; rates of nonfatal stroke were 4.1% vs 4.0% and those of fatal stroke were 0.5% vs 0.8%, in placebo vs pravastatin groups respectively. However, the HR for transient ischemic attack was borderline decreased of 0.75 (rates 3.5% vs 2.7%; 95% CI 0.55-1.00, P=0·051) in the pravastatin group. Furthermore, pravastatin reduced the risk of the composite primary endpoint by 15%. When the primary endpoint was separated into its coronary and cerebrovascular components, there was a 19% reduction in coronary events, but no discernible effect on cerebrovascular events. New cancer diagnoses were more frequent on pravastatin than on placebo (HR 1.25, 95%CI 1.04—1.51, P=0.020). However, when authors incorporated this finding in a meta-analysis of all pravastatin and all statin trials, they showed no overall increase in cancer risk. Mortality from coronary disease fell by 24% (P=0.043) in the pravastatin group. Pravastatin had non-significant effect on cognitive function or disability.

According to this study findings, pravastatin given for 3 years reduced the risk of coronary disease in elderly individuals. However, the effect on cerebrovascular risk was not relevant. PROSPER trial suggested to extent to elderly individuals the treatment strategy currently used in middle aged people.

Three RCTs Specifically Addressed the Effects of Statins in Patients with Renal Disease[33-35]

Die Deutsche Diabetes Dialyse (4D)[33]

The German Diabetes and Dialysis Study (4D) showed that atorvastatin had no statistically significant effect on cardiovascular death, nonfatal myocardial infarction, and stroke in patients with diabetes receiving hemodialysis.

The 4D was a multicenter, randomized, double-blind, prospective study aimed to investigate the benefit of statins in patients with type 2 diabetes mellitus and receiving hemodialysis, who were at high risk for cardiovascular disease and death. In 4D, 1,255 subjects with type 2 diabetes mellitus and receiving maintenance hemodialysis for less than two years were randomly assigned to receive 20 mg of atorvastatin per day or matching placebo at 178 centers in Germany. The primary endpoint was a composite of death from cardiac causes, nonfatal myocardial infarction, and stroke. Secondary endpoints included death from all causes and all cardiac and cerebrovascular events combined. Data were recorded at four weeks and then every six months.

After four weeks of treatment, the median level of LDL-C was reduced by 42% among patients receiving atorvastatin, and by 1.3% among those receiving placebo. During a median follow-up period of four years, 469 patients (37%) reached the primary endpoint, without statistical differences between atorvastatin and placebo groups: relative risk, 0.92; 95 %CI 0.77 to 1.10; P=0.37). Atorvastatin had non-significant effect on the individual components of the primary endpoint, except that the relative risk of fatal stroke was unexpectedly increased among those receiving the drug 2.03 (95 %CI 1.05 to 3.93; P=0.04). For all strokes and nonfatal stroke, risk was similar: relative risk 1.33; 95%CI 0.90–1.97; P=0.15 and relative risk 1.04; 95%CI 0.64–1.69; P=0.89, respectively. Atorvastatin significantly reduced the rate of all cardiac events combined (relative risk, 0.82; 95 %CI 0.68 to 0.99; P=0.03) but not all cerebrovascular events combined (relative risk, 1.12; 95 %CI 0.81 to 1.55; P=0.49) or total mortality (relative risk, 0.93; 95% CI 0.79 to 1.08; P=0.33).

From this trial, the complete absence of a stroke benefit and the increase in fatal strokes contributed considerably to the finding that the, in patients with diabetes and renal failure, treatment effect of atorvastatin on the primary endpoint was less than predicted.

A Study to Evaluate the Use of Rosuvastatin in Subjects on Regular Hemodialysis (AURORA)[34]

A Study to Evaluate the Use of Rosuvastatin in Subjects on Regular Hemodialysis (AURORA) was a randomized, double-blind, placebo-controlled, multicenter trial to evaluate the benefit of statins in high risk patients who were undergoing hemodialysis. Men and women 50 to 80 years of age who had end-stage renal disease and had been treated with regular hemodialysis or hemofiltration for at least 3 months were recruited from 280 centers in 25 countries. Eligible patients were randomly assigned (in blocks of four in a 1:1 ratio) to receive rosuvastatin, 10 mg daily, or matching placebo. The primary endpoint was the time to a major cardiovascular event, defined as a nonfatal stroke, nonfatal myocardial infarction, or death from cardiovascular causes.

Secondary endpoints included all-cause mortality, cardiovascular event–free survival (i.e., freedom from nonfatal myocardial infarction, nonfatal stroke, death from cardiovascular causes, and death from any other cause), procedures performed for stenosis or thrombosis of the vascular access for long-term hemodialysis (arteriovenous fistulas and grafts only), and coronary or peripheral revascularization, death from cardiovascular causes, and death from non-cardiovascular causes.

2,776 patients were randomly assigned to double-blind treatment with rosuvastatin at a dose of 10 mg (1,391 patients) or placebo (1,385 patients).

After 3 months, the mean reduction in LDL cholesterol levels was 43% in patients receiving rosuvastatin, from a mean baseline level of 100 mg per deciliter (2.6 mmol per liter). During a median follow-up period of 3.8 years, the primary endpoint occurred in 396 patients assigned to receive rosuvastatin (9.2 events per 100 patient-years) and in 408 patients assigned to receive placebo (9.5 events per 100 patient-years) with non-significant effect of statins treatment (HR for the primary endpoint in the rosuvastatin group vs. the placebo group, 0.96; 95% CI, 0.84 to 1.11; P=0.59). No significant effect of rosuvastatin therapy as compared with placebo was also observed for each of the endpoint components. The respective event rates were 1.2 and 1.1 per 100 patient-years for nonfatal stroke (P=0.42), 7.2 and 7.3 per 100 patient-years for death from cardiovascular causes (P=0.97), and 2.1 and 2.5 per 100 patient-years for nonfatal myocardial infarction (P=0.23). A per-protocol analysis of patients who continued to receive active study medication until they reached a study endpoint confirmed the lack of an effect of rosuvastatin on the primary composite endpoint.

The lack of an effect of rosuvastatin therapy on the primary endpoint was consistent in all tested subgroups, including patients with diabetes, preexisting cardiovascular disease, hypertension, a high LDL cholesterol level, or an elevated high-sensitivity C-reactive protein level. Subgroup analyses according to the overall time on hemodialysis therapy or the overall time on renal-replacement therapy also did not influence the response to therapy.

Adverse events were similarly reported in 1,338 patients who received rosuvastatin (96.3%) and in 1,332 patients who received placebo (96.7%). Serious adverse events were reported in 1140 patients who received rosuvastatin (82.1%) and in 1,159 patients who received placebo (84.1%). Most patients reported multiple events; a total of 36,780 adverse events and 9.017 serious adverse events were reported during the study, with non-significant difference between treatment groups.

Given the lack of a treatment effect of rosuvastatin on the primary endpoint, the study then examined the relationship between lipid levels and cardiovascular endpoints within the trial. There was no relationship between the primary cardiovascular endpoint and either baseline LDL cholesterol levels (HR per 1 mg per deciliter [0.03 mmol per liter], 1.00; 95% CI, 0.82 to 1.29; P=0.83) or LDL cholesterol levels at 3 months (HR 0.95; 95% CI, 0.83 to 1.09; P=0.48).

According to this randomized trial, in patients undergoing hemodialysis, the initiation of treatment with rosuvastatin lowered the LDL cholesterol level but had non-significant effect on the composite endpoint of nonfatal stroke, death from cardiovascular causes, or nonfatal myocardial infarction.

Study of Heart and Renal Protection (SHARP)[35]

The Study of Heart and Renal Protection (SHARP) trial aimed to assess the efficacy and safety of the combination of simvastatin plus ezetimibe in patients without cardiac history but with moderate-to-severe kidney disease.

This randomized double double-blind trial included 9,270 patients with chronic kidney disease (3,023 on dialysis and 6,247 not) with no known history of myocardial infarction or coronary revascularization. Patients were randomly assigned to simvastatin 20 mg plus ezetimibe 10 mg daily versus matching placebo. The prespecified outcome was first major atherosclerotic event (nonfatal myocardial infarction or coronary death, non-hemorrhagic stroke, or any arterial revascularization procedure).

4,650 patients were assigned to receive simvastatin plus ezetimibe and 4,620 to placebo. Allocation to simvastatin plus ezetimibe yielded an average LDL cholesterol difference of 0.85 mmol/L (with about two-thirds compliance) during a median follow-up of 4.9 years and produced a significant 17% proportional reduction in major atherosclerotic events (526 [11.3%] simvastatin plus ezetimibe vs 619 [13.4%] placebo; rate ratio [RR] 0.83, 95% CI 0.74–0.94; logrank test P=0.0021). There were significant reductions in non-hemorrhagic stroke (2.8% vs 3.8%; RR 0.75, 95% CI 0.60–0.94; P=0·01) and arterial revascularization procedures (6.1% vs 7.6%; RR 0.79, 95% CI 0.68–0.93; P=0.0036). Non-significantly fewer patients allocated to simvastatin plus ezetimibe had a nonfatal myocardial infarction or died from coronary heart disease (4.6% vs 5.0%; RR 0.92, 95% CI 0.76–1.11; P=0.37).

After weighting for subgroup-specific reductions in LDL cholesterol, there was no good evidence that the proportional effects on major atherosclerotic events differed from the summary rate ratio in any subgroup examined, and, in particular, they were similar in patients on dialysis and those who were not.

The risk of myopathy was only two per 10,000 patients per year of treatment with simvastatin plus ezetimibe (0.2% vs 0·1%). There was no evidence of excess risks of hepatitis (0.5% vs 0.4%), gallstones (2.3% vs 2.3%), or cancer (9.4% vs 9.5%, P=0.89) and there was non-significant excess of death from any non-vascular cause (14.4% vs 13.2%, P=0.13).

This trial therefore showed that reduction of LDL cholesterol with simvastatin 20 mg plus ezetimibe 10 mg daily safely reduced the incidence of major atherosclerotic events in patients with advanced chronic kidney disease with different severity.

When the SHARP results are compared with those of the previous statin trials in renal patients (4D, AURORA) showing no benefit from statins in renal patients, it appears that the absence of significant reductions in earlier trials could have been due both to the much smaller number and the much smaller proportion of vascular events in their primary outcomes that were related to atherosclerosis and, hence, preventable by lowering of LDL cholesterol.

RCTs Reporting on Stroke Risk with Statins Use for Secondary Prevention

Scandinavian Simvastatin Survival Study (4S)[36,37]

The Scandinavian Simvastatin Survival Study (4S) was one of the oldest trials assessing the benefit of effective cholesterol lowering in secondary prevention settings. The 4S was designed to evaluate the effect of cholesterol lowering with simvastatin on mortality and morbidity in patients with CHD. 4,444 patients with angina pectoris or previous myocardial infarction and serum cholesterol of 5.5-8.0 mmol/L on a lipid-lowering diet were randomized to double-blind treatment with simvastatin (10-40mg/d) or placebo. The primary endpoint was total mortality. The secondary endpoint (analyzed by time of first event) was major coronary event. The tertiary endpoints (analyzed by time of first event) were any coronary events, death or any atherosclerotic event (coronary, cerebrovascular and peripheral), incidence of myocardial revascularization procedures, and incidence of hospital admission for acute cardiac events. Over the 5.4 years median follow-up period, simvastatin produced mean changes in total cholesterol, LDL-C, and HDL-C of -25%, -35%, and +8%, respectively, with few adverse effects. Significantly more patients died in the placebo group (12%), compared with the simvastatin group (8%). The relative risk of death in the simvastatin group was 0.7 (95% CI 0.58-0.85, P=0.0003). The 6-year probabilities of survival in the placebo and simvastatin groups were 87.6% and 91.3%, respectively. There were 189 coronary deaths in the placebo group and 111 in the simvastatin group (relative risk 0.58, 95% CI 0.46-0.73), while non-cardiovascular causes of death accounted for 49 and 46 deaths, respectively. 622 patients (28%) in the placebo group and 431 (19%) in the simvastatin group had one or more major coronary events: the relative risk was 0.66 (95% CI 0.59-0.75, $P < 0.00001$), and the respective probabilities of escaping such events were 70.5% and 79.6%. A post-hoc analysis on fatal plus nonfatal cerebrovascular events showed a significant reduction in the simvastatin group: there were 98 patients with events in the placebo group and 70 in the simvastatin group, relative risk 0.70 (95% CI 0.52-0.96; P=0.024). The overall frequency of adverse events was similar in the two groups, including similar rates of cancer. A single case of rhabdomyolysis was recorded in the simvastatin group. Increase in creatine kinase more than ten times the upper limit of normal range occurred in 1 and 6 patients in the placebo and simvastatin group respectively.

This study showed that long-term treatment with simvastatin was safe , decreased cardiac and cerebrovascular events (fatal and nonfatal) and improved survival in CHD patients.

Cholesterol and Recurrent Events (CARE)[38]

The Cholesterol and Recurrent Events (CARE) trial was the first large-scale secondary prevention trial performed in US of cholesterol reduction with an HMG-CoA reductase inhibitor after myocardial infarction in which stroke was a prespecified endpoint. Patients were randomized to double blind 40 mg pravastatin daily vs placebo. Patients were recruited from 80 participating centers, 13 in Canada and 67 in the United States. In the CARE study the effect of lowering cholesterol on the incidence of vascular events was assessed in patients with a baseline low total cholesterol level. Men and postmenopausal women were eligible if they had had an acute myocardial infarction between 3 and 20 months before randomization, were 21 to 75 years of age, and had plasma total cholesterol levels of less than 240 mg per deciliter, LDL cholesterol levels of 115 to 174 mg per deciliter, fasting triglyceride levels of less than 350 mg per deciliter (4.0 mmol per liter), fasting glucose levels of no more than 220 mg per deciliter (12.2 mmol per liter), left ventricular ejection fractions of no less than 25%, and no symptomatic congestive heart failure.

Primary endpoint was fatal coronary event or a nonfatal myocardial infarction. To further elucidate the relationship between pravastatin treatment and cerebrovascular outcome in this population, the CARE Endpoints Committee developed categorical stroke definitions at the outset of the study and subsequently performed a detailed review of all reported cerebrovascular events.

There were 4,159 subjects (86% male, 14% female) randomized to the pravastatin (n=2,081) or placebo (n=2,078) arms of the trial. Baseline lipids were identical in the placebo and treatment arms, with total serum cholesterol of 209+/-17 mg/dL, LDL cholesterol of 139+/-15 mg/dL, HDL cholesterol of 39+/-9 mg/dL, and triglycerides of 155+/-61 mg/dL.

As reported in the CARE study, compared with placebo controls, total serum cholesterol was reduced by 20% (42 mg/dL), LDL cholesterol was reduced by 32% (44 mg/dL), HDL cholesterol was raised by 5% (2 mg/dL), and triglycerides was reduced by 14% (22 mg/dL) in pravastatin-treated patients (P<0.001 for all effects).

In overall 4,159 patients, the primary endpoint of the study, coronary artery disease–related death or nonfatal myocardial infarction, was reduced by 24% in pravastatin-treated patients compared with those on placebo.

In addition, investigator-reported stroke incidence significantly declined in patients assigned to pravastatin.

Risk factors for stroke were similar at baseline. The prevalence of hypertension, diabetes mellitus, current smoking, congestive heart failure, and left ventricular ejection fractions were no different between placebo and treatment groups. In addition, at randomization, 83% of patients in both groups were currently taking aspirin on a regular basis, with an additional 2% taking another form of platelet inhibitor. There was a history of prior stroke in 2.9% of placebo and 3.0% of pravastatin-treated patients, with 4.8% and 5.3%, respectively, of subjects having experienced either stroke or Transient Ischemic Attack (TIA) in the past (P=NS for both).

Over a median 5-year follow-up period, first incident stroke of any type occurred in 52 patients assigned to pravastatin and 76 placebo patients, representing a 32% reduction in relative risk (95%CI, 4% to 52%, P=0.03). Similarly, strokes or TIAs were experienced by 92 patients receiving pravastatin compared with 124 on placebo, for a relative risk reduction of 27% (95%CI 4% to 44%, P=0.02). There was a treatment-associated reduction in all stroke categories, although there was inadequate power to test for significance because of the limited number of outcome events in each class. A non-significant 21% (95%CI -20% to 48%, P=0.268) risk reduction for ischemic (atherosclerotic or tandem arterial pathology) strokes was observed. There was no increase in intracerebral hemorrhages on pravastatin, with 6 events occurring in placebo-treated patients compared with 2 on pravastatin therapy. Only 6 fatal strokes were documented, which included 5 patients on pravastatin versus 1 on placebo. In univariate analysis, age > 60 years, absence of a history of hypertension, diabetes, prior stroke, or TIA, and a left ventricular ejection fraction >40% were all associated with enhanced reduction of stroke or TIA with pravastatin. However, when evaluated by stepwise regression, both stroke and stroke or TIA incidence were reduced independently of potential covariates (age, sex, history of hypertension, current use of cigarettes, diabetes, left ventricular ejection fraction, history of stroke or TIA, and baseline lipid values).

Pravastatin reduced both stroke and stroke or TIA incidence in patients with higher lipid levels, including total, LDL, and HDL cholesterol and triglycerides. There was non-significant event reduction in patients with lower baseline levels. Further division of baseline LDL cholesterol into quintile (lowest quintile at <125 mg/dL, middle 3 quintile at 125 to 150 mg/dL inclusive, upper quintile at <150 mg/dL), revealed a trend toward a greater reduction in stroke and stroke or TIA with increasing LDL cholesterol, which became more evident at levels <150 mg/dL. Above this cutpoint, patients on pravastatin exhibited a 44% reduction in stroke (214 to 73, P=NS) and a 54% reduction in stroke or TIA (17 to 74, P=0.009). However, a test for interaction between the treatment effect in the 3 LDL cholesterol groups was of only borderline significance (P=0.07).

In conclusion, the CARE trial showed that pravastatin significantly reduced stroke and stroke or TIA incidence after myocardial infarction in patients with average serum cholesterol levels despite the high concurrent use of antiplatelet therapy.

Long-Term Intervention with Pravastatin in Ischemic Disease (LIPID)[39]

The Long-term Intervention with Pravastatin in Ischemic Disease (LIPID) trial investigated the effects of pravastatin on mortality in patients with coronary heart disease and a broad range of cholesterol levels. In a double-blind, randomized trial, the effects of pravastatin (40 mg daily) with those of a placebo were compared over a mean follow-up period of 6.1 years in 9,014 patients who were 31 to 75 years of age. Patients had a history of myocardial infarction or hospitalization for unstable angina and initial plasma total cholesterol levels of 155 to 271 mg per deciliter. Both groups received advice on following a cholesterol-lowering diet. The primary study outcome was mortality from coronary heart disease. Secondary outcomes were stroke; non-hemorrhagic stroke; death from any cause, death from cardiovascular causes and death from nonfatal myocardial infarction; coronary revascularization; hospital days; serum lipid levels; and the relation between changes in lipid levels to the occurrence of cardiovascular endpoints.

Patients in the LIPID trial who received pravastatin (40mg daily) achieved reductions of 24% in CHD mortality, 22% in total mortality and 19% in the incidence of stroke (P=0.048) in comparison with patients who received placebo. Death from coronary heart disease occurred in 8.3% of the patients in the placebo group (N=373) and 6.4% of those in the pravastatin group (N=287), a significant relative reduction in risk of 24% (95% CI 12 to 35; P<0.001). Overall mortality was 14.1% in the placebo group (N=633) and 11.0% in the pravastatin group (N=498) with a significant relative reduction in risk of 22 % (95% CI 13 to 31; P<0.001). The incidence of any stroke was significantly lower in the pravastatin group stroke: 3.7% in the pravastatin group vs 4.5% in the placebo group (19% reduction in risk, 95% CI 0-34; P=0.048). Furthermore the rate of all cardiovascular outcomes was consistently lower among patients assigned to receive pravastatin; these outcomes included myocardial infarction (29% reduction in risk, P<0.001), death from coronary heart disease or nonfatal myocardial infarction (24 % reduction in risk, P<0.001), and coronary revascularization (20% reduction in risk, P<0.001). The effects of treatment were similar for all predefined subgroups. There were no clinically significant adverse events of treatment with pravastatin. Of relevance, 82% of participants were taking aspirin; therefore, pravastatin reduced the risk of adverse events even in patients who were already receiving antiplatelet therapy.

The results of this trials suggested that pravastatin therapy reduced mortality from coronary heart disease, overall mortality and any stroke rate, as compared with the rates in the placebo group, as well as the incidence of all prespecified cardiovascular events in patients with a history of myocardial infarction or unstable angina who had a broad range of initial cholesterol levels.

Gruppo Italiano Per Lo Studio Della Sopravvivenza Nell'infarto Miocardico (GISSI)[40]

The aim of the Gruppo Italiano per lo Studio della Sopravvivenza nell'Infarto miocardico (GISSI) study was to assess the efficacy of a low-dose pravastatin regimen (20mg/d) in patients with acute myocardial infarction and hypercholesterolemia (total blood cholesterol level >200mg/dL). Overall 4,271 recent myocardial infarction patients (<6months) were randomized to low-dose pravastatin or no statins treatment. The publication of results from other trials prompted the Data Safety and Monitoring Board and the Steering Committee to change the protocol and later to stop randomization with a decreased statistical power. Mainly because of the on-course modification of the study protocol, 402/2,133 (18.8%) patients in the control group started a cholesterol-lowering treatment during follow-up. Conversely, 296/2,138 (13.8%) patients permanently stopped taking their tablets. Side effects, however, were the reason for discontinuing therapy in 57 (2.7%) patients in the pravastatin group, and patient reluctance to continue accounted for most of the remainder. After excluding control patients who had started a cholesterol-lowering treatment during follow-up, the following changes of median lipid concentrations in the control group over the whole course were observed: total cholesterol -1.9%; LDL cholesterol -2.9%; triglycerides -2.0%; HDL cholesterol +1.4%. The analysis carried out excluding patients randomized to pravastatin treatment and actually not assuming the drug clearly indicated the cholesterol-lowering efficacy of low-dose pravastatin.

No relevant differences in mortality or stroke endpoints between the two arms of the trial were found. During the study, 256 (6.0%) patients either died or had a nonfatal stroke or a myocardial infarction, 136 (6.4%) in the control group and 120 (5.6%) in the pravastatin group (relative risk 0.90, 95% CI 0.71-1.15, P = 0.41); 160 patients died, 88 (4.1%) in the control group and 72 (3.4%) in the pravastatin group (relative risk 0.84, 94% CI 0.61-1.14, P = 0.26). The reduction of cardiovascular events was more evident in the by-treatment analysis, with coronary heart disease deaths being significantly decreased (RR 0.60, 95% CI 0.38-0.96, P = 0.04). There reduction of strokes remained non-significant: Relative risk reduction -9% (range -104 to 42).

Despite the decreased statistical power due to its premature stopping, the results of the GISSI suggested that a low-dose treatment with pravastatin (20 mg daily) might be effective in reducing blood lipids, and underlined the importance of long-term compliance with treatments in the search for a maximal effective dosage.

RCTs Reporting on Stroke Risk with Aggressive Statin Regimen for Secondary Prevention

Stroke Prevention by Aggressive Reduction in Cholesterol Levels (SPARCL)[41,42,43]

The Stroke Prevention by Aggressive Reduction in Cholesterol Levels (SPARCL) trial was the first and only trial specifically designed to investigate the effect of secondary prevention of stroke in patients with cerebrovascular disease from statins use. SPARCL a randomized, double-blind, placebo-controlled trial, showed that treatment with aggressive high-dose (80mg) atorvastatin per day reduced the risk of stroke and coronary events in 4,731 patients with recent stroke and TIA and no known CHD. This benefit was found despite only

78% adherence to randomized treatment by the end of the trial. However, since more patients in the placebo group discontinued study treatment and began open-label, non-study statins therapy than patients in the atorvastatin group (25.4% versus 11.4%), this could have led to an underestimate of the potential of benefit of treatment.

The primary hypothesis of the SPARCL trial was that treatment with 80 mg atorvastatin per day would reduce the combined risk of fatal and nonfatal stroke in patients with a recent stroke or TIA. Eligible patients were men and women older than 18 years and having had an ischemic or hemorrhagic stroke or TIA (all diagnosed by a neurologist within 30 days of the event) 1 to 6 months before randomization. Patients with hemorrhagic stroke could be included if they were deemed by the investigator to be at risk for ischemic stroke or CHD. Patients had to be ambulatory (modified Rankin score <3) and have a LDL-C level >2.6 and <4.9 mmol/L (>100 and <190 mg/dL). The exclusion criteria included having atrial fibrillation, mechanical prosthetic heart valves, CHD, or subarachnoid hemorrhage.

The SPARCL primary outcome was the time from randomization to the first occurrence of a nonfatal or fatal stroke. There were 7 prespecified secondary composite outcomes: stroke or TIA; major coronary event (cardiac death, nonfatal myocardial infarction, or resuscitated cardiac arrest); major cardiovascular event (stroke plus any major coronary event); acute coronary event (major coronary event or unstable angina); any CHD event (acute coronary event plus coronary revascularization procedure, unstable angina or angina/ischemia requiring emergent hospitalization); revascularization procedure (coronary, carotid, or peripheral); and any cardiovascular event (any of the former plus clinically significant peripheral vascular disease). Individual components of the composite endpoints and all-cause mortality were also prespecified secondary outcomes. After 6 years of follow-up 265 patients in the atorvastatin group had a fatal or nonfatal stroke compared with 311 in the control group. There was a significant 16% relative risk reduction in time to first occurrence of stroke with atorvastatin (Adjusted HR 0.84, 95%CI 0.71-0.99). For the secondary endpoint of time to stroke or TIA, there was a significant 23% relative risk reduction (HR 0.77; 95%CI 0.67-0.88) with 375 events in the atorvastatin group and 476 in the controls. Moreover, there was a 35% reduction of coronary events (HR 0.65; 95%CI 0.49-0.87).

In an analysis restricted to patients included in SPARCL with a carotid stenosis at baseline, statins treatment was associated with a 33% reduction in the risk of stroke (HR 0.67, 95% CI 0.47–0.94, P=0.02).

A post-hoc analysis of the SPARCL analyzed the relationship between lipid levels and stroke risks. There were 55,045 LDL-C measurements obtained during the trial (mean of 11.6 measurements per patient); 32.7% of the measurements corresponded to no change or an increase in LDL-C, 39.4% to a <50% decrease, and 27.9% to a > 50% decrease. Almost all (96%) of > 50% decreases in LDL-C were from patients randomized to atorvastatin treatment (88% of patients randomized to atorvastatin).

Compared with no change or an increase, patients with > 50% reductions in LDL-C had a 31% reduction (HR=0.69; 95% CI, 0.55 to 0.87; P=0.0016) in the combined risk of nonfatal and fatal stroke (the SPARCL primary endpoint), including a 30% reduction in nonfatal stroke (HR=0.7; 95% CI, 0.55 to 0.89; P=0.004). Whereas ischemic strokes were reduced by 33% (P=0.0018), there was no increase in hemorrhagic stroke (HR=1.04; 95% CI, 0.61 to 1.78; P=0.8864), although the confidence intervals around the point estimate were wide. Further adjustment for age, gender time-varying systolic blood pressure, cigarette smoking, diabetes, compliance to study drug, and antihypertensive and antiplatelet agents use did not modify these findings.

Compared with LDL-C > 2.6 mmol/L (> 100 mg/dL), achieving an LDL-C level <1.8 mmol/L (<70 mg/dL) was associated with a 28% reduction in the risk of stroke (P=0.0018) without an increase in the risk of hemorrhagic stroke (P=0.3358).

Another post-hoc analysis of SPARCL data was performed to determine whether men and women similarly benefited from randomization to statins treatment. There were no sex-based treatment differences in lipid profiles between men and women (LDL-cholesterol, P=0.986; total cholesterol, P=0.452; HDL-cholesterol, P=0.126; triglycerides, P=0.8437; Apo A1, P=0.135; Apo B, P=0.955). Men and women had similar treatment associated benefits for each study endpoint (ie, there were non-significant treatment by sex interactions for the combined risk of nonfatal and fatal stroke, nonfatal stroke, fatal stroke, stroke or TIA, major cardiac events, major cardiovascular events, revascularization procedures, or any CHD event). The treatment by sex interaction term for all cause mortality was marginally significant (P=0.06). The second set of analyses using Cox regression models with stratification to control for additional potential confounders provided almost identical results.

In conclusion, according to SPARCL, stroke and other cardiovascular events are similarly reduced with atorvastatin 80mg/d in men and women with recent stroke or TIA.

Phase Z of the A to Z Trial[44]

The A to Z trial was an international trial consisting of 2 overlapping phases. Phase A was an open- label non-inferiority trial comparing enoxaparin with unfractionated heparin in patients with non–ST-elevation acute coronary syndrome (ACS) who were treated with tirofiban and aspirin. Phase Z was designed to evaluate a strategy of early initiation of intensive treatment with simvastatin in ACS patients compared with a delayed, less intensive strategy. Specifically, Phase Z was a double-blind trial comparing 2 statin regimens in patients with ACS: a strategy of early initiation of intensive treatment with simvastatin (40mg/d followed by 80mg/d) was compared with a delayed less invasive strategy (placebo for 4 months followed by 20mg/d of simvastatin). Patients between the ages of 21 and 80 years with either non–ST-elevation ACS or ST-elevation MI were eligible for enrollment if they had a total cholesterol level of 250 mg/dL (6.48 mmol/L) or lower. Initially, patients were entered into phase Z only if they presented with non–ST-elevation ACS, were stabilized during phase A of the trial for at least 12 consecutive hours within 5 days after symptom onset, and met at least 1 high-risk characteristics. The protocol was then amended to allow patients with non-ST elevation ACS who were not enrolled in phase A and patients with ST-elevation MI to enter directly into phase Z. The primary efficacy endpoint of the trial was a composite of cardiovascular death, nonfatal MI, readmission for ACS and stroke. Secondary endpoints included individual components of the primary endpoint, revascularization due to documented ischemia, all-cause mortality, new-onset congestive heart failure (requiring admission or initiation of heart failure medications), and cardio-vascular rehospitalization.

4,497 patients were enrolled in phase Z of the A to Z trial at 322 centers in 41 countries: 2,265 patients were assigned to receive 40 mg/d of simvastatin for 1 month followed by 80mg/d thereafter and 2,232 were assigned to receive placebo for 4 months followed by 20mg/d of simvastatin.

Treatment was discontinued prematurely in 711 patients (32%) in the placebo plus delayed 20mg of simvastatin group and in 765 (34%) in the simvastatin aggressive strategy group (40mg/d and then 80mg/d). The median follow-up period was 721 days.

In the placebo plus simvastatin group, median LDL cholesterol levels increased by 11% during the 4-month placebo period from 111 mg/dL (2.87 mmol/L) to 124 mg/dL (3.21 mmol/L) and then decreased to 77 mg/dL (1.99mmol/L) at month 8 after the initiation of 20 mg of simvastatin (31% change from baseline). In the simvastatin only group, the median LDL cholesterol levels decreased by 39% to 68 mg/dL (1.76 mmol/L) over the first month during treatment with 40 mg/d of simvastatin and then decreased an additional 6% to 62 mg/dL (1.61 mmol/L) at month 4 following the increase to the 80 mg/d of simvastatin. The primary endpoint of cardiovascular death, MI, readmission for ACS, and stroke occurred without significant difference in 343 patients (16.7%) in the placebo plus simvastatin group compared with 309 (14.4%) in the simvastatin only group (HR 0.89; 95% CI, 0.76-1.04; P=0.14). Furthermore, non-significant differences were observed between treatment groups with regard to the secondary endpoints of stroke, MI, readmission for ACS, or revascularization due to documented ischemia.

Stroke rates were 1.8% in the placebo plus delayed simvastatin vs 1.3% in the aggressive simvastatin only group, a difference that was non-significant (HR 0.79, 95% CI 0.48-1.30; P=0.36).

In a post-hoc analysis, no difference between treatment groups in the primary endpoint was evident over the first 4 months following randomization, which corresponded to the placebo-controlled comparison period (HR, 1.01; 95% CI 0.83-1.25; P= 0.89). However, from 4 months through the end of the study, the primary endpoint was significantly reduced from 9.3% in the placebo plus simvastatin group to 6.8% in the simvastatin only group (HR, 0.75; 95%CI, 0.60-0.95; P=0.02).

The trial did not achieve the prespecified endpoint at 4 months. It suggested that among patients with ACS, the early initiation of an aggressive simvastatin regimen resulted in a favorable trend toward reduction of major cardiovascular events.

Aggressive Lipid-Lowering Initiation Abates New Cardiac Events (ALLIANCE)[45]

The Aggressive Lipid-Lowering Initiation Abates New Cardiac Events (ALLIANCE) study was a prospective, randomized trial, to evaluate outcomes attributable to different lipid treatment strategies in a predefined CHD patient group.

During the trial, patients were randomized to receive either an aggressive lipid-lowering regimen using atorvastatin or "usual care" as deemed appropriate by the patient's regular physicians. The study was designed and executed as a "real-world" trial to determine if an aggressive, focused approach to hyperlipidemia would outperform current physician practice in CHD patients.

Eligible subjects were men or women >18 years of age with known CHD defined as a history of acute MI (>3 months before screening), percutaneous transluminal coronary angioplasty (>6 months before screening), coronary artery bypass graft surgery (>3 months before screening), or unstable angina (>3 months before screening). Inclusion LDL-C levels were between 110mg/dL (2.8mmol/L) and 200mg/dL (5.2mmol/L) for patients receiving lipid-lowering medication and between 130 mg/dL (3.4mmol/L) and 250mg/dL (6.5mmol/L) for patients receiving no lipid-regulating therapy.

CHD patients with hyperlipidemia were randomized to either an aggressive treatment arm using atorvastatin or usual care and followed for 51.5 months on average. Atorvastatin-group patients were titrated to LDL-C goals of <80mg/dl (2.1mmol/L) or a maximum atorvastatin dose of 80mg/day. Combination lipid therapy was not allowed. After dose titration was completed, subjects were followed every six months. Usual-care patients received any treatment deemed appropriate by their regular physicians. Approximately two-thirds of patients were on lipid-regulating agents at baseline. The primary efficacy parameter was time to first cardiovascular event. Primary cardiovascular events included cardiac death, nonfatal MI, resuscitated cardiac arrest, cardiac revascularization, and unstable angina requiring hospitalization. Secondary outcomes included non-cardiac death, peripheral revascularization, hospitalization for congestive heart failure, and stroke. Of 3,451 patients screened at 16 centers, 2,442 were randomized, with 1,217 assigned to the atorvastatin group and 1,225 to the usual care group.

A total of 958 patients in the atorvastatin group and 941 in the usual care group completed endpoint assessments. In the atorvastatin group, the median dose of atorvastatin received by patients over the course of the study was 40.5mg/day; 545 patients (45%) received 80 mg/day.

The mean LDL-C levels at baseline (on pre-randomization lipid-lowering treatment) were 147mg/dL (3.8 mmol/L) in the atorvastatin group and 146 mg/dL (3.8 mmol/L) in the usual care group. At the end of the study, LDL-C levels had decreased by 34.3% to 95 mg/dl (2.5 mmol/L) in the atorvastatin group and by 23.3% to 111mg/dL (2.9 mmol/L) in the usual care group ($P < 0.0001$).

At study completion, 72.4% of patients in the focused group had achieved their goal (LDL-C <100 mg/dL [2.6 mmol/L]) compared with 40.0% of those receiving usual care ($P< 0.001$).

The patients in the atorvastatin group also demonstrated significantly greater reductions in total cholesterol than those in the usual care group ($P< 0.0001$). Reductions in triglycerides and increases in high-density lipoprotein cholesterol were moderate in both groups.

A total of 289 (23.7%) patients in the atorvastatin group compared with 333 (27.7%) patients in the usual care group experienced a primary outcome (HR, 0.83; 95% CI 0.71 to 0.97, P=0.02). This reduction in morbidity was largely due to fewer nonfatal myocardial infarctions (4.3% vs. 7.7%, P= 0.0002). Levels of LDL-C were reduced more (34.3% vs. 23.3%, P=0.0001) and National Cholesterol Education Program goals (LDL-C <100 mg/dl) more likely met at end-of-study visits (72.4% vs. 40.0%) in patients receiving atorvastatin compared with those receiving usual care.

Trends favoring the aggressively treated group did not reach statistical significance for all the components of the primary composite and secondary endpoints. In particular, stroke, that was a secondary endpoint, occurred in 35 (2.9%) in the aggressive atorvastatin group vs in 39 (3.2%) in the usual care group (HR 0.87, 95%CI 0.55-1.38; P=0.552).

The occurrence of serious adverse events was similar in the atorvastatin (40%) and the usual care groups (42%). In both treatment arms, the most common reported serious adverse events were chest pain, atrial fibrillation pneumonia, cellulitis and gastrointestinal hemorrhage.

Subgroup analyses by gender, age, and race showed efficacy results consistent with the overall population. No significant interactions between treatment and gender, age, or race were observed.

From this trial, an aggressive, focused statins therapy management strategy outperformed usual care in clinic patients with CHD, but the effects on stroke prevention were uncertain.

Greek Atorvastatin and Coronary Heart Disease Evaluation (GREACE)[46]

The Greek Atorvastatin and Coronary Heart Disease Evaluation (GREACE) was a prospective, intention-to-treat randomized study performed in Greece to assess the effect of atorvastatin on morbidity and mortality of patients with established CHD. A total of 1,600 consecutive patients were randomized either to atorvastatin or to 'usual' medical care.

All patients with LDL-C >100mg/dL (2.6mmol/L), after a 6-week period on hypolipidaemic diet were enrolled into the study. In the atorvastatin group, the starting dose was 10 mg/day. The dose of atorvastatin was titrated up to 80mg/day for patients not reaching the LDL-C goal of <100 mg/dL with lower dosages. The patients on 'usual' care received whatever drug treatment was prescribed by their physician. The primary endpoints of the study in both groups were total and coronary mortality, as well as nonfatal myocardial infarction, unstable angina, congestive heart failure, revascularization and stroke. The secondary endpoints were the safety and efficacy of hypolipidemic drug treatment as well as the cost-effectiveness of atorvastatin. All patients were followed up for a mean period of 3 years.

The mean dosage of atorvastatin was 24 mg/day. Statins reduced total cholesterol by 36%, LDL-C by 46%, triglycerides by 31%, and non-high-density lipoprotein cholesterol (non-HDL-C) by 44%, while it increased HDL-C by 7%; all these changes were significant. The LDL-C treatment goal was reached by 95% (n = 759) of patients on atorvastatin.

During the study 196 (24.5%) CHD patients on 'usual' care had a CHD recurrent event or died vs. 96 (12%) CHD patients on atorvastatin; RR 0.49, 95% CI 0.27–0.73, P<0.0001. In detail, after 3 years of follow-up, the composite endpoint of death, nonfatal myocardial infarction, unstable angina, coronary heart failure, revascularization or stroke, was significantly lowered by 51%, the incidence of stroke was significantly decreased by 47% and all the components of the primary endpoint were significantly reduced in the atorvastatin group. Atorvastatin reduced, in comparison to 'usual' care, total mortality (RR 0.57, 95%CI 0.39–0.78, P= 0.0021), coronary mortality (RR 0.53, 95%CI 0.29–0.74, P= 0.0017), coronary morbidity (RR 0.46, 95%CI 0.25–0.71, P< 0.0001), and stroke (RR 0.53, 95%CI 0.30–0.82, P= 0.034). Furthermore, all analyzed subgroups of patients (women, those with diabetes mellitus, arterial hypertension, age 60 to 75 years, congestive heart failure, recent unstable angina or prior revascularization) benefited from treatment with atorvastatin. Withdrawal of patients because of side-effects from the atorvastatin group was low (0.75%) and similar to that of the 'usual' care group (0.4%).

From this secondary prevention statins Greek trial, it was suggested that long-term treatment of CHD patients with atorvastatin to achieve lipid targets significantly reduced total and coronary mortality, coronary morbidity and stroke, in comparison to patients receiving 'usual' medical care. Treatment with atorvastatin was well tolerated.

Incremental Decrease in End Points through Aggressive Lipid Lowering (IDEAL)[47]

The Incremental Decrease in End Points Through Aggressive Lipid Lowering (IDEAL) study was a multicenter, prospective, randomized, open-label, blinded trial to compare the effects of two strategies of lipid lowering on the risk of cardiovascular diseases among patients with a previous MI. The objective was that an intensive lowering of LDL-C with atorvastatin at the highest recommended dose would yield incremental benefit compared with the moderate, most widely used dose of simvastatin.

Patients were randomly assigned to receive a high dose of atorvastatin (80mg/d) or usual dose simvastatin (20mg/d). The trial was carried out at 190 ambulatory cardiology and private specialist centers in Denmark, Finland, Iceland, the Netherlands, Norway, and Sweden.

Men and women aged 80 years or younger with a history of a definite myocardial infarction and who qualified for statins therapy according to national guidelines at the time of recruitment, were eligible. Patients were followed up at the centers after 12 and 24 weeks and every 6 months thereafter. If, at 24 weeks, plasma total cholesterol level was higher than 190 mg/dL (5.0 mmol/L), the dose of simvastatin could be increased to 40 mg/d. The dose of atorvastatin could be decreased to 40 mg/d for adverse events.

The primary clinical outcome was time to first occurrence of a major coronary event, defined as coronary death, hospitalization for nonfatal acute myocardial infarction, or cardiac arrest with resuscitation. There were 3 prespecified composite secondary outcomes: (1) major cardiovascular events [(any primary event plus stroke (the diagnosis of stroke required evidence of a neurological deficit, usually localized, lasting 24 hours or until death, usually confirmed by diagnostic imaging)]; (2) any CHD event (any primary event, any coronary revascularization procedure, or hospitalization for unstable angina); (3) any cardiovascular events (any of the former plus hospitalization with a primary diagnosis of congestive heart failure and peripheral arterial disease, defined as new clinical diagnosis or hospitalization for such disease). In addition, individual components of the composite endpoints were also prespecified as secondary outcomes, as was all-cause mortality.

Overall 8,888 patients were randomized, 4,439 assigned to high dose atorvastatin arm and 4,449 assigned to usual dose simvastatin At the end of the study, 1,034 (23%) patients were prescribed simvastatin, 40mg/d. In patients allocated to receive atorvastatin, 80mg/d, 250 (6%) had their dosage reduced to 40 mg/d by 24 weeks; in 587 patients (13%), the final dose was 40 mg.

Patients in the simvastatin group who were not taking a statin at the time of randomization had, on average, a reduction in LDL-C of 33% after 12 weeks. In the group allocated to atorvastatin, 80 mg/d, statin-naive patients had a mean reduction in LDL-C of 49%. During treatment, mean LDL-C levels were 104 mg/dL (2.7 mmol/L) in the simvastatin group and 81mg/dL (2.1 mmol/L) in the atorvastatin group. Total cholesterol and triglyceride levels were also significantly lower in the atorvastatin group compared with the simvastatin group, whereas HDL-C levels were slightly but significantly higher in the simvastatin group.

The primary endpoint of major coronary events (coronary death, acute myocardial infarction, or cardiac arrest with resuscitation) occurred in 463 patients (10.4%) in the simvastatin group and in 411 (9.3%) in the atorvastatin group. This corresponded to a non-significant relative risk reduction of 11% with atorvastatin, 80 mg/d (HR, 0.89; 95% CI, 0.78-1.01; $P = 0.07$).

The composite secondary endpoint of any major cardiovascular event including stroke was indeed significantly reduced in the atorvastatin group (HR, 0.87; 95% CI, 0.78-0.98; P=0.02). Fatal and nonfatal strokes occurred in 174 patients (3.9%) treated with simvastatin and 151 patients (3.4%) treated with atorvastatin, a difference that was not statistically relevant: HR 0.87; 95%CI 0.70-1.08; P= 0.20). Hemorrhagic strokes occurred in 6 patients in each treatment group.

The risk of death from any cause was similar in both study groups (HR, 0.98 95% CI, 0.85-1.13; P = 0.80).

There were non-significant differences in the frequency of serious clinical adverse experiences between the 2 trial groups. There were, however, more patients in the atorvastatin group who discontinued study medication because of investigator-reported adverse effects. Elevation of liver enzyme levels occurred more frequently in the atorvastatin group, but this was not related to any increased incidence of clinical liver disease. Myalgia occurred more frequently in the atorvastatin group, but myopathy rates were exceedingly low in both the atorvastatin and simvastatin groups.

In this study of patients with previous MI, intensive lowering of LDL-C did not result in a significant reduction in the primary outcome of major coronary events or stroke, but did reduce the risk of composite secondary vascular endpoints including both any cardiac and stroke events. Patients with MI may benefit from intensive lowering of LDL-C without an increase in non-cardiovascular mortality or other serious adverse reactions.

Myocardial Ischemia Reduction with Aggressive Cholesterol Lowering (MIRACL)[48]

The Myocardial Ischemia Reduction with Aggressive Cholesterol Lowering (MIRACL) study tested the hypothesis that treatment with atorvastatin (80mg/d), initiated soon after presentation with unstable angina or non–Q-wave acute MI, reduced the occurrence of early, recurrent ischemic events, including stroke and death. It was conducted at 122 centers in Europe, North America, South Africa, and Australasia. Eligible patients were adults aged 18 years or older with chest pain or discomfort of at least 15 minutes' duration that occurred at rest or with minimal exertion within the 24-hour period preceding hospitalization and represented a change from their usual angina pattern.

Patients were monitored for ischemic events for 16 weeks after randomization. The primary combined endpoint was death, nonfatal acute MI, cardiac arrest with resuscitation, or recurrent symptomatic myocardial ischemia with objective evidence requiring emergency re-hospitalization. Secondary endpoints were the occurrence of each primary endpoint component as well as nonfatal stroke, new or worsening congestive heart failure requiring hospitalization, worsening angina requiring re-hospitalization but without new objective evidence of ischemia, coronary revascularization by surgical or percutaneous means, time to first occurrence of any primary or secondary endpoint, and percentage changes in blood lipid levels from baseline to end of study.

The trial enrolled 3,086 patients; 1,538 were randomly assigned to receive 80mg atorvastatin and 1,548 to receive placebo.

At the time of randomization, serum lipid levels were nearly identical in both groups with mean LDL cholesterol level of 124 mg/dL (3.2 mmol/L), mean triglycerides level of 184 mg/dL (2.0 mmol/L), and mean HDL cholesterol level of 46 mg/dL (1.2 mmol/L). At 6 weeks, reductions in total and LDL cholesterol and triglycerides with atorvastatin were reached. At the end of the study, LDL cholesterol had increased by an adjusted mean of 12% to 135 mg/dL (3.5 mmol/L) in the placebo group and decreased by an adjusted mean of 40% to 72 mg/dL (1.9 mmol/L) in the atorvastatin group. Triglycerides increased by an adjusted mean of 9% to 187 mg/dL (2.1 mmol/L) in the placebo group and decreased by an adjusted mean of 16% to 139 mg/dL (1.6 mmol/L) in the atorvastatin group. Changes in HDL cholesterol during the study were minor in both groups.

During the 16-week study period, a primary endpoint event occurred in 228 patients (14.8%) in the atorvastatin group and 269 patients (17.4%) in the placebo group, an absolute difference of 2.6%. Atorvastatin treatment significantly reduced the risk of the primary combined endpoint (RR, 0.84; 95% CI, 0.70-1.00; P=.048). Stroke was a secondary endpoint and there were significant differences between groups for incidence of nonfatal stroke, which occurred in 9 patients in the atorvastatin group, compared with 22 patients in the placebo group (RR, 0.41; 95% CI, 0.20-0.87; P = 0.02) and either fatal or nonfatal stroke, which occurred in 12 patients in the atorvastatin group, compared with 24 patients in the placebo group (RR, 0.50; 95% CI, 0.26-0.99; P=0.045).

There were no significant differences in risk of death, nonfatal acute MI, or cardiac arrest with resuscitation between the atorvastatin group and the placebo group, coronary revascularization procedures, worsening heart failure, worsening angina.

These results suggested that for patients with acute coronary syndrome, lipid-lowering therapy with high dosage atorvastatin, 80 mg/d, reduced recurrent ischemic stroke and cardiac events in the first 16 weeks.

Study of the Effectiveness of Additional Reductions in Cholesterol and Homocysteine (SEARCH)[49]

The Collaborative Group Study of the Effectiveness of Additional Reductions in Cholesterol and Homocysteine (SEARCH) trial aimed to establish efficacy and safety of more intensive statins treatment in secondary prevention for patients at high cardiovascular risk.

SEARCH was a double-blind randomized trial that investigated long-term treatment with 80 mg versus 20 mg simvastatin daily in a large population of patients with a history of myocardial infarction.

Participants were either currently on or had clear indication for statins therapy, and had a total cholesterol concentration of at least 3.5 mmol/L if already on a statin or 4.5 mmol/L if not. The primary endpoint was major vascular events, defined as coronary death, myocardial infarction, stroke, or arterial revascularization.

12,064 individuals (10,012 men and 2,052 women) with a history of myocardial infarction and an average age of 64.2 years, were randomly assigned to treatment groups: 6,031 participants were allocated 80mg simvastatin daily, and 6,033 allocated 20mg simvastatin daily. During a mean follow-up of 6.7 years, allocation to 80mg simvastatin produced an average 0.35 mmol/L greater reduction in LDL cholesterol compared with allocation to 20 mg. Major vascular events occurred in 1,477 (24.5%) participants allocated to 80mg simvastatin versus 1,553 (25.7%) of those allocated to 20mg, corresponding to a non-significant 6% proportional reduction (RR 0.94, 95% CI 0.88–1.01; P=0.10).

Compared with 20mg simvastatin, allocation to 80mg simvastatin was associated with proportional non-significant reductions in major coronary events of 4%, in any stroke of 9% , and in non-coronary revascularizations of 23%.

There were 209 (3.5%) strokes in the 80mg simvastatin and 230 (3.8%) in the 20mg simvastatin group for a RR of 0.91 (95%CI 0.77–1.08; P= 0.30). The effect on any stroke reflected RRs of 0.91 (95%CI 0.75–1.10) for nonfatal stroke and of 0.85 (95%CI 0.60–1.21) for fatal stroke, with no apparent effect on definite hemorrhagic stroke (0.4% vs 0.4%) and RR of 0.91 (95%CI 0.77–1.09) for the residual of presumed ischemic stroke (3.9% vs 4.2%).

Compared with two (0.03%) cases of myopathy in patients taking 20 mg simvastatin daily, there were 53 (0.9%) cases in the 80 mg group.

The reduction in major vascular events with a further 0·35 mmol/L reduction in LDL cholesterol in this trial was consistent with previous trials. Myopathy was increased with 80 mg simvastatin daily, but intensive lowering of LDL cholesterol could be achieved safely with other regimens.

Pravastatin or Atorvastatin Evaluation and Infection Therapy–Thrombolysis in Myocardial Infarction (PROVE IT–TIMI 22)[50]

The Pravastatin or Atorvastatin Evaluation and Infection Therapy–Thrombolysis In Myocardial Infarction (PROVE IT–TIMI 22) trial enrolled 4,162 patients to evaluate whether high-dose atorvastatin 80mg would reduce first events, recurrent cardiovascular events, and total events, compared with pravastatin 40mg during the 2-year follow-up in patients after an acute coronary syndrome.

The primary endpoint was a composite of death from any cause, stroke, MI, unstable angina, or revascularization. The first analysis of PROVE IT–TIMI 22 data showed that more intensive lipid lowering with high-dose atorvastatin reduced the first occurrence of the primary endpoint compared with moderate lipid lowering with pravastatin: first primary endpoint events were reduced by 16% with atorvastatin 80mg versus pravastatin 40mg (n=464 vs. n=537, respectively; P=0.005) the rates of the primary endpoint were 26.3% in the pravastatin group and 22.4% in the atorvastatin group.

After a mean follow-up of 24 months, additional events were also reduced by 19% with atorvastatin 80mg (n=275 vs. n=340, respectively; P=0.009). Overall, there were 138 fewer primary efficacy events with atorvastatin 80mg versus pravastatin 40mg (RR: 0.85, 95% CI: 0.77 to 0.94, P=0.001).

When examining the individual components of the primary composite endpoint, the majority of additional events reduced in the atorvastatin 80mg group were unstable angina events requiring rehospitalization and revascularization, with a similar number of deaths, MI, and strokes. Strokes were infrequent and overall occurred in 21 of the pravastatin 40mg group and 25 of the atorvastatin 80mg group (P=0.529).

Authors concluded that maintaining low levels of low-density lipoprotein cholesterol was central to prevent additional atherosclerotic development and subsequent cardiovascular events. A more intensive low-density lipoprotein cholesterol lowering strategy with atorvastatin 80mg reduced both first and subsequent primary endpoint events compared with pravastatin 40mg after acute coronary syndrome.

TNT (Treating to New Targets)[51,52]

The Treating to New Targets (TNT) Study was a double blinded randomized trial designed to assess the effects on cerebrovascular and cardiovascular events of treating patients with stable coronary disease with LDL-C levels substantially below 100mg/dl.

In this randomized trial 10,001 patients with documented coronary disease and with an LDL-C level<130 mg/dl were randomly assigned to double-blind therapy with either 10mg or 80mg atorvastatin per day and followed for a median of 4.9 years. The primary predefined outcome was the occurrence of a major cardiovascular event, defined as death from coronary heart disease, nonfatal non-procedure-related myocardial infarction, resuscitated cardiac arrest, or fatal or nonfatal stroke.

Secondary outcomes were a major coronary event (the primary endpoint without stroke), a cerebrovascular event, hospitalization for congestive heart failure, peripheral artery disease, death from any cause, any cardiovascular event, and any coronary event.

Mean LDL-C levels were 101 mg/dL in 10mg atorvastatin and 77 mg/dL in 80 mg group. In addition to the relevant reduction in major cardiovascular events (HR 0.78, 95% CI 0.69 to 0.89; P =0.0002), the primary endpoint of the trial, patients in the 80mg arm experienced a significant reduction in cerebrovascular events and stroke (fatal and nonfatal). During the follow-up period, 272 patients (2.7%) experienced a stroke, including 30 who experienced a fatal stroke. A TIA occurred in 197 patients, and a total of 448 (4.5%) experienced a cerebrovascular event (stroke or TIA). Stroke was significantly reduced by 25% in the 80mg compared with the 10mg group (2.3% vs 3.1% HR 0.75, 95% CI 0.59 to 0.86; P = 0.021). All cerebrovascular events were also reduced in the 80mg arm (HR 0.77, 95% CI 0.64 to 0.93; P = 0.007). Overall, 54% of the strokes were ischemic, 25% were embolic, 12% were hemorrhagic, and in 9% the cause was unknown. For each type of stroke the incidence was lower in the 80mg group than in the 10mg group. The incidence of hemorrhagic stroke was similar in the 80mg and 10mg groups, 16 and 18 respectively, and the hemorrhagic strokes were distributed evenly across quintiles of achieved LDL-C during treatment.

Each 1mg/dL reduction in LDL-C with treatment was associated with a 0.6% relative risk reduction in cerebrovascular events (P= 0.002) and a 0.5% relative risk reduction in stroke (P=0.041). According to this study. among patients with established coronary disease, treating to an LDL-cholesterol substantially below 100 mg/dl with 80 mg/day atorvastatin reduced both stroke and cerebrovascular events by an additional 20% to 25% compared with the 10mg/day dose. An increase in hemorrhagic stroke was not seen at low LDL-C levels.

RCTs with Active Comparators

Five RCTs on the benefit of statins use for secondary prevention did not test statins use vs placebo but compared two different statin regimens and therefore are considered as "active comparator" trials. The aim was to evaluate whether more aggressive statins use would increase benefit with respect to less aggressive statins. All these trials (Ato Z, IDEAL, SEARCH, TIMI, TNT)[44,47,49,50,51,52] used a more aggressive drug strategy vs a lower dose regimen and have been reviewed above (see "RCTs reporting on Stroke Risk with Aggressive Statin Regimen for Secondary Prevention"). Cumulative analyses of these trials have also been performed in systematic reviews (see "Meta-analyses"). Results are summarized in Table II.

2. Perioperative and Long-Term Outcome in Carotid Stenosis with the Use of Statins

Providing optimal medical management during the perioperative period is critical to minimize the rate of complications and ensure patients to achieve superior benefit following carotid interventions. Several studies have recently showed notably improvements in postoperative outcomes of patients taking a statin medication undergoing vascular surgery and specifically carotid interventions.[53,54,55,56,57,58,59]

The Statins for Risk Reduction in Surgery (StaRRs) Study[53]

The Statins for Risk Reduction in Surgery (StaRRS) showed that use of statins was highly protective against perioperative cardiac complications in patients undergoing vascular surgery. In this retrospective study O'Neil-Callahan et al, analyzed outcomes of patients treated at a tertiary referral center to evaluate the potential beneficial effect of statins in preventing perioperative nonfatal and fatal complications in patients undergoing non-cardiac vascular surgery. The main objective was to address whether the use of statins in patients undergoing carotid endarterectomy (CEA) or other non- cardiac procedures was associated with a reduced risk of perioperative cardiac complications and whether this benefit was independent of other candidate predictors of these outcomes.

Univariate and multivariate analyses with propensity score balancement for the use of statins were performed to identify predictors of perioperative complications and medications that might confer a protective effect. A total of 1,163 hospitalizations on 997 patients were retrieved and included in the study analysis. Overall, statins were given in about half the cases (n 526, 45.2%). Complications occurred in 157 of 1,163 eligible hospitalizations and were significantly fewer in patients receiving statins (9.9%) than in those not receiving statins (16.5%), corresponding to a 6.6% unadjusted difference in the risk of complications with statins (NNT=15). The difference was mostly accounted by myocardial ischemia and congestive heart failure. When comparing complication rate in statins vs non statins, the OR was 0.56 (95% CI 0.39 to 0.79, P=0.0012), and a similar and statistically significant OR estimate was seen for the combined endpoint of death, MI, and myocardial ischemia (OR 0.56, 95% CI 0.31 to 0.99, P=0.046).

The beneficial effect of statins use was similar in univariate (OR 0.56, 95%CI 0.39-0.79; P=0.0012) and adjusted analyses in the final multivariate model that also accounted for age, gender, body mass index, type of operation, acuity of operation, left ventricular dysfunction, and diabetes mellitus (OR 0.52, 95%CI 0.35-0.76, P=0.001). No other pharmacologic intervention (beta-blockers, ACE-inhibitors, aspirin) was retained as an independent predictor of the complication rate in the multivariate model. In particular, when beta-blockers were also considered with forced entry in the multivariate model, the protective effect of statins remained unchanged (OR 0.52, 95% CI 0.35 to 0.77), whereas beta-blockers alone had no clear effect (OR 0.96, 95% CI 0.66 to 1.40).

According to propensity score, the use of statins was still associated with a halving of the odds of having a complication in the most representative quartiles groups (OR 0.48, 95% CI 0.2 to 90.80, P = 0.005).

Baltimore Experiences[54,55]

The group of Baltimore (Johns Hopkins Hospital) extensively analyzed the use of statins in CEA patients and showed that perioperative statins use could reduce the incidence of cerebrovascular events and mortality among patients undergoing CEA.

The Johns Hopkins Hospital's authors first observed that patients receiving statins or diuretics were less likely to present for CEA with symptoms of stroke or TIA. These data raised the question of whether the preoperative use of these medications protected patients with carotid stenosis from developing symptomatic disease and contributed to improved outcomes among patients undergoing CEA. Authors performed a retrospective case-control study to analyze the influence of statins and diuretics in all the patients who presented for CEA to see whether preoperative medication use or patient characteristics were associated with the presence of symptomatic cerebrovascular disease at the time of operation.

Cases were identified by reviewing the medical history of each patient who presented for CEA during the time period and finding documentation of recent symptoms attributed to ipsilateral carotid stenosis, including evidence of stroke, TIA, or amaurosis fugax. Asymptomatic controls were selected at a 1.5:1 ratio from age-matched patients who presented for CEA within the same month of surgery without any clinical symptoms of cerebrovascular disease. The exposure variables for the analysis included recent medication use of statins, beta-blockers, diuretics, angiotensin-converting enzyme inhibitors, and calcium channel blockers.

A total of 1,561 patients presented for CEA between 1994 and 2004, were included: 660 (42%) patients had documented symptoms of stroke or TIA at the time of CEA and 991 (58%) patients without any clinical symptoms. Among patients with clinical symptoms, 226 (34%) were certified by a neurologist to have evidence of a stroke, whereas the remaining 434 (66%) patients were documented to have evidence of TIA.

At the time of operation, 1,172 (75%) patients were taking at least 1 cardiovascular medication. There were 657 (42%) patients taking a statin drug, 627 (40%) patients taking a beta-blocker, 424 (27%) patients taking a diuretic, 391 (25%) patients taking an angiotensin-converting enzyme inhibitor, and 421 (27%) patients taking a calcium channel blocker.

The mean age and sex distribution were similar between cases and controls, although symptomatic patients were more likely to have an ulcerative plaque (18% symptomatic vs 11% asymptomatic; P < 0.01) and a lower mean percentage of ipsilateral carotid stenosis than asymptomatic patients. Compared with asymptomatic controls, patients presenting for CEA with symptoms of stroke or TIA were less likely to have hyperlipidemia (43% vs 55%; P<0.01) or a history of coronary artery disease (43% vs 54%; P <0.01) and were less likely to be receiving statins (35% vs 47%; P < 0.01), beta-blockers (34% vs 44%; P <0.01), and diuretics (22% vs 31%; P <0 .01). After controlling for potential interaction and confounding by using propensity score adjustment and logistic regression analysis, preoperative use of statins (adjusted OR, 0.72; 95% CI, 0.56-0.92; P =0 .01) and diuretics (adjusted OR, 0.74; 95% CI, 0.58-0.95; P=0.02) were independently associated with a lower likelihood of having cerebrovascular symptoms at the time of CEA.[54]

In an additional study, the group of Baltimore retrospectively investigated whether statins use reduced the incidence of perioperative stroke and mortality among symptomatic and asymptomatic patients undergoing CEA.[55] 1,566 patients (987 men and 579 women; mean age, 72 years) were included . The indication for CEA was symptomatic disease in 660 (42%)

cases. Six hundred fifty-seven (42%) patients received a statin medication for at least 1 week before surgery. Statins use was associated with a reduction in perioperative strokes (1.2% vs 4.5%; P <0.01), TIA (1.5% vs 3.6%; P < 0.01), all-cause mortality (0.3% vs 2.1%; P < 0.01), and median [interquartile range] length of hospitalization (2 days [2-5 days] vs 3 days [2-7 days]; P <0.05). Adjusting for all demographics and comorbidities in multivariate analysis, statins use independently reduced the odds of stroke threefold (OR, 0.35 [95%CI 0.15-0.85]; P<0.05) and death fivefold (OR, 0.20 [95%CI 0.04-0.99]; P < 0.05).

Authors thereby confirmed the benefit of statins use in patients undergoing surgery for carotid stenosis: perioperative statins use may reduce the incidence of cerebrovascular events and mortality among patients undergoing CEA.

Canadian Experience[56]

Kenendy et al, further confirmed a protective effect of statins therapy in symptomatic patients pre-treated at the time of CEA. Authors collected data from a chart review of a large sample of patients (n=3,360) undergoing CEA in Western Canada. Outcomes of patients on statins versus those not on statins were compared using logistic regression to account for differences in patient characteristics, and propensity score methods to account for factors influencing patient allocation to statins.

Eight hundred and fifteen of 2,031 symptomatic patients and 665 of 1,252 asymptomatic patients were on a statin at the time of hospital admission. Authors found that statins use by symptomatic patients was associated with reduced in-hospital mortality (adjusted OR 0.25 [95%CI 0.07 to 0.90] and in-hospital ischemic stroke or death (adjusted OR 0.55 [95% CI 0.32 to 0.95], but not in-hospital cardiac outcomes, (adjusted OR 0.87 [95%CI 0.49 to 1.54], respectively). The improvement in outcomes was robust when tested using propensity score matching. This association was not seen in asymptomatic patients on statins (adjusted OR, in-hospital mortality 0.54 [95%CI 0.13 to 2.24]; in-hospital ischemic stroke or death OR 1.34 [95% CI 0.61 to 2.93]; in-hospital cardiac outcomes, OR 1.37 [95%CI 0.73 to 2.58]).
Other studies investigated the use of statins in carotid stenting (CAS) patients.

Groschel et al, Experience[57]

Groschel et al, specifically analyzed the effect of statins use on patients undergoing CAS. This retrospective study was restricted to periprocedural outcomes and symptomatic patients. Overall, 180 patients with symptomatic carotid stenosis were reviewed. The frequency of cardiovascular complications (composite of stroke, myocardial infarction, and death within 30 days after CAS) between 127 patients without preprocedural statins treatment and that of 53 patients with preprocedural statins treatment at CAS were compared.

The 30-day outcome for all major stroke and death was three of 180 (2%) patients. The incidence of cardiovascular events (composite of stroke, myocardial infarction, and death within 30 days after CAS) was significantly different between patients with preprocedural statins treatment (2 of 53 [4%]) and those without preprocedural statins treatment (19 of 127 [15%], P<0.05). The mean length of stay in the intensive care unit was 1.13 days +/- 0.5 in patients with and 1.75 days +/- 2 in patients without preprocedural statins treatment (P <0.05).

These higher complication rates among patients without preprocedural statins treatment were not mediated by adjustment for age, sex, other baseline characteristics, degree of carotid stenosis, use of cerebral protection devices, or the year in which CAS was performed.

At multiple logistic regression analysis preprocedural statins therapy was identified as the only independent negative predictor (OR, 0.2; 95% CI 0.02, 0.8; P<.05) of cardiovascular events after CAS.

These results suggested that periprocedural statins treatment was associated with a reduction of periprocedural cardiovascular complications after CAS in patients with symptomatic carotid stenosis.

Italian Experience[58]

Data from an Italian experience, suggested that statins use was associated not only with decreased perioperative risks but also with reduced late ischemic strokes and mortality rates in patients undergoing CAS (either symptomatic or not). Authors reviewed outcomes of 1,083 consecutive CAS (29% females, mean age 71.5 years; 24.7% symptomatic) to investigate whether statins use was associated with decreased perioperative and late risks of stroke, mortality, and restenosis after CAS. 465 (43%) patients were on statins medication at the time of CAS. Statins use was associated with a reduction of perioperative stroke and death (OR 0.327, 95%CI 0.13-0.80, P =0.016) according to multivariable analysis. Statins effect was more significant in reducing stroke and death in symptomatic patients (OR 0.13; P = 0.032) and in males (OR 0.27, P = 0.01). At 5 years, survival (87.2% vs 78.3%; P =0.009) and ischemic stroke-free interval (88.9% vs 99.7%; P = 0.02) rates were higher in the statins group of patients. Adjusting for propensity score and covariates in Cox regression analyses, statins use was independently associated with reduced long-term mortality risk (HR 0.56, 95% CI 0.32-0.97; P =0.039) and borderline associated with decreased late ischemic stroke risk (HR 0.14; 95% CI 0.018-1.08, P= 0.059). There was no effect on restenosis rates. Authors suggested that statins therapy should be considered part of the best medical treatment in current CAS practice.

Other studies raised concerns regarding that the benefit of statins use may be lower in women with vascular disease.

Bushnell et al, Experience[59]

To assess whether there were sex-specific differences in stroke incidence severity, and mortality associated with statins use in vascular patients, Bushnell et al, pooled data from subjects enrolled in 3 trials of oral glycoprotein IIb/IIIa inhibitors for CHD. Stroke outcomes were compared among 8,191 baseline statin users versus 14,752 nonusers. Stroke severity was assessed retrospectively with the Canadian Neurological Scale (CNS) based on records with scoreable neurological examinations.

According to baseline characteristics of included patients across these 3 trials, Authors found that statins nonusers were more likely to be women, current smokers and have atrial fibrillation and a history of stroke. A total of 217 subjects had strokes (0.95%). Authors found that statin users had a lower risk of stroke in unadjusted (HR, 0.69; 95% CI 0.51 to 0.92) and risk-adjusted models (HR, 0.72; 95% CI 0.53 to 0.97). There was no difference in stroke mortality with statins use (P=0.8). CNS scores could be assigned to 106 of the subjects, with no difference in severity among statin users and nonusers (median CNS=10.5 in users versus CNS=9.75 in nonusers; P=0.14).

Women had more severe strokes than men (median CNS=10.5 in men versus 9.5 in women; Poisson regression P=0.035). Furthermore, women had more severe strokes after adjustment for statins use (P=0.03) and the combination of statins use, atrial fibrillation, and age (P=0.03).

Authors concluded that in patients with vascular disease, statins use might be associated with a reduced risk of stroke but not severity or mortality. Women had more severe strokes than men, a difference that was not explained by baseline characteristics or statins use.

3. Subclinical Carotid Disease. IMT and Carotid Palque Regression with Statins Use

Evidence form epidemiology and clinical studies has shown IMT to be a strong predictor for development of carotid plaque and cholesterol (and LDL) to be key factors for development of atherosclerosis. Several clinical studies with statins have shown delayed progression or even regression of subclinical carotid disease assessed by measurements of IMT. Most of these studies were designed to determine whether control of LDL cholesterol would retard the progression of IMT or asymptomatic carotid plaques.[1] A reduction in IMT has been documented especially with aggressive lowering lipid levels in various trials.[44,47,49,50,51,52]

The true mechanisms of statins on promoting carotid plaque regression are unclear , however one of the best-characterized effects of statins therapy is an improvement in endothelial function, which can occur through a cholesterol-dependent or a cholesterol-independent mechanism. This last mechanism by which statins improve endothelial function is thought to involve a nitric oxide (NO) dependent process since NO regulates the paracrine anti-atherosclerotic functions of the endothelium. Statins can thereby reduce serum cholesterol levels and inflammation, the effects on each of these processes appear to be independent of one another.

Amarenco et al, in a meta-analysis of statins studies showed that each 10% reduction in LDL with statins was estimated to reduce the carotid IMT by 0.73% per year (95% CI 0.27 to 1.19).[3,4] Statins induced LDL reduction has been significantly correlated to plaque volume reduction and inversely correlated with arterial reverse remodeling associated with plaque regression.[60,61,62,63]

Crisby et al, Experience[60]

Crisby et al, investigated the effect of 3 months of pravastatin treatment on composition of human carotid plaques removed during CEA to assess changes in plaque composition leading to lesion stability in humans.[60] Plaques from patients with symptomatic carotid stenosis and receiving pravastatin 40mg/day for 3 months showed less oxidized LDL immunoreactivity ($P<0.001$), fewer macrophages ($P<0.05$), fewer T cells ($P<0.05$), less matrix metalloproteinases-2 immunoreactivity ($P<0.05$), greater level of tissue inhibitor of metalloproteinases-2 ($P< 0.05$) and higher collagen content ($P<0.005$) when compared to plaques from patients without statins use. Thereby, the use of pravastatin decreased lipids, lipid oxidation, inflammation, MMP-2, and cell death and increased TIMP-1 and collagen content in human carotid plaques, confirming its plaque-stabilizing effect in humans.[60]

In a study of 137 patients who underwent CEA , the plaques removed at operation from patients who were taking statins had significantly lower levels of matrix metalloproteinase-1 and 9 and interleukin-6 when compared to plaques from patients without statins.[61]

The efficacy in lipid lowering effect from statins use and atherosclerotic plaque regression has been investigated with noninvasive imaging studies (echo and Magnetic Resonance Imaging) also in aortic and coronary plaques.[62,63] Aortic studies have shown that with use of simvastatin LDL cholesterol decreased by 23% ($P<0.05$) in 6 months, aortic plaque regression (plaque volume/area reduction) was significantly related to LDL cholesterol reduction ($P<0.02$ and $P<0.005$, respectively), and luminal volume increase was inversely related to LDL cholesterol reduction ($P<0.04$).[62]

Other work also supported the importance of fibrous cap thinning with symptomatic carotid disease and statins. Statins seem also to reduce the vascular expression of adhesion molecules that participate in cellular recruitment to plaque and promoting plaque stability and reduce platelet reactivity, probably due to a decreased thromboxane A2 production.[64,65] These mechanisms within the plaque are likely to translate into a reduction of plaque disruption, thrombosis and related carotid events.

Conclusion

Over the past decades, statins have been proven to significantly decrease coronary events in primary and secondary prevention trials. Recent clinical trials have indicated that statins significantly reduce stroke risk in patients with vascular, non-cardiac, disease. Specifically, the benefits provided by statins in patients with carotid disease are confirmed by clinical and imaging data. In RCTs specifically focused on secondary prevention of stroke (SPARCL)[41,42,43] the treatment with atorvastatin significantly reduced the risk of recurrent cerebrovascular events in patients with recent stroke or TIA.

Mounting evidence supports a link between statins exposure and improved outcomes in patients with carotid stenosis receiving or not a revascularization procedure, even though the mechanisms behind the statin effects are not totally defined.

Even though meta-analysis of RCTs on statins show that each 1mmol/L (39mg/dL) decrease in LDL cholesterol may correspond to a reduction of relative risk for stroke of more than 20%, it is unknown whether these findings might be due to the cholesterol reduction or to pleiotropic effects from statins (including improved endothelial function, decreased platelet aggregation, reduced vascular inflammation). Ongoing research should better clarify this issue as well as should identify how to optimize dosage and duration of statins treatment in these patients.

References

[1] Sacco RL, Liao JK. Drug Insight: statins and stroke. *Nat. Clin. Pract. Cardiovasc. Med.* 2005;2:576-584.

[2] Goldstein LB, Bushnell CD, Adams RJ, Appel LJ, Braun LT, Chaturvedi S, Creager MA, Culebras A, Eckel RH, Hart RG, Hinchey JA, Howard VJ, Jauch EC, Levine SR, Meschia JF, Moore WS, Nixon JV, Pearson TA; American Heart Association Stroke Council; Council on Cardiovascular Nursing; Council on Epidemiology and Prevention; Council for High Blood Pressure Research, Council on Peripheral Vascular Disease, and Interdisciplinary Council on Quality of Care and Outcomes Research. Guidelines for the primary prevention of stroke: a guideline for healthcare professionals from the American Heart Association/American Stroke Association. *Stroke.* 2011;42:517-584.

[3] Amarenco P, Labreuche J. Lipid management in the prevention of stroke: review and updated meta-analysis of statins for stroke prevention. *Lancet Neurol.* 2009;8:453-463.

[4] Amarenco P, Labreuche J, Lavallée P, Touboul PJ. Statins in stroke prevention and carotid atherosclerosis: systematic review and up-to-date meta-analysis. *Stroke.* 2004;35:2902-2909.

[5] O'Regan C, Wu P, Arora P, Perri D, Mills EJ. Statin therapy in stroke prevention: a meta-analysis involving 121,000 patients. *Am. J. Med.* 2008;121: 24-33.

[6] Cholesterol Treatment Trialists' (CTT) Collaboration, Baigent C, Blackwell L, Emberson J, Holland LE, Reith C, Bhala N, Peto R, Barnes EH, Keech A, Simes J, Collins R. Efficacy and safety of more intensive lowering of LDL cholesterol: a meta-analysis of data from 170,000 participants in 26 randomised trials. *Lancet.* 2010;376:1670-81.

[7] Taylor F, Ward K, Moore TH, Burke M, Davey Smith G, Casas JP, Ebrahim S. Statins for the primary prevention of cardiovascular disease. *Cochrane Database Syst. Rev.* 2011:CD004816.

[8] Thavendiranathan P, Bagai A, Brookhart MA, Choudhry NK. Primary prevention of cardiovascular diseases with statin therapy: a meta-analysis of randomized controlled trials. *Arch. Intern. Med.* 2006;166:2307-13.

[9] Brugts JJ, Yetgin T, Hoeks SE, Gotto AM, Shepherd J, Westendorp RG, de Craen AJ, Knopp RH, Nakamura H, Ridker P, van Domburg R, Deckers JW. The benefits of statins in people without established cardiovascular disease but with cardiovascular risk factors: meta-analysis of randomised controlled trials. *BMJ.* 2009;338:b2376.

[10] Brugts JJ, Deckers JW. Statins and all-cause mortality in high-risk primary prevention of patients with cardiovascular risk factors. *Arch. Intern. Med.* 2010;170:2041-2044.

[11] Spector R, Snapinn SM.Statins for secondary prevention of cardiovascular disease: the right dose. *Pharmacology.* 2011;87:63-9.

[12] Hackam DG, Woodward M, Newby LK, Bhatt DL, Shao M, Smith EE, Donner A, Mamdani M, Douketis JD, Arima H, Chalmers J, MacMahon S, Tirschwell DL, Psaty BM, Bushnell CD, Aguilar MI, Capampangan DJ, Werring DJ, De Rango P, Viswanathan A, Danchin N, Cheng CL, Yang YH, Verdel BM, Lai MS, Kennedy J, Uchiyama S, Yamaguchi T, Ikeda Y, Mrkobrada M. Statins and intracerebral hemorrhage: collaborative systematic review and meta-analysis. *Circulation.* 2011;124:2233-42.

[13] Preiss D, Seshasai SR, Welsh P, Murphy SA, Ho JE, Waters DD, DeMicco DA, Barter P, Cannon CP, Sabatine MS, Braunwald E, Kastelein JJ, de Lemos JA, Blazing MA, Pedersen TR, Tikkanen MJ, Sattar N, Ray KK. Risk of incident diabetes with intensive-dose compared with moderate-dose statin therapy: a meta-analysis. *JAMA.* 2011;305:2556-64.

[14] Prospective Studies Collaboration, Lewington S, Whitlock G, Clarke R, Sherliker P, Emberson J, Halsey J, Qizilbash N, Peto R, Collins R. Blood cholesterol and vascular mortality by age, sex, and blood pressure: a meta-analysis of individual data from 61 prospective studies with 55,000 vascular deaths. *Lancet.* 2007;370:1829-39.

[15] Kizer JR, Madias C, Wilner B, Vaughan CJ, Mushlin AI, Trushin P, Gotto AM Jr, Pasternak RC. Relation of different measures of low-density lipoprotein cholesterol to risk of coronary artery disease and death in a meta-regression analysis of large-scale trials of statin therapy. *Am. J. Cardiol.* 2010;105:1289-96.

[16] Kang S, Wu Y, Li X. Effects of statin therapy on the progression of carotid atherosclerosis: a systematic review and meta-analysis. *Atherosclerosis.* 2004;177: 433-42.

[17] West of Scotland Coronary Prevention Study Group. Influence of pravastatin and plasma lipids on clinical events in the West of Scotland Coronary Prevention Study (WOSCOPS).*Circulation.* 1998;97:1440-5.

[18] Shepherd J, Cobbe SM, Ford I, Isles CG, Lorimer AR, MacFarlane PW, McKillop JH, Packard CJ; West of Scotland Coronary Prevention Study Group. Prevention of coronary heart disease with pravastatin in men with hypercholesterolemia. 1995. *Atheroscler Suppl.* 2004;5:91-7.

[19] A.M. Gotto. Establishing the benefit of statins in low-to-moderate—risk primary prevention: The Air Force/Texas Coronary Atherosclerosis Prevention Study (AFCAPS/TexCAPS). *Atheroscler Suppl.* 2007;8:3-8.

[20] ALLHAT Officers and Coordinators for the ALLHAT Collaborative Research Group. The Antihypertensive and Lipid-Lowering Treatment to Prevent Heart Attack Trial. Major outcomes in moderately hypercholesterolemic, hypertensive patients randomized to pravastatin vs usual care: The Antihypertensive and Lipid-Lowering Treatment to Prevent Heart Attack Trial (ALLHAT-LLT).*JAMA.* 2002;288: 2998-3007.

[21] Margolis KL, Dunn K, Simpson LM, Ford CE, Williamson JD, Gordon DJ, Einhorn PT, Probstfield JL; ALLHAT Collaborative Research Group. Coronary heart disease in moderately hypercholesterolemic, hypertensive black and non-black patients randomized to pravastatin versus usual care: the antihypertensive and lipid lowering to prevent heart attack trial (ALLHAT-LLT). *Am. Heart J.* 2009;158:948-55.

[22] Sever PS, Dahlöf B, Poulter NR, Wedel H, Beevers G, Caulfield M, Collins R, Kjeldsen SE, Kristinsson A, McInnes GT, Mehlsen J, Nieminen M, O'Brien E, Ostergren J; ASCOT investigators. Prevention of coronary and stroke events with atorvastatin in hypertensive patients who have average or lower-than-average cholesterol concentrations, in the Anglo-Scandinavian Cardiac Outcomes Trial--Lipid Lowering Arm (ASCOT-LLA): a multicentre randomised controlled trial. *Lancet.* 2003;361:1149-58.

[23] Sever PS, Poulter NR, Dahlof B, Wedel H, Beevers G, Caulfield M, Collins R, Kjeldsen SE, Kristinsson A, McInnes G, Mehlsen J, Nieminen MS, O'Brien ET, Ostergren J; ASCOT Investigators. The Anglo-Scandinavian Cardiac Outcomes Trial

lipid lowering arm: extended observations 2 years after trial closure. *Eur. Heart J.* 2008;29:499-508.

[24] Colhoun HM, Betteridge DJ, Durrington PN, Hitman GA, Neil HA, Livingstone SJ, Thomason MJ, Mackness MI, Charlton-Menys V, Fuller JH; CARDS investigators. Primary prevention of cardiovascular disease with atorvastatin in type 2 diabetes in the Collaborative Atorvastatin Diabetes Study (CARDS): multicentre randomised placebo-controlled trial. *Lancet.* 2004 21-27;364:685-96.

[25] Everett BM, Glynn RJ, MacFadyen JG, Ridker PM. Rosuvastatin in the prevention of stroke among men and women with elevated levels of C-reactive protein: justification for the Use of Statins in Prevention: an Intervention Trial Evaluating Rosuvastatin (JUPITER). *Circulation.* 2010;121:143-50.

[26] Sasaki J, Arakawa K, Iwashita M, Matsushita Y, Kono S; Kyushu Lipid Intervention Study (KLIS)Group. Reduction in serum total cholesterol and risks of coronary events and cerebral infarction in Japanese men: the Kyushu Lipid Intervention Study. *Circ. J.* 2003;67:473-8.

[27] Nakamura H, Arakawa K, Itakura H, Kitabatake A, Goto Y, Toyota T, Nakaya N, Nishimoto S, Muranaka M, Yamamoto A, Mizuno K, Ohashi Y; MEGA Study Group. Primary prevention of cardiovascular disease with pravastatin in Japan (MEGA Study): a prospective randomised controlled trial. *Lancet.* 2006;368:1155-63.

[28] Knopp RH, d'Emden M, Smilde JG, Pocock SJ.Efficacy and safety of atorvastatin in the prevention of cardiovascular endpoints in subjects with typ e 2 diabetes: the Atorvastatin Study for Prevention of Coronary Heart Disease Endpoints in non-insulin-dependent diabetes mellitus (ASPEN). *Diabetes Care.* 2006;29:1478-85.

[29] Heart Protection Study Collaborative Group. MRC/BHF Heart Protection Study of cholesterol lowering with simvastatin in 20,536 high-risk individuals: a randomised placebo-controlled trial. *Lancet.* 2002;360:7-22.

[30] Collins R, Armitage J, Parish S, Sleight P, Peto R; Heart Protection Study Collaborative Group. Effects of cholesterol-lowering with simvastatin on stroke and other major vascular events in 20536 people with cerebrovascular disease or other high-risk conditions. *Lancet.* 2004;363:757-67.

[31] Heart Protection Study Collaborative Group, Bulbulia R, Bowman L, Wallendszus K, Parish S, Armitage J, Peto R, Collins R.Effects on 11-year mortality and morbidity of lowering LDL cholesterol with simvastatin for about 5 years in 20,536 high-risk individuals: a randomised controlled trial. *Lancet.* 2011;378:2013-20.

[32] Shepherd J, Blauw GJ, Murphy MB, Bollen EL, Buckley BM, Cobbe SM, Ford I, Gaw A, Hyland M, Jukema JW, Kamper AM, Macfarlane PW, Meinders AE, Norrie J, Packard CJ, Perry IJ, Stott DJ, Sweeney BJ, Twomey C, Westendorp RG; PROSPER study group. PROspective Study of Pravastatin in the Elderly at Risk. Pravastatin in elderly individuals at risk of vascular disease (PROSPER): a randomised controlled trial. *Lancet.* 2002;360:1623-30.

[33] Wanner C, Krane V, März W, Olschewski M, Mann JF, Ruf G, Ritz E; German Diabetes and Dialysis Study Investigators. Atorvastatin in patients with type 2 diabetes mellitus undergoing hemodialysis. *N. Engl. J. Med.* 2005;353:238-48.

[34] Fellström BC, Jardine AG, Schmieder RE, Holdaas H, Bannister K, Beutler J, Chae DW, Chevaile A, Cobbe SM, Grönhagen-Riska C, De Lima JJ, Lins R, Mayer G, McMahon AW, Parving HH, Remuzzi G, Samuelsson O, Sonkodi S, Sci D,

Süleymanlar G, Tsakiris D, Tesar V, Todorov V, Wiecek A, Wüthrich RP, Gottlow M, Johnsson E, Zannad F; AURORA Study Group. Rosuvastatin and cardiovascular events in patients undergoing hemodialysis. *N. Engl. J. Med.* 2009;360:1395-407.

[35] Baigent C, Landray MJ, Reith C, Emberson J, Wheeler DC, Tomson C, Wanner C, Krane V, Cass A, Craig J, Neal B, Jiang L, Hooi LS, Levin A, Agodoa L, Gaziano M, Kasiske B, Walker R, Massy ZA, Feldt-Rasmussen B, Krairittichai U, Ophascharoensuk V, Fellström B, Holdaas H, Tesar V, Wiecek A, Grobbee D, de Zeeuw D, Grönhagen-Riska C, Dasgupta T, Lewis D, Herrington W, Mafham M, Majoni W, Wallendszus K, Grimm R, Pedersen T, Tobert J, Armitage J, Baxter A, Bray C, Chen Y, Chen Z, Hill M, Knott C, Parish S, Simpson D, Sleight P, Young A, Collins R; SHARP Investigators. The effects of lowering LDL cholesterol with simvastatin plus ezetimibe in patients with chronic kidney disease (Study of Heart and Renal Protection): a randomised placebo-controlled trial. *Lancet.* 2011;377 :2181-92.

[36] Pedersen TR, Kjekshus J, Berg K, Haghfelt T, Faergeman O, Faergeman G, Pyörälä K, Miettinen T, Wilhelmsen L, Olsson AG, Wedel H; Scandinavian Simvastatin Survival Study Group. Randomised trial of cholesterol lowering in 4444 patients with coronary heart disease: the Scandinavian Simvastatin Survival Study (4S). 1994. *Atheroscler Suppl.* 2004;5:81-7.

[37] Simvastatin Survival Study Group. Randomised trial of cholesterol lowering in 4444 patients with coronary heart disease: the Scandinavian Simvastatin Survival Study (4S). *Lancet.* 1994; 344: 1383-89.

[38] Plehn JF, Davis BR, Sacks FM, Rouleau JL, Pfeffer MA, Bernstein V, Cuddy TE, Moyé LA, Piller LB, Rutherford J, Simpson LM, Braunwald E. Reduction of stroke incidence after myocardial infarction with pravastatin: the Cholesterol and Recurrent Events (CARE) study. The Care Investigators. *Circulation.* 1999;99:213-23.

[39] The Long-Term Intervention with Pravastatin in Ischaemic Disease Study Group. Prevention of cardiovascular events and death with pravastatin in patients with coronary heart disease and a broad range of initial cholesterol levels. *N. Engl. J. Med.* 1998;339:1349-57.

[40] Marchioli R, Barzi F, Bomba E, Chieffo C, Di Gregorio D, Di Mascio R, Franzosi MG, Geraci E, Levantesi G, Maggioni AP, Mantini L, Marfisi RM, Mastrogiuseppe G, Mininni N, Nicolosi GL, Santini M, Schweiger C, Tavazzi L, Tognoni G, Tucci C, Valagussa F; GISSI-Prevenzione Investigators. Early protection against sudden death by n-3 polyunsaturated fatty acids after myocardial infarction: time-course analysis of the results of the Gruppo Italiano per lo Studio della Sopravvivenza nell'Infarto Miocardico (GISSI)-Prevenzione. *Circulation.* 2002;105:1897-903.

[41] Amarenco P, Goldstein LB, Szarek M, Sillesen H, Rudolph AE, Callahan A 3rd, Hennerici M, Simunovic L, Zivin JA, Welch KM; SPARCL Investigators. Effects of intense low-density lipoprotein cholesterol reduction in patients with stroke or transient ischemic attack: the Stroke Prevention by Aggressive Reduction in Cholesterol Levels (SPARCL) trial. *Stroke.* 2007;38:3198-204.

[42] Stroke Prevetion by Aggressive Reduction in Cholestrol Levels (SPARCL) Investigators, Karam JG, Loney-Hutchinson L, McFarlane SI. High-dose atorvastatin after stroke or transient ischemic attack: The Stroke Prevention by Aggressive Reduction in Cholesterol Levels (SPARCL) Investigators. *J. Cardiometab Syndr.* 2008;3:68-9.

[43] Sillesen H, Amarenco P, Hennerici MG, Callahan A, Goldstein LB, Zivin J, Messig M, Welch KM; Stroke Prevention by Aggressive Reduction in Cholesterol Levels Investigators. Atorvastatin reduces the risk of cardiovascular events in patients with carotid atherosclerosis: a secondary analysis of the Stroke Prevention by Aggressive Reduction in Cholesterol Levels (SPARCL) trial. *Stroke.* 2008;39:3297-302.

[44] De Lemos JA, Blazing MA, Wiviott SD, Lewis EF, Fox KA, White HD, Rouleau JL, Pedersen TR, Gardner LH, Mukherjee R, Ramsey KE, Palmisano J, Bilheimer DW, Pfeffer MA, Califf RM, Braunwald E; A to Z Investigators. Early intensive vs a delayed conservative simvastatin strategy in patients with acute coronary syndromes: phase Z of the A to Z trial. *JAMA.* 2004;292:1307-16.

[45] Koren MJ, Hunninghake DB; ALLIANCE Investigators. Clinical outcomes in managed-care patients with coronary heart disease treated aggressively in lipid-lowering disease management clinics: the alliance study. *J. Am. Coll. Cardiol.* 2004;44:1772-9.

[46] Athyros VG, Papageorgiou AA, Mercouris BR, Athyrou VV, Symeonidis AN, Basayannis EO, Demitriadis DS, Kontopoulos AG. Treatment with atorvastatin to the National Cholesterol Educational Program goal versus 'usual' care in secondary coronary heart disease prevention. The GREek Atorvastatin and Coronary-heart-disease Evaluation (GREACE) study. *Curr Med Res Opin.* 2002;18:220-8.

[47] Pedersen TR, Faergeman O, Kastelein JJ, Olsson AG, Tikkanen MJ, Holme I, Larsen ML, Bendiksen FS, Lindahl C, Szarek M, Tsai J; Incremental Decrease in End Points Through Aggressive Lipid Lowering (IDEAL) Study Group.High-dose atorvastatin vs usual-dose simvastatin for secondary prevention after myocardial infarction: the IDEAL study: a randomized controlled trial. *JAMA.* 2005;294:2437-45.

[48] Schwartz GG, Olsson AG, Ezekowitz MD, Ganz P, Oliver MF, Waters D, Zeiher A, Chaitman BR, Leslie S, Stern T; Myocardial Ischemia Reduction with Aggressive Cholesterol Lowering (MIRACL) Study Investigators.Effects of atorvastatin on early recurrent ischemic events in acute coronary syndromes: the MIRACL study: a randomized controlled trial. *JAMA.* 2001;285:1711-8.

[49] Study of the Effectiveness of Additional Reductions in Cholesterol and Homocysteine (SEARCH) Collaborative Group, Armitage J, Bowman L, Wallendszus K, Bulbulia R, Rahimi K, Haynes R, Parish S, Peto R, Collins R.Intensive lowering of LDL cholesterol with 80 mg versus 20 mg simvastatin daily in 12,064 survivors of myocardial infarction: a double-blind randomised trial.*Lancet.* 2010;376:1658-69.

[50] Murphy SA, Cannon CP, Wiviott SD, McCabe CH, Braunwald E. Reduction in recurrent cardiovascular events with intensive lipid-lowering statin therapy compared with moderate lipid-lowering statin therapy after acute coronary syndromes from the PROVE IT-TIMI 22 (Pravastatin or Atorvastatin Evaluation and Infection Therapy-Thrombolysis In Myocardial Infarction 22) trial. *J Am Coll Cardiol.* 2009;54:2358-62.

[51] Waters DD, LaRosa JC, Barter P, Fruchart JC, Gotto AM Jr, Carter R, Breazna A, Kastelein JJ, Grundy SM. Effects of high-dose atorvastatin on cerebrovascular events in patients with stable coronary disease in the TNT (treating to new targets) study. *J. Am. Coll. Cardiol.* 2006;48: 1793-9.

[52] Shepherd J, Kastelein JJ, Bittner V, Deedwania P, Breazna A, Dobson S, Wilson DJ, Zuckerman A, Wenger NK; Treating to New Targets Investigators. Effect of intensive lipid lowering with atorvastatin on renal function in patients with coronary heart

disease: the Treating to New Targets (TNT) study. *Clin. J. Am. Soc. Nephrol.* 2007;2:1131-9.

[53] O'Neil-Callahan K, Katsimaglis G, Tepper MR, Ryan J, Mosby C, Ioannidis JP, Danias PG. Statins decrease perioperative cardiac complications in patients undergoing noncardiac vascular surgery: the Statins for Risk Reduction in Surgery (StaRRS) study. *J. Am. Coll. Cardiol.* 2005;45:336-42.

[54] Brooke BS, McGirt MJ, Woodworth GF, Chang DC, Roseborough GS, Freischlag JA, Perler BA. Preoperative statin and diuretic use influence the presentation of patients undergoing carotid endarterectomy: results of a large single-institution case-control study. *J. Vasc. Surg.* 2007;45:298-303.

[55] McGirt MJ, Perler BA, Brooke BS, Woodworth GF, Coon A, Jain S, Buck D, Roseborough GS, Tamargo RJ, Heller J, Freischlag JA, Williams GM. 3-hydroxy-3-methylglutaryl coenzyme A reductase inhibitors reduce the risk of perioperative stroke and mortality after carotid endarterectomy. *J. Vasc. Surg.* 2005;42:829-36.

[56] Kennedy J, Quan H, Buchan AM, Ghali WA, Feasby TE. Statins are associated with better outcomes after carotid endarterectomy in symptomatic patients. *Stroke.* 2005;36:2072-2076.

[57] Gröschel K, Ernemann U, Schulz JB, Nägele T, Terborg C, Kastrup A. Statin therapy at carotid angioplasty and stent placement: effect on procedure-related stroke, myocardial infarction, and death. *Radiology.* 2006;240:145-51.

[58] Verzini F, De Rango P, Parlani G, Giordano G, Caso V, Cieri E, Isernia G, Cao P. Effects of statins on early and late results of carotid stenting. *J. Vasc. Surg.* 2011;53:71-9.

[59] Bushnell CD, Griffin J, Newby LK, Goldstein LB, Mahaffey KW, Graffagnino CA, Harrington RA, White HD, Simes RJ, Califf RM, Topol EJ, Easton JD. Statin use and sex-specific stroke outcomes in patients with vascular disease. *Stroke.* 2006;37:1427-31.

[60] Crisby M, Nordin-Fredriksson G, Shah PK, Yano J, Zhu J, Nilsson J. Pravastatin treatment increases collagen content and decreases lipid content, inflammation, metalloproteinases, and cell death in human carotid plaques: implications for plaque stabilization. *Circulation.* 2001;103:926-33.

[61] Molloy KJ, Thompson MM, Jones JL, Schwalbe EC, Bell PR, Naylor AR, Loftus IM. Unstable carotid plaques exhibit raised matrix metalloproteinase-8 activity. *Circulation.* 2004;110:337-43.

[62] Lima JA, Desai MY, Steen H, Warren WP, Gautam S, Lai S. Statin-induced cholesterol lowering and plaque regression after 6 months of magnetic resonance imaging-monitored therapy. *Circulation.* 2004;110:2336-41.

[63] Nicholls SJ, Borgman M, Nissen SE, Raichlen JS, Ballantyne C, Barter P, Chapman MJ, Erbel R, Libby P. Impact of statins on progression of atherosclerosis: rationale and design of SATURN (Study of Coronary Atheroma by InTravascular Ultrasound: effect of Rosuvastatin versus AtorvastatiN). *Curr Med Res Opin.* 2011;1119-29.

[64] Paciaroni M, Hennerici M, Agnelli G, Bogousslavsky J.Statins and stroke prevention. *Cerebrovasc Dis.* 2007;24:170-82.

[65] Paciaroni M, Bogousslavsky J. Statins and stroke prevention. *Expert Rev. Cardiovasc Ther.* 2009;7:231-43.

In: Statins
Editors: Benedetta La Grua and Alessandro Molinelli

ISBN: 978-1-62081-367-6

Chapter II

Statins: Their Pleiotropic Effects beyond Lowering Cholesterol

Shouji Shimoyama*
Gastrointestinal Unit, Settlement Clinic, Tokyo, Japan

Abstract

3-hydroxy-3-methylglutaryl (HMG)-CoA reductase is a rate-limiting enzyme of the mevalonate pathway for cholesterol synthesis. Statins inhibit this enzyme, thus having functions for lowering cholesterol. There is also a growing body of evidence that statins have pleiotropic effects, independent of lowering cholesterol. These pleiotropic effects are partly exerted by inhibiting synthesis of isoprenoids, which are downstream molecules of the mevalonate pathway, involved in the activation of small GTPases that eventually modulate an intracellular signal cascade. These effects include: (i) anti-atherosclerosis and plaque stabilizating effects by inhibiting various steps of athelogenic and plaque formation cascades; (ii) inhibiting inflammation, which plays a pivotal role in the pathogenesis of atherosclerosis; (iii) neovascularizing or increasing blood flow in ischemic tissue, leading to cardio- and neuroprotective effects and subsequent improvements of vascular dementia; (iv) favorable effects on such neurodegenerative diseases as Alzheimer disease and Parkinson disease; (v) improving bone health through stimulation of bone formation and osteoclast inhibition ; (vi) improving renal dysfunction and preventing the progression of chronic kidney diseases; and finally (vii) negative or at least neutral effects on the development of some kinds of cancers. This chapter highlights current knowledge on the potential mechanisms for statin-mediated pleiotropic effects. Since these pleiotropic effects are significant on the aging-related or lifestyle-related diseases which have increasingly attracted global health concern, e.g. metabolic, neurological, and neoplastic diseases, this chapter will help researchers to develop new treatment strategies that incorporate statins as comprehensively effective agents, ultimately leading to prevent or regress such diseases.

* Address of corresponding author and for reprints: Shouji Shimoyama, M.D., Gastrointestinal Unit, Settlement Clinic, 4-20-7, Towa, Adachi-ku, Tokyo, 120-0003, Japan, Tel: +81-3-3605-7747 Fax: +81-3-3605-0244,e-mail address: shimoyama@apost.plala.or.jp.

Key Words: Statins, Pleiotropic effect, Vascular inflammation, Isoprenylation, Nitric oxide, Alzheimer disease, Parkinson disease, Chronic kidney disease, Osteoporosis, Malignancy

1. Introduction

Statins are potent inhibitors of 3-hydroxy 3-methylglutaryl-CoA (HMG-CoA) reductase, the rate-controlling enzyme at the apex of the mevalonate pathway. Statins inhibit this enzyme and exhibit a subsequent potent effect associated with a lowering of cholesterol; thus they have gained the cornerstone of hypercholesterolemia medical treatment. Besides lowering cholesterol, statins also inhibit endoproduct synthesis for a diverse array of mevalonate pathways. Subsequently, these actions exert a wide spectrum of biological effects, including: reducing endothelial dysfunction, inhibiting inflammatory responses, stabilizing atherosclerotic plaques, and modulating cell signal cascades. Therefore, statins exert "pleiotropic effects", a term used to collectively refer to the effects independent of and beyond lowering cholesterol.

There are several reviews of statins' pleiotropic effects that focus on the biological events during atherogenesis [1, 2]. However, considering that the end products of the mevalonate pathway are important for the intracellular growth signal transduction responsible for cell growth, proliferation, migration, and survival, as well as for many other substrates responsible for the development of a variety of diseases, it is hypothesized that statins may manifest beneficial effects on many organs not restricted to vessels, and evidence has been accumulated to support this hypothesis. This chapter reviews recent knowledge on statins' pleiotropic effects on a wide spectrum of diseases and organs, within and beyond vessels.

2. Vascular Pathobiology during Atherogenesis

Although atherosclerosis is a resultant of incredibly complex processes, a brief summary of the biological events during atherosclerosis is provided, first, for the better understanding of the pleiotropic effects associated with statins. Atherosclerotic plaque formation comprises a hierarchy of biological phenomena, starting with endothelial injury and the subsequent inflammatory cell recruiting. An early step of atherogenesis is an altered endothelial permeability. After endothelial injury occurs, inflammatory cascade ensues with monocytes, macrophages, lymphocytes, and platelets recruited at the injured site, followed by a penetration of these cells into the subendothelial spaces [3-5].

Factors that attract these cells include: intracellular adhesion molecules (ICAMs), vascular-cell adhesion molecules (VCAMs), and monocytes chemoattractant protein-1 (MCP-1), as well as cytokines such as the tumor-necrosis factor (TNF) and interleukins (ILs) [5, 6]. Macrophages and lymphocytes secrete inflammatory cytokines that can modify endothelial function. Platelet aggregability is increased by various factors such as impaired platelet-derived nitric oxide and oxidative stress [7].

Once circulatory low-density lipoproteins (LDL) are trapped in a vessel wall, they can undergo oxidation to form an oxidized LDL (oxLDL) at the subendothelial space [8, 9]. Platelets promote cholesterol accumulation via LDL-C receptor-mediated endocytosis [3].

OxLDL is able to convert monocytes to activated macrophages and promote macrophage proliferation [10]. Activated macrophages take up the oxLDL, or lipid-laden platelets,, migrate into the intima through their scavenger receptors and become foamy cells [3, 8, 9]. In addition, OxLDL on platelets and endothelial cells promotes platelet aggregation [11] or endothelial dysfunction [12].

Additionally, vascular smooth muscle cells (VSMCs) migrate from the media to the intima at the injury site, a process which is stimulated by various kinds of cytokines [5]. Serum lipoproteins also accumulate in the injured intima. The continued accumulation of these cells and serum lipids together forms a "fatty streak" —a region of intimal thickening as the earliest event in the atherosclerotic plaque formation processes.

When vascular injury conditions such as hyperlipidemia or other risk factors continue, the inflammatory responses will then also continue. VSMCs and circulating monocytes continue to infiltrate into the lesion, and the cytokines formed by the activated macrophages themselves and other cells participating in this process potentiate to cause a remodeling of the fatty streak to form a fibrous cap which is composed of VSMCs and the extracellular matrix proteins they secrete [5].

Macrophages in the cap not only continue to make cytokines, but they also make matrix metalloproteinases (MMPs) and tissue factors (TF) [13, 14]. MMPs, which are proteolytic enzymes that weaken the fibrous cap through collagen degradation, and TF, which is a strong activator of blood coagulation that also causes plaque instability [15], both contribute to disrupt the cap. Then, all types of vascular cells, such as endothelial cells, VSMCs, and macrophages, undergo apoptosis [16], the processes which play a key role on the pathogenesis of vascular remodeling and plaque vulnerability, ultimately causing rupture [17, 18].

Once the plaque has ruptured, the fibrous cap is exposed to blood, the further vicious cycle of blood cell aggregation and coagulation begins, and atherosclerotic plaques develop. The encroachment of the vessel, with the culmination of cellular and molecular events, ensues with terminal events such as myocardial or cerebral infarctions.

Taking the whole athelogenic process into account, increased apoptosis may either prevent VSMCs accumulation and halt the progression of vascular wall thickening orpromote plaque destabilization and rupture by thinning out the fibrous cap. Therefore, it is unknown whether the induction of apoptosis in VSMCs by statins is beneficial or harmful, and the clinical importance of the apoptosis process remains to be elucidated (see section 4.1).

Importantly, inflammation is a central event engaged throughout the entire atherosclerotic cascade process , starting from the fatty streak formation with inflammatory cell aggregation and ending with plaque destabilization manifesting clinical events. The lineage of cellular events is a result of a complex cascade, involving many kinds of circulating and vascular cells, enzymes, and cytokines which interplay each other. This networking is critical to determine the directions the lesion will take.

Therefore, the degree and nature of inflammation, as well as the cytokine expression caused by different cell types, may determine whether a lesion will progress, remain static, or undergo regression. The statins' ability to modify these events is the nature of their pleiotropic effects, and the fundamental mechanisms of this modification will be discussed below.

3. Key Biological Events of Statins That Explain Their Pleiotropic Effects

Through HMG-CoA reductase inhibition, statins prevent the synthesis of isoprenoid intermediates such as farnesyl pyrophosphate (FPP) and geranylgeranyl pyrophosphate (GGPP), downstream products of mevalonate pathway. These intermediates act as lipid anchors for the post-translational modifications of a variety of guanosine triphosphate (GTP)-binding proteins such as Ras and Ras-like proteins (e.g., Rho, Rab, Rac, and Cdc42, etc.) [19]. The post-translational modification (isoprenylation) allows for the translocation of these proteins from the cytoplasm to the cell membrane. This membrane localization is an initial event for the activation of GTP-binding proteins, which cycles between the inactive, switch-off GDP-bound state and the active, switch-on GTP-bound state. Ras prenylation is dependent on farnesylation whereas Rho prenylation is dependent on geranylgeranylation.

Activated Ras eventually initiates a series of mitogenic signaling cascades such as Raf/MAPK (mitogen activated protein kinase, also known as extracellular signal-regulated kinases; ERKs), Rac/Rho (Ras-homologous), and PI3K/Akt (phosphatidylinositol 3-kinase/v-akt murine thymoma viral oncogene homolog 1, also known as PKB). Activation of these cascades eventually activates a variety of downstream target genes relevant to cell proliferation [20]; regulation of the cytoskeleton and morphologic changes that increase cell invasive properties [21]; antiapoptosis that prevents cellular senescence, and motility-dependent cell dissemination [22]; all of which ultimately promote cell growth, proliferation, migration, angiogenesis, and survival [20]. Rho regulates the reorganization of intracellular actin cytoskeleton and membrane trafficking [19]. Rac1 increases oxidative stress sensitivity, and Rac1 and Cdc42 regulate cell shape and membrane ruffles through the formation of lamellipodia and filopodia [23]. Considering that Ras and Rho act as cornerstone molecules which transmit signals from upstream of receptor tyrosine kinases to downstream messenger proteins, the inhibition of both FPP and GGPP production by statins leads to accumulate inactive Ras and Rho; hinders hierarchical signal transduction cascades; and, ultimately, modulates aforementioned various biological events, which are fundamental molecular mechanisms of pleiotropic effects of statins.

4. Statins' Pleiotropic Effects

4.1. Anti-Atherogenic and Plaque Stabilization Effects (Figure)

Endothelium-derived nitric oxide (NO) is relevant to vascular health. It inhibits several components of the atherogenic process including monocyte adhesion to the endothelial surface [24], platelet aggregation [25], and VSMC proliferation [26]. NO can also inhibit oxidative modification of LDL (ox-LDL) [27] and *vice versa* [28].

Several lines of evidence have implicated anti-atherogenic connections between statins and the upregulation of endothelial nitric oxide synthase (eNOS). First, since Rho acts as a negative regulator of eNOS expressions [23, 29, 30], statins' inhibition of GGPP production and subsequent inactivation of Rho results in an eNOS expression increase. Furthermore, statins upregulate eNOS by stabilizing eNOS mRNA or inhibiting the oxLDL-induced downregulation of eNOS [31]. Second, statins stimulate the PI3K/Akt pathway [32], a direct activator of eNOS [33]. The PI3K/Akt pathway mediates growth factor- and anchorage-dependent survival signals in endothelial cells [34] and promotes endothelial cell migration [35], the effects which are essential for the differentiation of endothelial cells into vasculature structures. Third, statins suppress caveolin-1 production, a negative regulator of eNOS leading to a direct inhibition of NO production [36-39]. Finally, statins induce the Kruppel-like factor-2 (KLF-2), resulting in a subsequent eNOS expression in endothelial cells. This KLF-2 induction is dependent on Rho pathway inhibition [40]. In addition, KLF-2 is a key regulator of vascular barrier functioning; thus KLF-2 induction by statins may maintain endothelial barrier integrity and reduce vascular permeability [41]. Furthermore, NO is a potent vasodilator. Benefits of increased blood flow by an increased eNOS expression on ischemic tissue will be discussed below (see section 4.3).

Underlying biological events of statins that exert its pleiotropic effects on improvement of endothelial function.

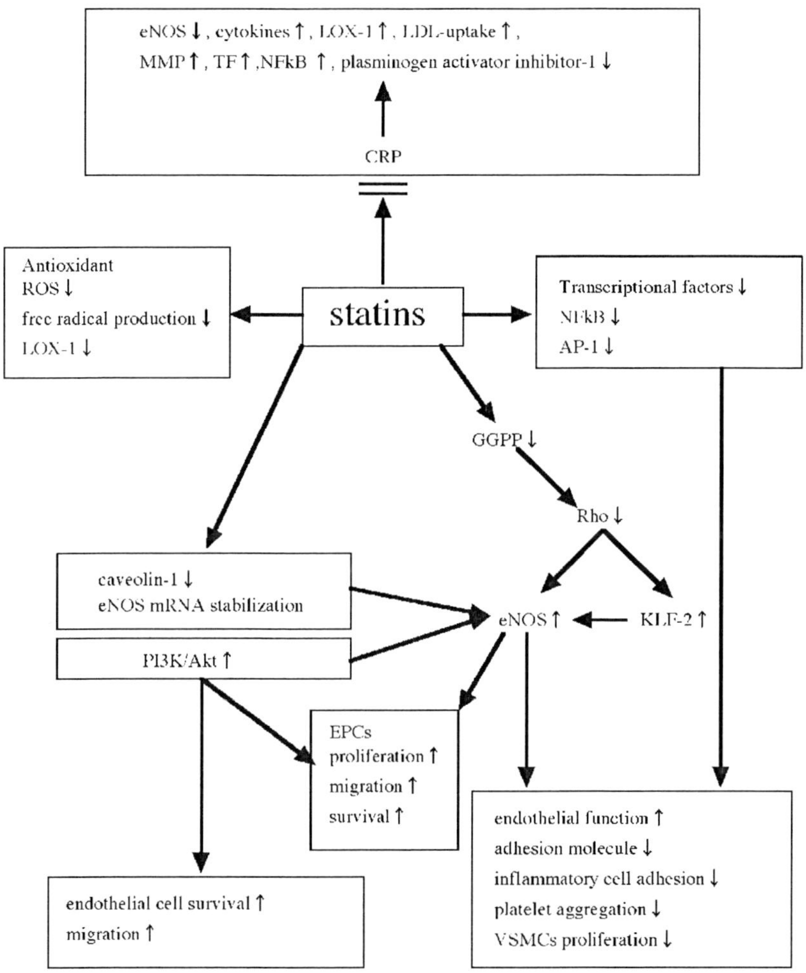

Figure 1.

Another potential mechanism by which statins exert anti-atherogenic properties is through antioxidant effects [42]. Stains attenuate production of reactive oxygen species (ROS) [43], free radical production [44], and platelet aggregability through improvement of redox state of platelets [7]. Statins are able to downregulate the receptor to oxLDL (LOX-1) on macrophages or endothelial cells, resulting in a subsequent reduced uptake of oxLDL in these cells [45, 46].

As described in section 2, migration and proliferation of VSMCs and inflammatory cells are major components of atherogenesis, and statins interfere with this process. The inactivation of Ras and Rho by statins, and the subsequent inhibition of MAPK signaling cascade, attenuates macrophage proliferation [10]. Statins induce the apoptosis of inflammatory cells [47] and VSMCs [47, 48]. Taken together, statins are able to combat the foamy cell production and eventual fibrous cap formation through inhibiting many participants responsible for its formation. However, the effects of statins on vascular cell apoptosis seem to be dependent on the types of statins. Lipophilic statins are able to stimulate apoptosis of VSMCs, whereas hydrophilic statins are anti-apoptotic [49, 50].

Plaque rupturing is a major cause of acute ischemic events. This rupturing causes the activation of platelet and coagulation cascades with subsequent thrombus formations, and, ultimately, blood vessel occlusion. MMPs and TF produced by activated macrophages may weaken the fibrous cap leading to plaque instability, eventually causing a rupture and enhanced thrombogenicity [13]. Statins inhibit MMPs and TF production from activated macrophages [13] and may attenuate their proteolytic and thrombogenic activities; thus they have the potential to stabilize atherosclerotic plaque [13, 51, 52]. The plaque stabilizing properties of statins, therefore, are mediated through the combined effects of decreasing lipid levels, macrophage accumulation reductions, decreased MMPs and TF production, and increased collagen content in the plaque [51, 52]. Accordingly, in the MIRACL trial, the risk of reducing ischemic events was achieved by an early atorvastatin administration. Interestingly, these salutary effects were observed at first month of the treatment initiation and did not appear to depend on the baseline LDL-C levels [53], suggesting that atorvastatin possesses anti-atherogenic properties beyond cholesterol lowering. The SATURN trial has very recently demonstrated an atheroma volume regression by atorvastatin and rosuvastatin [54].

4.2. Anti-Inflammatory Effects with Anti-Atherogenesis (Figure)

Since inflammation plays a pivotal role in the pathogenesis of atherosclerosis, the ability of statins to modulate immune response is gaining increasing interest. Statins attenuate the expression of cytokines or adhesion molecules, such as: a monocytes chemotactic protein [55], IL-8 [56], ICAM-1 [57], TNF-α [58], nuclear factor kappa-B (NFκB) [58], IL-6 [59], VCAM-1 [60]. In addition, statins also downregulate NFκB [61] and activator protein-1 (AP-1) [62], which are regulators of gene transcription involved in a large series of inflammatory processes. These anti-inflammation effects are also mediated by the inhibition of adhesion molecules and endothelial NO production [63].

The C-reactive protein has traditionally been used as a marker of inflammation, and high sensitivity CRP (hs-CRP) reflects low-grade systemic inflammation. In addition, it is regarded as a partaker in the pathogenesis of atherosclerosis. Furthermore, CRP activates endothelial cells and macrophages to express adhesion molecules, cytokines, and TF, as well as enhances LDL-C uptake [64]. CRP causes a direct reduction in eNOS expression [65, 66], augments key adhesion molecules and inflammatory cytokines [67], enhances LDL-C uptake by macrophages [67], increases expression of oxLDL receptor (LOX-1) on endothelial cells [68], increases plasminogen activator inhibitor-1 activity resulting in an impaired fibrinolytic capacity [69], releases TF through NFκB activation [70], and induces MMPs from macrophages [71] or endothelial cells [72]. Therefore, there is a paradigm shift in which CRP is merely no longer an indicator of inflammation, but CRP is recognized as an initiator of several pathogenic pathways that can cause atherogenic changes; thus the inhibition of CRP production may be antiatherogenic.

This fundamental logic has been confirmed by the several clinical studies. The REVERSAL trial observed CRP reduction by statins although the degree of reduction was different between statins [73]. Pravastatin (PRINCE trial) [74] and lovastatin (AFCAPS/TexCAPS trial) [75] reduced CRP concentration, and patients with CRP above the median benefited from lovastatin therapy even in the absence of overt dyslipidemia. [75]. In the PROVE-IT/TIMI22 trial, patients that achieved dual goals of LDL-C <70mg/dL and CRP (<2mg/L) by atorvastatin or pravastatin had significant coronary event risk reduction [76, 77]. Finally, in the JUPITER trial, patients with normal LDL-C (<3.4mmol/L) but elevated CRP (>2mg/L) levels were randomized to receive 20mg/day rosuvastatin or placebo [78]. Strikingly, rosuvastatin achieved a 44% risk reduction in the primary end point under this accrual condition (e.g., normal LDL-C level), and the subset of patients that mostly benefited from this drug was that which achieved both low LDL-C (<1.8mmol/L) and low CRP levels (65% risk reduction for patients with CRP<2mg/L, and there 79% risk reduction for patients with CRP<1mg/L) [79]. Furthermore, when hs-CRP levels were similar between statin-treated and placebo-treated patients, the improvement of endothelial functioning was also similar [80]. These results suggest that increased CRP concentration is associated with increased risk of cardiovascular events even with normal LDL-C levels, and statin therapy could specifically reduce this risk by reducing the CRP level. Interestingly, a small molecule inhibitor of CRP reduced cardiovascular events in rats suggesting that the lowering CRP effect is not only a mere reflection of inflammation reduction, but that CRP may deteriorate an acute myocardial infarction and ischemic stroke [81].

4.3. Neovascularization and Increased Blood Flow (Figure)

As introduced in section 4.1, statins prompt angiogenesis beneficial in the ischemic tissues. Cerivastatin enhanced eNOS activity, capillary density, and collateral flow in the ischemic mice model, whereas these effects disappeared in eNOS deficient mice [82]. Interestingly, the augmented blood flow that occurred in ischemic tissue was not observed in cancers, suggesting that statins may not promote tumor neovascularization [83]. These angiogenic effects of statins seemed dose-dependent (angiogenic at lower concentrations and antiangiogenic at higher concentrations [84]) whereas other investigators showed even higher statins concentrations being angiogenic [82].

Several lines of evidence have implicated that statins also enhance neovascularization by stimulating endothelial progenitor cells (EPCs). EPCs originating from the bone marrow were isolated from the peripheral blood [85], and they may participate in vascular healing [86] and neovascularization in ischemic tissues [87]. Statins inhibit isoprenylation, activate PI3K/Akt pathway, and enhance eNOS expression, leading to promote EPCs proliferation, migration, and survival [88-90], as well as prevent senescence of EPCs [91] and endothelial cells [92]; thus statins have a therapeutic potential for the vasculogenesis of ischemic tissues. Accordingly, statins can reduce infarct size and ameliorate ischemic stroke through PI3K/Akt activation [93] or through an increase in eNOS expression [94, 95]. Very recently, NO-donating atorvastatin has been shown to improve circulating angiogenic cell function [96].

Such an inhibition of endothelial senescence and increased blood flow by statins contributes to brain health by preventing the progression of vascular dementia as a result of cerebral infarction. The three isoforms of NOS — endothelial, neuronal, and inducible NOS (designated as eNOS, nNOS, and iNOS, respectively) — have been characterized in brain cells [97]. Immediately after brain ischemia, eNOS produces NO which is protective because of its vasodilation effect; however, when ischemia develops, NO is released from nNOS and later iNOS, which is harmful because it contributes to brain damage. Therefore, both the upregulation of eNOS and the inhibition of iNOS by statins are considered as neuroprotective [98]. In addition, statins' anti-inflammatory ability and antioxidant effects, as well as its being able maintain endothelial function, are all contributors to neuroprotection in the ischemic brain [98].

Taken together, statins can offer conditions shifting from vasoconstriction to vasodilatation leading to enhanced angiogenesis, synaptogenesis, and neurogenesis. Clinically, patients already taking statins at the time of stroke onset had lower likelihood of stroke severity [99], experienced less worsening during hospitalization [100], exhibited decreased post-stroke mortality [100], and received benefits for their long-term functional outcome [101]. In the same sense, the discontinuation of statins after an ischemic stroke was associated with higher risk of dependency, earlier neurologic deterioration, and poor survival [102]. The improved stroke outcome was independent of the baseline LDL-C level [103], suggesting that statins possess a pleiotropic anti-ischemic function. These observations have prompted to conduct a novel phase I dose-escalating lovastatin study (NeuSTART study) [104]. Currently, no randomized trials have been available to assess the role of statins in the treatment of vascular dementia (see section 4.4, ref. [144]).

4.4. Neurodegenerative Disorders

Recent evidence has stimulated the discussions of statins as potential novel drugs for neurodegenerative disorders. Alzheimer disease (AD) is one of the most common forms of dementia, and an accumulation of amyloid-β in the brain has been found to be a significant responsible factor associated with the earlier onset of the disease. Amyloid-β, a peptide derived by a sequential proteolytic cleavage of amyloid precursor protein (APP) by β- and γ-secretase [105], accumulates in, and is a main constituent of, senile plaques that cause neurotoxicity and neurodegeneration.

AD has multiple connections with lipids [106]. Cholesterol levels are associated with β-secretase activity and subsequent amyloid-β peptide deposit formation and secretion [105]; thus cholesterol exacerbates amyloid-β associated neurotoxicity [106, 107]. On the other hand, cholesterol levels inversely correlated with the nonamyloidgenic α-cleavage of APP

[105, 108]. Autopsy studies confirmed the experimental findings of an association between dyslipidemia and AD-related pathology [109, 110].

Another responsible factor for AD is polymorphism of apolipoprotein E (APOE), a lipid transport protein. It is coded by a gene that exhibits allele variants ε2, ε3, and ε4, which respectively code for three APOE isoforms, APOE2, APOE3, and APOE4. The ApoEε4 genotype is associated with raised LDL-C [111, 112] and has been found to be the most highly ranked locus in regulating LDL-C levels at the whole genome level [113]. APOEε4 promotes the efflux of cholesterol from neurons less effectively than APOEε2 and APOEε3 [114]. In addition, APOE4 binds with amyloid-β with high activity and specificity [115], and is associated with aggregation [106] and less amyloid-β clearance [116]. Accordingly, possession of one or more copies APOEε4 was known to increase the risk of developing AD or of cognitive decline [117], whereas neuritic degeneration was absent in the ApoE null phenotype [118]. Furthermore, APOE4, in combination with atherosclerosis, was substantially associated with a higher risk of cognitive decline [119], vascular dementia [120], and AD [120]. Therefore, there may be an interplay and genetic link between cholesterol and amyloid-β through the APOE variant for establishing AD. Given the lack of effective therapy for AD and its association with aging, AD gains one of the most pressing health concerns worldwide.

Statins may be a candidate for AD treatment, partly through its lipid reduction and partly, but more fundamentally, through its direct effects on amyloid-β metabolism or APOE4. For example, decreased amyloid-β secretion was a result of an inhibition associated with the isoprenylation of GTP-binding proteins such as Rac [121], Rab [122, 123], and Rho [123, 124], the effects being independent of lowering cholesterol [125]. Statins could exert a neuroprotective effect by preventing atherothrombotic events in the brain via inhibiting macrophage functioning, platelet aggregation, and cytokine expression [126] as well as by reducing amyloid-β formation in hipoccampal neurons [127]. Statins' ability to reduce AD risk or cognitive decline in the ApoEε4 allele carriers was more prominently than [128, 129], or at least equal to [130], those in the nonApoEε4 allele carriers. These findings could be a mechanistic basis why statins are associated with less dementia risk.

However, not all clinical and epidemiological studies support these mechanisms. The prevalence of AD in patients taking statins was 60-73% lower as compared with patients taking other medications for cardiovascular disease [131], although the prevalence of AD was different between statins. Patients with a statin therapy resulted in having a significant reduction in developing dementia [132, 133], better mental status performance [134], slower cognitive functioning deterioration [135], and greater decreased amyloid-β levels [136]. Simvastatin also reduced amyloid-β production in normocholesterolemic, mild AD patients [137]. These effects could be explained by the statins' pleiotropic properties rather than cholesterol lowering [133, 134] since other lipid-lowering agents could not demonstrate the same effects [128]. However, the previous [138-140] and more recent [141, 142] RCTs failed to find any significant clinical benefit associated with statins on cognitive functioning. Collectively, several meta-analyses found that effects of statins were null on the prevention of dementia or AD [143, 144], but seemingly marginally positive on the treatment of dementia [145].

The pitfalls why all statins do not create equal results on dementia may be the differences in lipophilicity, patient age, baseline cholesterol levels, and concomitant drugs affecting xenobiotics, although the agreement in the literature is not always complete. Lipophilic statins more effectively pass the blood-brain barrier than hydrophilic statins [146, 147]. Since cholesterol in the central nervous system originates mainly from *in situ* synthesis [148], the in situ inhibition of cholesterol production in the central nervous system may be more rational against AD; thus lipophilic statins are theoretically more effective than hydrophilic statins. One population-based study, however, found that statins' could exert AD risk reduction regardless of their lipophilicity [130]. Carriers of ApoEε4 experience greater LDL-C reduction as compared with wild type ApoE carriers [149]. In this regard, several conceivable determinants of AD patients most likely to be beneficial from statins have been proposed: aged between 65 and 74 years; ApoEε4 phenotype; normocholesterolemia; and, sparingly, users of drugs that inhibit CYP3A4 [150].

Another neurodegenerative disorder is Parkinson disease (PD), caused by the death of dopaminergic neurons in the substantia nigra. Its clinical manifestation includes resting tremor, rigidity, slowness of movement, and postural instability. Several lines of mechanisms are postulated in the pathogenesis of PD. Neuroinflammatory events, such as accumulation of inflammatory cytokines, oxidative stress, and apoptotic-related proteins, are recognized as responsible factors for the pathogenesis and progression of PD [151, 152]. Two kinds of isoforms of NOS, iNOS and nNOS, are potentially implicated in the neurodegeneration occurring in PD [153]. APOEε2, not APOEε4, is positively associated with the higher prevalence of sporadic PD [154]; the findings being in sharp contrast to AD, in which APOEε4 is a major susceptibility gene whereas APOEε2 is protective for the disease.

The current dopaminergic treatments improve the motor symptoms for patients with early stage PD, while they are also associated with disabling side effects and do not halt the progression of the disease. Therefore, there is a pressing need for establishing the disease's preventive treatments. The idea of investigating the possibility of statins to produce neuroprotection, to reduce PD risk, and to prevent worsening of the disease comes to us from the fact that statins reduce oxidant production [151], protect dopaminergic neurons from subsequent inflammatory damage [151], and influence directly on the dopaminergic system [155, 156].

People taking statins exhibited a lower incidence of PD [157]. Statin users experienced delayed onset and slower development of PD, but fibrate users did not [158]. The risk reduction of PD may have a dose-response relationship because long-term statin users showed the strongest protective association [159] although there are some differences in efficacy between statins. As described in this section, this phenomenon may partly be due to the different ability to cross the blood-brain barrier between statins, depending on their lipophilicity [146]. However, by contrast, there exists some opposing findings of lower LDL-C [160] or total cholesterol [161] levels correlated with increased PD risk. One plausible explanation for the ambiguity regarding the connection between cholesterol and PD lies in the cause and effect association that, although higher cholesterol levels facilitate the onset of the disease, once the disease sets in, cholesterol levels start decreasing because of an overall degenerative process, such as nausea, vomiting, loss of appetite, and constipation.

Although promising, clinical studies to date have been unable to draw definitive conclusions whether statins are effective against AD and PD. The inconclusive results necessitate further studies with different statins in the long-term follow-up period to clarify whether statins have therapeutic potential in slowing down the development in AD and PD.

4.5. Chronic Kidney Disease (CKD)

The correlation between lipid reduction and the preservation of kidney function suggests that dyslipidemia is a risk factor for progression of CKD [162]. CKD may progress via the direct toxic effects of lipids and the inflammation mechanisms commonly seen in the systemic vasculature.

Lipoproteins accumulate in glomerular cells, mesangial cells, and mesangial matrix; the subsequent progression of renal microinjury stimulates cytokine expression, induces podocyte apoptosis and loss of nephrin (an adhesion molecule specific for the glomerular slit diaphragm), and decreases PI3K/Akt activity, collectively altering the glomerular size-selective barrier to proteins that cause albuminuria [163].

The vicious circle between worsening the renal function and dyslipidemia makes it imperative that dyslipidemia should be aggressively treated with currently available therapies. In this regard, discussions concerning statin use in CKD patients seem to have two aspects: one is whether statins can prevent cardiovascular events in CKD patients, and another is whether statins can improve renal function in CKD patients or prevent acute rejection in patients undergoing renal transplantation. Since this chapter deals with statins' pleiotropic effects, the discussion in this section specifically highlights on the latter topic.

The underlying mechanisms of statins' salutary effects on CKD have been investigated *in vitro* and *in vivo*. Statins inhibit mesangial cell proliferation [164, 165], improve renal dynamics [166] through increase in NO and eNOS [167], and prevent glomerular hypertrophy [168] and inflammatory processes [169]. The sum of cellular and molecular responses leads to ameliorate renal diseases.

Table 1 lists the results of various clinical trials investigating the effects of statins on CKD or graft rejection. Statins resulted in a slower decline of the glomerular filtration rate (GFR) [170, 171], slower decline or improvement in creatinine clearance [171-173], reduction in proteinuria [171, 174], prevention of kidney function loss [174, 175], and increase in estimated GFR [176, 177].

However, some RCTs observed the opposite results. There was no improvement in albuminuria [178] or eGFR [179].

Furthermore, active therapy was not associated with any less deterioration in CKD [180] or kidney function [181] than with the placebo. Subsequent meta-analyses revealed that statins may have a protective effect on the progression of renal dysfunction and proteinuria [182-184] and the degree of protection was greater according to the greater baseline albuminuria or proteinuria [185], suggesting that the more severe CKD patients may receive a greater benefit from statins.

Whether or not statins protect the renal allograft is unknown, and the evidence to support the therapeutic efficacy of statins in renal transplantation setting is mixed. Renal transplant recipients treated with statins experienced better graft survival [186], better renal function [187], less collagen deposition [187], and reduced episodes of acute and chronic renal rejection [188] as compared with those untreated by stains. However, other studies could not find such benefits [189, 190].

Two meta-analyses demonstrated no significant differences in the risk of acute rejection between kidney transplant recipients receiving statin and those receiving placebo [183, 191].

Table 1. Effect of statin on kidney function in CKD or transplant patients. Results of RCTs and metaanalyses

Study type (name) [reference]	Statin	number of patients		Effects
		Treatment arm	Reference arm	
CKD patients				
Subanalysis of RCT (CARE) [170]	pravastatin	345	345	reduced decline in GFR
RCT [171]	atorvastatin	28	28	slower decline in GFR, reduced proteinuria, slow creatinie clearance
RCT [172]	fluvastatin	80	50	10-15% increase in creatinin clearance
RCT (GREACE) [173]	atorvastatin	783	703	improve renal function
RCT (PLANET-I,II) [174]	atorvastatin	NA	NA	reduction in proteinuria, slower decline in eGFR
3 RCTs combined* [175]	pravastatin	1702	1700	reduction in kidney function loss by 34%
Subanalysis of postmarketing study (LIVES) [176]	pitavastatin	958	NA	improve eGFR
5 placebo controlled trials combined [177]	rosuvastatin	377	148	improvement in eGFR
RCT (PREVEND-IT) [178]	pravastatin	433	431	no reduction in albuminuria
RCT (JUPITER) [179]	rosuvastatin	1638	1629	no improvement in eGFR
RCT (SHARP) [180]	simvastatin, ezetimibe	4650	4620	no reduction of CKD progression
Post-hoc analysis of RCT (AFCAPS/TexCAPS) [181]	lovastatin	145	159	no efficacy on decreasing kidney function loss
metaanalysis [182]		281	267	no improvement in creatinine clearance
metaanalysis [182]		156	155	decreased proteinuria
metaanalysis [183]		311		reduced proteinuria
metaanalysis [183]		548		no improvement in GFR
metaanalysis [184]		683	640	reduction in the rate of kidney function loss
metaanalysis [185]		702	682	reduced albuminuria, proteinuria
Transplant patients				
RCT (ALERT) [189]	fluvastatin	1050	1052	no effects on graft loss, doubling serum creatinine, and decline in GFR
RCT [190]	simvastatin	53	52	no improvement in graft survival
metaanalysis [183]		324	315	no reduction in allograft rejection
metaanalysis [191]		324	315	no reduction in allograft rejection

CKD; chronic kidney disease, RCT; randomized controlled trial, GFR; glomerular filtration rate. eGFR: estimated glomerular filtration rate, NA; not available.
*WOSCOPS, CARE, LIPID.

4.6. Osteoporosis and Bone Fracture

Statins appear to modulate bone formation, inflammation, and angiogenesis, thus providing an exciting new direction for research on the statins' pleiotropic effects on bone. Since the causes of bone fracture are complicated by the other confounding factors, such as falls, neuromuscular competence, and cognitive impairment, the biochemical markers of bone turnover should be taken into account for the analyses of statins' effect on bone, including bone formation markers such as bone alkaline phosphatase and osteocalcin, as well as bone resorptive markers such as c-telopeptide of type I collagen (CTX) and n-telopeptide of type I collagen (NTX).

Since the first demonstration that relatively high doses of simvastatin could stimulate bone morphogenetic protein-2 (BMP-2) expression and bone formation while suppressing the number of osteoclasts [192], a number of observational studies or meta-analyses have been performed and produced inconsistent results concerning the association between statin use, and bone fracture or bone mineral density (BMD) [193]. Some observational studies reported that statin users experienced increased BMD and had a less likelihood of bone fracturing [194-196] with a dose-effect relationship [194]. The possibility that these protective effects against a fracture are a result of reducing cholesterol seems unlikely because such effects were not obtained by using non-statin cholesterol lowering drugs [195]. On the other hand, however, other observational studies failed to find such a salutary association [197, 198]. Investigations regarding the association between statins and bone metabolism also provided inconsistent results. Statins achieved a positive effect associated with decreasing CTX but had a null effect on bone formation [199], whereas another study found neither a change in bone formation markers nor CTX by statins [200]. The results of meta-analyses were also mixed, seemingly dependant on the types of studies included (Table 2). Significantly fewer bone fractures and increased BMD by statins were observed when meta-analyses included both observational studies and RCTs [201-204], whereas such significance disappeared when meta-analyses only analyzed RCTs [202-204]. A very recent meta-analysis [205], including only RCTs, also failed to demonstrate any preventive effects on fractures, any increase in BMD, and any beneficial effects on bone formation and absorptive markers [205].

Table 2. Effects of statin on bone. Results of metaanalyses

Analyzed study type [reference]	Number of patients		Effects	
	Treatment arm	Reference arm	Fracture	BMD
RCT and observational study [201]	NA	NA	NA	Total hip↑; Femoral neck ↑
RCT and observational study [202]	NA	NA	Overall ↓	NA
RCT and observational study [203]	NA	NA	Hip ↓ ; Vertebra→	Hip↑; Vertebra→
RCT and observational study [204]	NA	NA	Hip ↓ ; Nonspine ↓	NA
RCT only [205]	1255	1258	Overall→	NA
RCT only [205]	580	212	NA	Lumbar→; Total hip→

↑;increased, ↓ ;decreased, →; no effect
BMD; bone mineral density, NA; not available

The substantial variability in outcomes makes it difficult to ascertain whether statins could have a bone benefit. The reasons why the previous studies consistently provided contradictory results may be in the fact that statins' effect on bone health may differ according to the different skeletal sites, types of statins, and doses of statins. Increased BMD by statins was found in the forearm but not in lumbar, spine, hip, or femoral neck [206], suggesting the possibility of site-specific effects of statins. Which polarity of statins used may also produce different results [201, 202] because of the low uptake and poor distribution of the more hydrophilic statins beyond the liver to the periphery [207]. This may be a plausible explanation for discrepancies within some meta-analyses, where no positive effects on bone have been observed from hydrophilic statins [201]. Another explanation may be a lower bioavailability of statins at the bone microenvironment than expected, since only a small (5%) fraction of oral route statins may finally reach the peripheral circulation after they first pass metabolism [208].

Nevertheless, several underlying mechanisms are postulated why and how statins render bone health. First, statins inhibit Rho activity leading to enhance BMP-2 [209], a growth factor that directly enhances osteoblast differentiation and bone formation [210]. This effect also enhances osteocalcin [209], the major noncollagenous bone matrix protein and is considered as an osteoblastic differentiation marker [209]. Second, statins stimulate VEGF expression via activating the PI3K/Akt pathway to promote osteoblast differentiation [211]. In addition, VEGF stimulates BMP-2 [212] and *vice versa* [213]. Considering that vascular invasion is a prerequisite for calcification during bone formation [213], proangiogenic effects of statins that include initiating and activatinga cascade involving BMP-2 and VEGF, collectively, enhance bone health. Third, as described in section 4.3, the ability of statins to promote EPCs differentiation presumably permit them to give rise to osteoblast differentiation since progenitor cell lineages differentiating into endothelial and osteoblastic cells have recently been thought to overlap [214]. Finally, statins can suppress bone resorption by inhibiting isoprenoid formation in a similar way that has been described for some bisphosphonates. Nitrogen-containing bisphosphonates inhibit osteoclast activity and induce osteoclast apoptosis [215, 216] via inhibiting the isoprenoid biosynthesis pathway [217]. This may offer a reasonable argument that statins indeed possess anti-resorptive functions.

Therefore, theoretically, statins may have an anabolic effect on bones, making them a potentially interesting treatment option for osteoporosis. However, the doses of statins exerting bone health in animal models were higher than those prescribed to humans. It should be noted that currently available RCTs on this topic are still scanty in the literature so that larger scale RCTs are needed to conclusively assess the potential effects of statins on bone health.

4.7. Malignancy

The association of long-term statin use with cancer risk has recently become an interesting topic because early animal studies suggested that statins may possess a carcinogenic potential [218] through the extrahepatic compensatory induction of mevalonate synthesis that possibly promotes the growth of occult neoplastic cells [219]. However, a number of epidemiological studies, retrospective analyses, or randomized controlled trials have provided inconclusive results concerning the effects of statins on cancer. Some showed positive effects on reducing incidences of overall [220] or site-specific cancer such as colon [221], lung [222], prostate [223], pancreas [224], and kidney [225], whereas others showed neutral effects [226-228] or even an increase [139]. Subsequent meta-analyses have consistently proved that statins have neutral effects on cancer (Table 3) although there are some exceptions.

Table 3. Statins and cancer risk by site. Meta-analysis results

Site	Cancer risk (references)		
	Neutral	Decreased	Increased
Overall	[229-239]	[242]	
Esophagus	[231]		
Stomach	[230, 231, 240]	[229]	
Colorectal	[229-232, 241]		
Gastrointesinal tract	[231, 232, 242, 243]		
Liver or Hepatobiliary	[229, 231, 242]		
Pancreas	[231, 244]		
Lung or respiratory	[229-232, 242, 243]		
Breast	[229-232, 243, 245]		
Uterus, Ovary	[229, 231, 236]		
Kidney, Urinary tract	[231, 246]		
Prostate	[229-232, 247]		
Lymphoma, NHL	[229, 242]		
Skin, Melanoma	[230, 231*, 232, 242, 243, 246, 248, 249]		[231]**
Skin, Non melanoma		[242]	
Hematological	[231, 242, 243, 250]		

NHL; non Hodgkin lymphoma.
*mean risk, **median risk.

Table 4. Trials of single statin use for tumor treatment

Statin	Phase	Number of patients	Doses	Tumors	Results	Reference
lovastatin	I	88	2-45mg/kg/day	Various*	1 minor response	[257]
lovastatin	I	26	7.5mg/kg/day	Head and neck	no response	[258]
lovastatin	I/II	18	20-30mg/kg/day	Brain	1 partial response, 1 minor response	[259]
Table 4. (Continued)						
lovastatin	II	16	35mg/kg/day	Stomach	no response	[260]
pravastatin	III	83	40mg/day	Liver	better survival in pravastatin arm	[261]
pravastatin	III	recruiting	40mg/day	Esophagus, Stomach	awaiting	[262]
pravastatin	NA	19	40-80mg/day	Liver	survival not improved	[263]

ND; not described.
*Tumor sites and patient number (in parentheses) include prostate (38), central nervous system (24), breast (7), colorectal (4), ovary (4), sarcoma (3), lung (2), others (6).

The growing body of evidence suggests that statins may have a potential to prevent cancer. Statins inhibit the growth signal cascade via inactivating Ras and Rho through FPP and GGPP inhibition, resulting in interference with Ras/RhoA functional localization as well as inhibiting the downstream protein kinases interacting with them. In addition, statins inhibit the adhesion molecule expression involved in cancer cell adhesion, invasion, and migration [251]. Moreover, statins induce apoptosis through caspase-dependent mechanisms [252], and the induction of apoptosis results in the inhibition of cancer tumorigenesis [253-255]. Furthermore, statins inhibit angiogenesis, the PI3K/Akt pathway, and cancer cell apoptosis [256], the effects which sharply contrast with those of statins in cardiovascular or cerebrovascular diseases. This duality is complex and is probably related to the organ site, cell types, and diseases. Although real, the precise mechanisms of the opposing effects of statins on angiogenesis in ischemic tissue and cancer remain to be elucidated.

The above *in vitro* results have motivated researchers to conduct several small-scale cancer trials investigating the use of statins as therapeutic anticancer agents. It should be noted that statin concentrations showing antiproliferative or antiangiogenic effects in *in vitro* conditions are 10-100 times higher than those of the clinically relevant doses, thereby the required statin doses in the anticancer statin trials may be higher than those used against hypercholesterolemia in order to achieve plasma concentrations relevant to those in *in vitro* anticancer studies. Accordingly, the reported dosages of statins are sometimes higher than those in the clinical use (Table 4) with unsatisfactory or, at best, modest clinical efficacy. Results of pravastatin use at daily dose (40mg/day) were promising in one trial [261], but await in another [262]. However, pravastatin at even a higher (40-80mg) dose failed to provide such effect [263] (Table 4). It should be noted that the anti-tumor effects of statins, as observed *in vitro* at high concentrations, can not necessarily be extrapolated into a clinical situation; therefore, the research direction appears to be a possibility with the combined use of statins and other chemotherapeutic agents, with an anticipation of dose reduction for either or both drugs [264].

Conclusion

Scientists have accomplished significant progress in unfolding the newer aspects of statins. This chapter highlights a number of biological processes that involve statin and their subsequent clinical usefulness beyond lowering cholesterol. Biological functions of statins, which are no longer restricted to only lowering lipids, include: vascular health promotion, neuroprotection, antineoplastic and renal benefits, and bone formation. A number of studies bolster the hypothesis that statins may be able to mitigate the course of such diseases or reduce the probability of developing them. Research efforts towards this wonder and multifunctional drug should aim at a deeper understanding of the key cellular and molecular events involved with statins. Ultimately, such insights might also prove useful in designing new therapeutic strategies aimed at slowing, or even halting, the disease progression.

There are several points that deserve to be mentioned for further studies. There seems to be a continuous debate whether the nature of statins' pleiotropic effects is in lowering cholesterol or in inhibiting isoprenoid synthesis, with the subsequent GTP-binding protein inactivation. One possible study design to address this question may include adding statins in the presence of mevalonate, which realizes the blockade of cholesterol synthesis without impaired isoprenylation. This gives researchers a way to separately analyze the cholesterol- and isoprenoid-dependent effects of statins.

It is also true that studies on the pleiotropic effects of statins have provided contradictory results. The possible mechanisms behind such inconsistencies could include the disparity of statins' tissue distribution, methodology, and the design of statin studies. The statins' lipophilicity affects the blood-brain barrier permeability. A negative charge and different transporter system may also play a role. Indication and cessation bias have been alluded to by several investigators as confounding factors [265]. Dose consideration (the applied statin dose not reaching a therapeutic concentration in the target organ [266]]) should also be taken into account. In this regard, it should be recalled that statin concentrations or doses *in vitro* and *in vivo* studies are usually higher than those measured in the blood of statin-treated patients. Furthermore, cholesterol is a major component of cell membranes; thus it is essential for maintaining their structure. The real challenge is to maintain cholesterol homeostasis after using statins to minimize the unanticipated side effects in patients who do not suffer from cholesterol-related problems. Therefore, although statins have the potential to impact the clinical arena, the theoretical mechanisms of statins and the applicability of the experimental effects at the clinical level should be confirmed in the clinical studies. This requires many cases and controls, with an attention to confounding factors and stratification. Large patient cohorts with detailed clinical records enable us to systemically test for statins' real pleiotropic effects.

As longevity continues to rise, diseases of aging such as metabolic syndrome, cerebrovascular diseases with dementia, neurodegenerative disorders, CKD, osteoporosis, and malignancy loom large as a major threat to public health. Since diseases of aging usually require long-lasting treatment, the importance of the clinical benefit of statins with regard to their pleiotropic effects should be continuously discussed, especially with consideration of the efficacy and doses of statins in long-term use settings. In addition, one should keep in mind the cost of therapy as well as the clinical benefits and harms of any long- time therapy. Whatever side of this scientific debate one chooses, statins remain an important part of our clinical armamentarium. Under the collaboration of basic scientists with clinicians, the merit of continuing this debate lies in exploring the possibility to foster the novel therapies for a wide spectrum of diseases.

References

[1] Calabrò, P., & Yeh, E.T. (2005). The pleiotropic effects of statins. *Curr Opin Cardiol.* 20, 541-546.

[2] Takemoto, M., & Liao, J.K. (2001). Pleiotropic effects of 3-hydroxy-3-methylglutaryl coenzyme a reductase inhibitors. *Arterioscler Thromb Vasc Biol.* 21, 1712-1719.

[3] Siegel-Axel, D., Daub, K., Seizer, P., Lindemann, S., & Gawaz, M. (2008). Platelet lipoprotein interplay: trigger of foam cell formation and driver of atherosclerosis. *Cardiovasc Res.* 78, 8-17.

[4] Jonasson, L., Holm, J., Skalli, O., Bondjers, G., & Hansson, G.K. (1986). Regional accumulations of T cells, macrophages, and smooth muscle cells in the human atherosclerotic plaque. *Arteriosclerosis.* 6, 131-138.

[5] Ross, R. (1999). Atherosclerosis--an inflammatory disease. *N Engl J Med.* 340, 115-126.

[6] Gerszten, R.E., Garcia-Zepeda, E.A., Lim, Y.C., Yoshida, M., Ding, H.A., Gimbrone, M.A. Jr, Luster, A.D., Luscinskas, F.W., & Rosenzweig, A. (1999). MCP-1 and IL-8 trigger firm adhesion of monocytes to vascular endothelium under flow conditions. *Nature*. 398, 718-723.

[7] Haramaki, N., Ikeda, H., Takenaka, K., Katoh, A., Sugano, R., Yamagishi, S., Matsuoka, H., & Imaizumi, T. (2007). Fluvastatin alters platelet aggregability in patients with hypercholesterolemia: possible improvement of intraplatelet redox imbalance via HMG-CoA reductase. *Arterioscler Thromb Vasc Biol*. 27, 1471-1477.

[8] Matsuura, E., Hughes, G.R., & Khamashta, M.A. (2008). Oxidation of LDL and its clinical implication. *Autoimmun Rev*. 7, 558-566.

[9] Steinberg, D. (1997). Oxidative modification of LDL and atherogenesis. *Circulation*. 95, 1062-1071.

[10] Senokuchi, T., Matsumura, T., Sakai, M., Yano, M., Taguchi, T., Matsuo, T., Sonoda, K., Kukidome, D., Imoto, K., Nishikawa, T., Kim-Mitsuyama, S., Takuwa, Y., & Araki, E. (2005). Statins suppress oxidized low density lipoprotein-induced macrophage proliferation by inactivation of the small G protein-p38 MAPK pathway. *J Biol Chem*. 280, 6627-6633.

[11] Relou, I.A., Hackeng, C.M., Akkerman, J.W., & Malle, E. (2003). Low-density lipoprotein and its effect on human blood platelets. *Cell Mol Life Sci*. 60, 961-971.

[12] Li, D., & Mehta, J.L. (2000). Upregulation of endothelial receptor for oxidized LDL (LOX-1) by oxidized LDL and implications in apoptosis of human coronary artery endothelial cells: evidence from use of antisense LOX-1 mRNA and chemical inhibitors. *Arterioscler Thromb Vasc Biol*. 20, 1116-1122.

[13] Aikawa, M., Rabkin, E., Sugiyama, S., Voglic, S.J., Fukumoto, Y., Furukawa, Y., Shiomi, M., Schoen, F.J., & Libby, P. (2001). An HMG-CoA reductase inhibitor, cerivastatin, suppresses growth of macrophages expressing matrix metalloproteinases and tissue factor in vivo and in vitro. *Circulation*. 103, 276-283.

[14] Taubman, M.B., Fallon, J.T., Schecter, A.D., Giesen, P., Mendlowitz, M., Fyfe, B.S., Marmur, J.D., & Nemerson, Y. (1997). Tissue factor in the pathogenesis of atherosclerosis. *Thromb Haemost*. 78, 200-204.

[15] Lin, M.C., Almus-Jacobs, F., Chen, H.H., Parry, G.C., Mackman, N., Shyy, J.Y., & Chien, S. (1997). Shear stress induction of the tissue factor gene. *J Clin Invest*. 99, 737-744.

[16] Mallat, Z., & Tedgui, A. (2000). Apoptosis in the vasculature: mechanisms and functional importance. *Br J Pharmacol*. 130, 947-962.

[17] Walsh, K., Smith, R.C., & Kim, H.S. (2000). Vascular cell apoptosis in remodeling, restenosis, and plaque rupture. *Circ Res*. 87, 184-188.

[18] Bennett, M.R. (1999). Apoptosis of vascular smooth muscle cells in vascular remodelling and atherosclerotic plaque rupture. *Cardiovasc Res*. 41, 361-368.

[19] Van Aelst, L., & D'Souza-Schorey, C. (1997). Rho GTPases and signaling networks. *Genes Dev*. 11, 2295-2322.

[20] Graaf, M.R., Richel, D.J., van Noorden, C.J., & Guchelaar, H.J. (2004). Effects of statins and farnesyltransferase inhibitors on the development and progression of cancer. *Cancer Treat Rev*. 30, 609-641.

[21] Ridley, A.J. (2001). Rho family proteins: coordinating cell responses. *Trends Cell Biol*. 11, 471-477.

[22] Rodriguez-Viciana, P., Warne, P.H., Dhand, R., Vanhaesebroeck, B., Gout, I., Fry, M.J., Waterfield, M.D., & Downward, J. (1994). Phosphatidylinositol-3-OH kinase as a direct target of Ras. *Nature*. 370, 527-532.

[23] Laufs, U., & Liao, J.K. (2000). Targeting Rho in cardiovascular disease. *Circ Res*. 87, 526-528.

[24] Tsao, P.S., McEvoy, L.M., Drexler, H., Butcher, E.C., & Cooke, J.P. (1994). Enhanced endothelial adhesiveness in hypercholesterolemia is attenuated by L-arginine. *Circulation*. 89, 2176-2182.

[25] Radomski, M.W., Palmer, R.M., & Moncada, S. (1990). An L-arginine/nitric oxide pathway present in human platelets regulates aggregation. *Proc Natl Acad Sci U S A*. 87, 5193-5197.

[26] Garg, U.C., & Hassid, A. (1989). Nitric oxide-generating vasodilators and 8-bromo-cyclic guanosine monophosphate inhibit mitogenesis and proliferation of cultured rat vascular smooth muscle cells. *J Clin Invest*. 83, 1774-1777.

[27] Hogg, N., Kalyanaraman, B., Joseph, J., Struck, A., & Parthasarathy, S. (1993). Inhibition of low-density lipoprotein oxidation by nitric oxide. Potential role in atherogenesis. *FEBS Lett*. 334, 170-174.

[28] Liao, J.K., Shin, W.S., Lee, W.Y., & Clark, S.L. (1995). Oxidized low-density lipoprotein decreases the expression of endothelial nitric oxide synthase. *J Biol Chem*. 270, 319-324.

[29] Laufs, U., & Liao, J.K. (1998). Post-transcriptional regulation of endothelial nitric oxide synthase mRNA stability by Rho GTPase. *J Biol Chem*. 273, 24266-24271.

[30] Ni, W., Egashira, K., Kataoka, C., Kitamoto, S., Koyanagi, M., Inoue, S., & Takeshita, A. (2001). Antiinflammatory and antiarteriosclerotic actions of HMG-CoA reductase inhibitors in a rat model of chronic inhibition of nitric oxide synthesis. *Circ Res*. 89, 415-421.

[31] Laufs, U., La Fata, V., Plutzky, J., & Liao, J.K. Upregulation of endothelial nitric oxide synthase by HMG CoA reductase inhibitors. *Circulation*. 97, 1129-1135.

[32] Kureishi, Y., Luo, Z., Shiojima, I., Bialik, A., Fulton, D., Lefer, D.J., Sessa, W.C., & Walsh, K. (2000). The HMG-CoA reductase inhibitor simvastatin activates the protein kinase Akt and promotes angiogenesis in normocholesterolemic animals. *Nat Med*. 6, 1004-1010.

[33] Fulton, D., Gratton, J.P., McCabe, T.J., Fontana, J., Fujio, Y., Walsh, K., Franke, T.F., Papapetropoulos ,A., & Sessa, W.C. (1999). Regulation of endothelium-derived nitric oxide production by the protein kinase Akt. *Nature*. 399, 597-601.

[34] Fujio, Y., & Walsh, K. Akt mediates cytoprotection of endothelial cells by vascular endothelial growth factor in an anchorage-dependent manner. *J Biol Chem*. 274, 16349-16354.

[35] Morales-Ruiz, M., Fulton, D., Sowa, G., Languino, L.R., Fujio, Y., Walsh, K., & Sessa, W.C. (2000). Vascular endothelial growth factor-stimulated actin reorganization and migration of endothelial cells is regulated via the serine/threonine kinase Akt. *Circ Res*. 86, 892-896.

[36] Plenz, G.A., Hofnagel, O., & Robenek, H. (2004). Differential modulation of caveolin-1 expression in cells of the vasculature by statins. *Circulation*. 109, e7-8.

[37] Pelat, M., Dessy, C., Massion, P., Desager, J.P., Feron, O., & Balligand, J.L. (2003). Rosuvastatin decreases caveolin-1 and improves nitric oxide-dependent heart rate and

blood pressure variability in apolipoprotein E-/- mice in vivo. Circulation. 107, 2480-2486.

[38] Feron, O., Dessy, C., Desager, J.P., & Balligand, J.L. (2001). Hydroxy-methylglutaryl-coenzyme A reductase inhibition promotes endothelial nitric oxide synthase activation through a decrease in caveolin abundance. *Circulation*. 103, 113-118.

[39] Bucci, M., Gratton, J.P., Rudic, R.D., Acevedo, L., Roviezzo, F., Cirino, G., & Sessa, W.C. (2000). In vivo delivery of the caveolin-1 scaffolding domain inhibits nitric oxide synthesis and reduces inflammation. *Nat Med*. 6, 1362-1367.

[40] Sen-Banerjee, S., Mir, S., Lin, Z., Hamik, A., Atkins, G.B., Das, H., Banerjee, P., Kumar, A., & Jain, M.K. (2005). Kruppel-like factor 2 as a novel mediator of statin effects in endothelial cells. *Circulation*. 112, 720-726.

[41] Lin, Z., Natesan, V., Shi, H., Dong, F., Kawanami, D., Mahabeleshwar, G.H., Atkins, G.B., Nayak, L., Cui, Y., Finigan, J.H., & Jain, M.K. (2010). Kruppel-like factor 2 regulates endothelial barrier function. *Arterioscler Thromb Vasc Biol*. 30, 1952-1959.

[42] Wolfrum, S., Jensen, K.S., & Liao, J.K. (2003). Endothelium-dependent effects of statins. *Arterioscler Thromb Vasc Biol*. 23, 729-736.

[43] Rikitake, Y., Kawashima, S., Takeshita, S., Yamashita, T., Azumi, H., Yasuhara, M., Nishi, H., Inoue, N., & Yokoyama, M. (2001). Anti-oxidative properties of fluvastatin, an HMG-CoA reductase inhibitor, contribute to prevention of atherosclerosis in cholesterol-fed rabbits. *Atherosclerosis*. 154, 87-96.

[44] Wassmann, S., Laufs, U., Bäumer, A.T., Müller, K., Ahlbory, K., Linz, W., Itter, G., Rösen, R., Böhm, M., & Nickenig, G. (2001). HMG-CoA reductase inhibitors improve endothelial dysfunction in normocholesterolemic hypertension via reduced production of reactive oxygen species. *Hypertension*. 37, 1450-1457.

[45] Li, D.Y., Chen, H.J., & Mehta, J.L. (2001). Statins inhibit oxidized-LDL-mediated LOX-1 expression, uptake of oxidized-LDL and reduction in PKB phosphorylation. *Cardiovasc Res*. 52, 130-135.

[46] Draude, G., Hrboticky, N., & Lorenz, R.L. (1999). The expression of the lectin-like oxidized low-density lipoprotein receptor (LOX-1) on human vascular smooth muscle cells and monocytes and its down-regulation by lovastatin. *Biochem Pharmacol*. 57, 383-386.

[47] Kaneider, N.C., Reinisch, C.M., Dunzendorfer, S., Meierhofer, C., Djanani, A., & Wiedermann, C.J. (2001). Induction of apoptosis and inhibition of migration of inflammatory and vascular wall cells by cerivastatin. *Atherosclerosis*. 158, 23-33.

[48] Erl, W., Hristov, M., Neureuter, M., Yan, Z.Q., Hansson, G.K., & Weber, P.C. (2003). HMG-CoA reductase inhibitors induce apoptosis in neointima-derived vascular smooth muscle cells. *Atherosclerosis*. 169, 251-258.

[49] Knapp, A.C., Huang, J., Starling, G., & Kiener, P.A. (2000). Inhibitors of HMG-CoA reductase sensitize human smooth muscle cells to Fas-ligand and cytokine-induced cell death. *Atherosclerosis*. 152, 217-227.

[50] Blanco-Colio, L.M., Villa, A., Ortego, M., Hernández-Presa, M.A., Pascual, A., Plaza, J.J., & Egido, J. (2002). 3-Hydroxy-3-methyl-glutaryl coenzyme A reductase inhibitors, atorvastatin and simvastatin, induce apoptosis of vascular smooth muscle cells by downregulation of Bcl-2 expression and Rho A prenylation. *Atherosclerosis*. 161, 17-26.

[51] Crisby, M., Nordin-Fredriksson, G., Shah, P.K., Yano, J., Zhu, J., & Nilsson, J. (2001). Pravastatin treatment increases collagen content and decreases lipid content, inflammation, metalloproteinases, and cell death in human carotid plaques: implications for plaque stabilization. *Circulation*. 103, 926-933.

[52] Aikawa, M., Rabkin, E., Okada, Y., Voglic, S.J., Clinton, S.K., Brinckerhoff, C.E., Sukhova, G.K., & Libby, P. (1998). Lipid lowering by diet reduces matrix metalloproteinase activity and increases collagen content of rabbit atheroma: a potential mechanism of lesion stabilization. *Circulation*. 97, 2433-2444.

[53] Schwartz, G.G., Olsson, A.G., Ezekowitz, M.D., Ganz, P., Oliver, M.F., Waters, D., Zeiher, A., Chaitman, B.R., Leslie, S., Stern, T. & Myocardial Ischemia Reduction with Aggressive Cholesterol Lowering (MIRACL) Study Investigators. (2001). Effects of atorvastatin on early recurrent ischemic events in acute coronary syndromes: the MIRACL study: a randomized controlled trial. *JAMA*. 285, 1711-1718.

[54] Nicholls, S.J., Ballantyne, C.M., Barter, P.J., Chapman, M.J., Erbel, R.M., Libby, P., Raichlen, J.S., Uno, K., Borgman, M., Wolski, K., & Nissen, S.E. (2011). Effect of Two Intensive Statin Regimens on Progression of Coronary Disease. *N Engl J Med*. 2011 Nov 15. [Epub ahead of print]

[55] Ferro, D., Parrotto, S., Basili, S., Alessandri, C., & Violi, F. (2000). Simvastatin inhibits the monocyte expression of proinflammatory cytokines in patients with hypercholesterolemia. *J Am Coll Cardiol*. 36, 427-431.

[56] Ito, T., Ikeda, U., Yamamoto, K., & Shimada, K. (2002). Regulation of interleukin-8 expression by HMG-CoA reductase inhibitors in human vascular smooth muscle cells. *Atherosclerosis*. 165, 51-55.

[57] Shirakawa, I., Sata, M., Saiura, A., Kaneda, Y., Yashiro, H., Hirata, Y., Makuuchi, M., & Nagai, R. (2007). Atorvastatin attenuates transplant-associated coronary arteriosclerosis in a murine model of cardiac transplantation. *Biomed Pharmacother*. 61, 154-159.

[58] Zelvyte, I., Dominaitiene, R., Crisby, M., & Janciauskiene, S. (2002). Modulation of inflammatory mediators and PPARgamma and NFkappaB expression by pravastatin in response to lipoproteins in human monocytes in vitro. *Pharmacol Res*. 45, 147-154.

[59] Massy, Z.A., Kim, Y., Guijarro, C., Kasiske, B.L., Keane, W.F., & O'Donnell, M.P. (2000). Low-density lipoprotein-induced expression of interleukin-6, a marker of human mesangial cell inflammation: effects of oxidation and modulation by lovastatin. *Biochem Biophys Res Commun*. 267, 536-540.

[60] Wagner, A.H., Gebauer, M., Güldenzoph, B., & Hecker, M. (2002). 3-hydroxy-3-methylglutaryl coenzyme A reductase-independent inhibition of CD40 expression by atorvastatin in human endothelial cells. *Arterioscler Thromb Vasc Biol*. 22, 1784-1789.

[61] Guijarro, C., Kim, Y., Schoonover, C.M., Massy, Z.A., O'Donnell, M.P., Kasiske, B.L., Keane, W.F., & Kashtan, C.E. (1996). Lovastatin inhibits lipopolysaccharide-induced NF-kappaB activation in human mesangial cells. *Nephrol Dial Transplant*. 11, 990-996.

[62] Dichtl, W., Dulak, J,, Frick, M., Alber, H.F., Schwarzacher, S.P., Ares, M.P., Nilsson, J., Pachinger, O., & Weidinger, F. (2003). HMG-CoA reductase inhibitors regulate inflammatory transcription factors in human endothelial and vascular smooth muscle cells. *Arterioscler Thromb Vasc Biol*. 23, 58-63.

[63] Stalker, T.J., Lefer, A.M., & Scalia, R. (2001). A new HMG-CoA reductase inhibitor, rosuvastatin, exerts anti-inflammatory effects on the microvascular endothelium: the role of mevalonic acid. *Br J Pharmacol*. 133, 406-412.

[64] Yeh, E.T., & Willerson, J.T. (2003). Coming of age of C-reactive protein: using inflammation markers in cardiology. *Circulation*. 107, 370-371.

[65] Venugopal, S.K., Devaraj, S., Yuhanna, I., Shaul, P., & Jialal, I. (2002). Demonstration that C-reactive protein decreases eNOS expression and bioactivity in human aortic endothelial cells. *Circulation*. 106, 1439-1441.

[66] Verma, S., Wang, C.H., Li, S.H., Dumont, A.S., Fedak, P.W., Badiwala, M.V., Dhillon, B., Weisel, R.D., Li, R.K., Mickle, D.A., & Stewart, D.J. (2002). A self-fulfilling prophecy: C-reactive protein attenuates nitric oxide production and inhibits angiogenesis. *Circulation*. 106, 913-919.

[67] Verma, S., Li, S.H., Badiwala, M.V., Weisel, R.D., Fedak, P.W., Li, R.K., Dhillon, B., & Mickle, D.A. (2002). Endothelin antagonism and interleukin-6 inhibition attenuate the proatherogenic effects of C-reactive protein. *Circulation*. 105, 1890-1896.

[68] Li, L., Roumeliotis, N., Sawamura, T., & Renier, G. (2004). C-reactive protein enhances LOX-1 expression in human aortic endothelial cells: relevance of LOX-1 to C-reactive protein-induced endothelial dysfunction. *Circ Res*. 95, 877-883.

[69] Devaraj, S., Xu, D.Y., & Jialal, I. (2003). C-reactive protein increases plasminogen activator inhibitor-1 expression and activity in human aortic endothelial cells: implications for the metabolic syndrome and atherothrombosis. *Circulation*. 107, 398-404.

[70] Cirillo, P., Golino, P., Calabrò, P., Calì, G., Ragni, M., De Rosa, S., Cimmino, G., Pacileo, M., De Palma, R., Forte, L., Gargiulo, A., Corigliano, F.G., Angri,V., Spagnuolo, R., Nitsch, L., & Chiariello, M. (2005). C-reactive protein induces tissue factor expression and promotes smooth muscle and endothelial cell proliferation. *Cardiovasc Res*. 68, 47-55.

[71] Abe, N., Osanai, T., Fujiwara, T., Kameda, K., Matsunaga, T., & Okumura, K. (2006). C-reactive protein-induced upregulation of extracellular matrix metalloproteinase inducer in macrophages: inhibitory effect of fluvastatin. *Life Sci*. 78, 1021-1028.

[72] Montero, I., Orbe, J., Varo, N., Beloqui, O., Monreal, J.I., Rodríguez, J.A., Díez, J., Libby, P., & Páramo, J.A. (2006). C-reactive protein induces matrix metalloproteinase-1 and -10 in human endothelial cells: implications for clinical and subclinical atherosclerosis. *J Am Coll Cardiol*. 47, 1369-1378.

[73] Nissen, S.E., Tuzcu, E.M., Schoenhagen, P., Brown, B.G., Ganz, P., Vogel, R.A., Crowe, T., Howard, G., Cooper, C.J., Brodie, B., Grines, C.L., DeMaria, A.N., & REVERSAL Investigators. (2004). Effect of intensive compared with moderate lipid-lowering therapy on progression of coronary atherosclerosis: a randomized controlled trial. *JAMA*. 291, 1071-1080.

[74] Albert, M.A., Danielson, E., Rifai, N., Ridker, P.M., & PRINCE Investigators. (2001). Effect of statin therapy on C-reactive protein levels: the pravastatin inflammation/CRP evaluation (PRINCE): a randomized trial and cohort study. *JAMA*. 286, 64-70.

[75] Ridker, P.M., Rifai, N., Clearfield, M., Downs, J.R., Weis, S.E., Miles, J.S., Gotto, A.M. Jr, & Air Force/Texas Coronary Atherosclerosis Prevention Study Investigators. (2001). Measurement of C-reactive protein for the targeting of statin therapy in the primary prevention of acute coronary events. *N Engl J Med*. 344, 1959-1965.

[76] Ridker, P.M., Cannon, C.P., Morrow, D., Rifai, N., Rose, L.M., McCabe, C.H., Pfeffer, M.A., Braunwald, E., & Pravastatin or Atorvastatin Evaluation and Infection Therapy-Thrombolysis in Myocardial Infarction 22 (PROVE IT-TIMI 22) Investigators. (2005). C-reactive protein levels and outcomes after statin therapy. *N Engl J Med*. 352, 20-28.

[77] Ridker, P.M., Morrow, D.A., Rose, L.M., Rifai, N., Cannon, C.P., Braunwald, E. (2005). Relative efficacy of atorvastatin 80 mg and pravastatin 40 mg in achieving the dual goals of low-density lipoprotein cholesterol <70 mg/dl and C-reactive protein <2 mg/l: an analysis of the PROVE-IT TIMI-22 trial. *J Am Coll Cardiol*. 45, 1644-1648.

[78] Ridker, P.M., Danielson, E., Fonseca, F.A., Genest, J., Gotto, A.M. Jr, Kastelein, J.J., Koenig, W., Libby, P., Lorenzatti, A.J., MacFadyen, J.G., Nordestgaard, B.G., Shepherd, J., Willerson, J.T., Glynn, R.J. & JUPITER Study Group. (2008). Rosuvastatin to prevent vascular events in men and women with elevated C-reactive protein. *N Engl J Med*. 359, 2195-2207.

[79] Ridker, P.M., Danielson, E., Fonseca, F.A., Genest, J., Gotto, A.M. Jr, Kastelein, J.J., Koenig, W., Libby, P., Lorenzatti, A.J., Macfadyen, J.G., Nordestgaard, B.G., Shepherd, J., Willerson, J.T., Glynn, R.J., & JUPITER Trial Study Group. (2009). Reduction in C-reactive protein and LDL cholesterol and cardiovascular event rates after initiation of rosuvastatin: a prospective study of the JUPITER trial. *Lancet*. 373, 1175-1182.

[80] Schneider, M.P., Schmidt, B.M., John, S., & Schmieder, R.E. (2011). Effects of statin treatment on endothelial function, oxidative stress and inflammation in patients with arterial hypertension and normal cholesterol levels. *J Hypertens*. 29, 1757-1764.

[81] Pepys, M.B., Hirschfield, G.M., Tennent, G.A., Gallimore, J.R., Kahan, M.C., Bellotti, V., Hawkins, P.N., Myers, R.M., Smith, M.D., Polara, A., Cobb, A.J., Ley, S.V., Aquilina, J.A., Robinson, C.V., Sharif, I., Gray, G.A., Sabin, C.A., Jenvey, M.C., Kolstoe, S.E., Thompson, D., & Wood, S.P. (2006). Targeting C-reactive protein for the treatment of cardiovascular disease. *Nature*. 440, 1217-1221.

[82] Sata, M., Nishimatsu, H., Suzuki, E., Sugiura, S., Yoshizumi, M., Ouchi, Y., Hirata, Y., & Nagai, R. (2001). Endothelial nitric oxide synthase is essential for the HMG-CoA reductase inhibitor cerivastatin to promote collateral growth in response to ischemia. *FASEB J*. 15, 2530-2532.

[83] Sata, M., Nishimatsu, H., Osuga, J., Tanaka, K., Ishizaka, N., Ishibashi, S., Hirata, Y., & Nagai, R. (2004). Statins augment collateral growth in response to ischemia but they do not promote cancer and atherosclerosis. *Hypertension*. 43, 1214-1220.

[84] Weis, M., Heeschen, C., Glassford, A.J., & Cooke, J.P. (2002). Statins have biphasic effects on angiogenesis. *Circulation*. 105, 739-745.

[85] Asahara, T., Murohara, T., Sullivan, A., Silver, M., van der Zee, R., Li, T., Witzenbichler, B., Schatteman, G., & Isner, J.M. (1997). Isolation of putative progenitor endothelial cells for angiogenesis. *Science*. 275, 964-967.

[86] Griese, D.P., Ehsan, A., Melo, L.G., Kong, D., Zhang, L., Mann, M.J., Pratt, R.E., Mulligan, R.C., & Dzau, V.J. (2003). Isolation and transplantation of autologous circulating endothelial cells into denuded vessels and prosthetic grafts: implications for cell-based vascular therapy. *Circulation*. 108, 2710-2715.

[87] Asahara, T., Kawamoto, A., & Masuda, H. (2011). Concise review: circulating endothelial progenitor cells for vascular medicine. *Stem Cells*. 29, 1650-1655.

[88] Llevadot, J., Murasawa, S., Kureishi, Y., Uchida, S., Masuda, H., Kawamoto, A., Walsh, K., Isner, J.M., & Asahara, T. (2001). HMG-CoA reductase inhibitor mobilizes bone marrow--derived endothelial progenitor cells. *J Clin Invest.* 108, 399-405.

[89] Dimmeler, S., Aicher, A., Vasa, M., Mildner-Rihm, C., Adler, K., Tiemann, M., Rütten, H., Fichtlscherer, S., Martin, H., & Zeiher, A.M. (2001). HMG-CoA reductase inhibitors (statins) increase endothelial progenitor cells via the PI 3-kinase/Akt pathway. *J Clin Invest.* 108, 391-397.

[90] Aicher, A., Heeschen, C., Mildner-Rihm, C., Urbich, C., Ihling, C., Technau-Ihling, K., Zeiher, A.M., & Dimmeler, S. (2003). Essential role of endothelial nitric oxide synthase for mobilization of stem and progenitor cells. *Nat Med.* 9, 1370-1376.

[91] Assmus, B., Urbich, C., Aicher, A., Hofmann, W.K., Haendeler, J., Rössig, L., Spyridopoulos, I., Zeiher, A.M., & Dimmeler, S. (2003). HMG-CoA reductase inhibitors reduce senescence and increase proliferation of endothelial progenitor cells via regulation of cell cycle regulatory genes. *Circ Res.* 92, 1049-1055.

[92] Ota, H., Eto, M., Kano, M.R., Kahyo, T., Setou, M., Ogawa, S., Iijima, K., Akishita, M., & Ouchi, Y. (2010). Induction of endothelial nitric oxide synthase, SIRT1, and catalase by statins inhibits endothelial senescence through the Akt pathway. *Arterioscler Thromb Vasc Biol.* 30, 2205-2211.

[93] Chen, J., Zhang, Z.G., Li, Y., Wang, Y., Wang, L., Jiang, H., Zhang, C., Lu, M., Katakowski, M., Feldkamp, C.S., & Chopp, M. (2003). Statins induce angiogenesis, neurogenesis, and synaptogenesis after stroke. *Ann Neurol.* 53, 743-751.

[94] Engelhorn, T., Doerfler, A., Heusch, G., & Schulz, R. (2006). Reduction of cerebral infarct size by the AT1-receptor blocker candesartan, the HMG-CoA reductase inhibitor rosuvastatin and their combination. An experimental study in rats. *Neurosci Lett.* 406, 92-96.

[95] Sironi, L., Cimino, M., Guerrini, U., Calvio, A.M., Lodetti, B., Asdente, M., Balduini, W., Paoletti, R., & Tremoli, E. (2003). Treatment with statins after induction of focal ischemia in rats reduces the extent of brain damage. *Arterioscler Thromb Vasc Biol.* 23, 322-327.

[96] Mangialardi, G., Monopoli, A., Ongini, E., Spinetti, G., Fortunato, O., Emanueli, C., & Madeddu, P. (2011). Nitric oxide-donating statin improves multiple functions of circulating angiogenic cells. *Br J Pharmacol.* 164, 570-583.

[97] Moro, M.A., Cárdenas, A., Hurtado, O., Leza, J.C., & Lizasoain, I. (2004). Role of nitric oxide after brain ischaemia. *Cell Calcium.* 36, 265-275.

[98] Vaughan, C.J., & Delanty, N. (1999). Neuroprotective properties of statins in cerebral ischemia and stroke. *Stroke.* 30, 1969-1973.

[99] Greisenegger, S., Müllner, M., Tentschert, S., Lang, W., & Lalouschek, W. (2004). Effect of pretreatment with statins on the severity of acute ischemic cerebrovascular events. *J Neurol Sci.* 221, 5-10.

[100] Elkind, M.S., Flint, A.C., Sciacca, R.R., & Sacco, R.L. (2005). Lipid-lowering agent use at ischemic stroke onset is associated with decreased mortality. *Neurology.* 65, 253-258.

[101] Martí-Fàbregas, J., Gomis, M., Arboix, A., Aleu, A., Pagonabarraga, J., Belvís, R., Cocho, D., Roquer, J., Rodríguez, A., García, M.D., Molina-Porcel, L., Díaz-Manera, J., & Martí-Vilalta, J.L. (2004). Favorable outcome of ischemic stroke in patients pretreated with statins. *Stroke.* 35, 1117-1121.

[102] Blanco, M., Nombela, F., Castellanos, M., Rodriguez-Yáñez, M., García-Gil, M., Leira, R., Lizasoain, I., Serena, J., Vivancos, J., Moro, M.A., Dávalos, A., & Castillo, J. (2007). Statin treatment withdrawal in ischemic stroke: a controlled randomized study. *Neurology*. 69, 904-910.

[103] Yoon, S.S., Dambrosia, J., Chalela, J., Ezzeddine, M., Warach, S., Haymore, J., Davis, L., & Baird, A.E. (2004). Rising statin use and effect on ischemic stroke outcome. *BMC Med*. 2, 4.

[104] Elkind, M.S., Sacco, R.L., MacArthur, R.B., Fink, D.J., Peerschke, E., Andrews, H., Neils, G., Stillman, J., Corporan, T., Leifer, D., & Cheung, K. (2008). The Neuroprotection with Statin Therapy for Acute Recovery Trial (NeuSTART): an adaptive design phase I dose-escalation study of high-dose lovastatin in acute ischemic stroke. *Int J Stroke*. 3, 210-218.

[105] Simons, M., Keller, P., Dichgans, J., & Schulz, J.B. (2001). Cholesterol and Alzheimer's disease: is there a link? *Neurology*. 57, 1089-1093.

[106] Di Paolo, G., & Kim, T.W. (2011). Linking lipids to Alzheimer's disease: cholesterol and beyond. *Nat Rev Neurosci*. 12, 284-296.

[107] Fernández, A., Llacuna, L., Fernández-Checa, J.C., & Colell, A. (2009). Mitochondrial cholesterol loading exacerbates amyloid beta peptide-induced inflammation and neurotoxicity. *J Neurosci*. 29, 6394-6405.

[108] Bodovitz, S., & Klein, W.L. (1996). Cholesterol modulates alpha-secretase cleavage of amyloid precursor protein. *J Biol Chem*. 271, 4436-4440.

[109] Matsuzaki, T., Sasaki, K., Hata, J., Hirakawa, Y., Fujimi, K., Ninomiya, T., Suzuki, S.O., Kanba, S., Kiyohara, Y., & Iwaki, T. (2011). Association of Alzheimer disease pathology with abnormal lipid metabolism: the Hisayama Study. *Neurology*. 77, 1068-1075.

[110] Pappolla, M.A., Bryant-Thomas, T.K., Herbert, D., Pacheco, J., Fabra Garcia, M., Manjon, M., Girones, X., Henry, T.L., Matsubara, E., Zambon, D., Wolozin, B., Sano, M., Cruz-Sanchez, F.F., Thal, L.J., Petanceska, S.S., & Refolo, L.M. (2003). Mild hypercholesterolemia is an early risk factor for the development of Alzheimer amyloid pathology. *Neurology*. 61, 199-205.

[111] Sing, C.F., & Davignon, J. (1985). Role of the apolipoprotein E polymorphism in determining normal plasma lipid and lipoprotein variation. *Am J Hum Genet*. 37, 268-285.

[112] Panza, F., D'Introno, A., Colacicco, A.M., Capurso, C., Pichichero, G., Capurso, S.A., Capurso ,A., & Solfrizzi, V. (2006). Lipid metabolism in cognitive decline and dementia. *Brain Res Rev*. 51, 275-292.

[113] Diabetes Genetics Initiative of Broad Institute of Harvard and MIT, Lund University, and Novartis Institutes of BioMedical Research. (2007). Genome-wide association analysis identifies loci for type 2 diabetes and triglyceride levels. *Science*. 316, 1331-1336.

[114] Michikawa, M., Fan, Q.W., Isobe, I., & Yanagisawa, K. (2000). Apolipoprotein E exhibits isoform-specific promotion of lipid efflux from astrocytes and neurons in culture. *J Neurochem*. 74, 1008-1016.

[115] Saunders, A.M., Strittmatter, W.J., Schmechel, D., George-Hyslop, P.H., Pericak-Vance, M.A., Joo, S.H., Rosi, B.L., Gusella, J.F., Crapper-MacLachlan, D.R., Alberts,

M.J., et al. (1993). Association of apolipoprotein E allele epsilon 4 with late-onset familial and sporadic Alzheimer's disease. *Neurology*. 43, 1467-1472.
[116] Kim, J., Castellano, J.M., Jiang, H., Basak, J.M., Parsadanian, M., Pham, V., Mason, S.M., Paul, S.M., Holtzman, D.M. (2009). Overexpression of low-density lipoprotein receptor in the brain markedly inhibits amyloid deposition and increases extracellular A beta clearance. *Neuron*. 64, 632-644.
[117] Corder, E.H., Saunders, A.M., Strittmatter, W.J., Schmechel, D.E., Gaskell, P.C., Small, G.W., Roses, A.D., Haines, J.L., & Pericak-Vance, M.A. (1993). Gene dose of apolipoprotein E type 4 allele and the risk of Alzheimer's disease in late onset families. *Science*. 261, 921-923.
[118] Holtzman, D.M., Bales, K.R., Tenkova, T., Fagan, A.M., Parsadanian, M., Sartorius, L.J., Mackey, B., Olney, J., McKeel, D., Wozniak, D., & Paul, S.M. (2000). Apolipoprotein E isoform-dependent amyloid deposition and neuritic degeneration in a mouse model of Alzheimer's disease. *Proc Natl Acad Sci U S A*. 97, 2892-2897.
[119] Haan, M.N., Shemanski, L., Jagust, W.J., Manolio, T.A., & Kuller, L. (1999). The role of APOE epsilon4 in modulating effects of other risk factors for cognitive decline in elderly persons. *JAMA*. 282, 40-46.
[120] Hofman, A., Ott, A., Breteler, M.M., Bots, M.L., Slooter, A.J., van Harskamp, F., van Duijn, C.N., Van Broeckhoven, C., & Grobbee, D.E. (1997). Atherosclerosis, apolipoprotein E, and prevalence of dementia and Alzheimer's disease in the Rotterdam Study. *Lancet*. 349, 151-154.
[121] Désiré, L., Bourdin, J., Loiseau, N., Peillon, H., Picard, V., De Oliveira, C., Bachelot, F., Leblond, B., Taverne, T., Beausoleil, E., Lacombe, S., Drouin, D., & Schweighoffer, F. (2005). RAC1 inhibition targets amyloid precursor protein processing by gamma-secretase and decreases Abeta production in vitro and in vivo. *J Biol Chem*. 280, 37516-37525.
[122] McConlogue, L., Castellano, F., deWit ,C., Schenk, D., & Maltese, W.A. (1996). Differential effects of a Rab6 mutant on secretory versus amyloidogenic processing of Alzheimer's beta-amyloid precursor protein. *J Biol Chem*. 271, 1343-1348.
[123] Ostrowski, S.M., Wilkinson, B.L., Golde, T.E., & Landreth, G. (2007). Statins reduce amyloid-beta production through inhibition of protein isoprenylation. *J Biol Chem*. 282, 26832-26844.
[124] Zhou, Y., Su, Y., Li, B., Liu, F., Ryder, J.W., Wu, X., Gonzalez-DeWhitt, P.A., Gelfanova, V., Hale, J.E., May, P.C., Paul, S.M., & Ni, B. (2003). Nonsteroidal anti-inflammatory drugs can lower amyloidogenic Abeta42 by inhibiting Rho. *Science*. 302, 1215-1217.
[125] Cole, S.L., Grudzien, A., Manhart, I.O., Kelly, B.L., Oakley, H., & Vassar, R. (2005). Statins cause intracellular accumulation of amyloid precursor protein, beta-secretase-cleaved fragments, and amyloid beta-peptide via an isoprenoid-dependent mechanism. *J Biol Chem*. 280, 18755-18770.
[126] Hess, D.C., Demchuk, A.M., Brass, L.M., & Yatsu, F.M. (2000). HMG-CoA reductase inhibitors (statins): a promising approach to stroke prevention. *Neurology*. 54, 790-796.
[127] Simons, M., Keller, P., De Strooper, B., Beyreuther, K., Dotti, C.G., & Simons, K. (1998). Cholesterol depletion inhibits the generation of beta-amyloid in hippocampal neurons. *Proc Natl Acad Sci U S A*. 95, 6460-6464.

[128] Li, G., Shofer, J.B., Rhew, I.C., Kukull, W.A., Peskind, E.R., McCormick, W., Bowen, J.D., Schellenberg, G.D., Crane, P.K., Breitner, J.C., & Larson, E.B. (2010). Age-varying association between statin use and incident Alzheimer's disease. *J Am Geriatr Soc*. 58, 1311-1317.

[129] Sparks, D.L., Connor, D.J., Sabbagh, M.N., Petersen, R.B., Lopez, J., & Browne, P. (2006). Circulating cholesterol levels, apolipoprotein E genotype and dementia severity influence the benefit of atorvastatin treatment in Alzheimer's disease: results of the Alzheimer's Disease Cholesterol-Lowering Treatment (ADCLT) trial. *Acta Neurol Scand Suppl*. 185, 3-7.

[130] Haag, M.D., Hofman, A., Koudstaal, P.J., Stricker, B.H., & Breteler, M.M. (2009). Statins are associated with a reduced risk of Alzheimer disease regardless of lipophilicity. The Rotterdam Study. *J Neurol Neurosurg Psychiatry*. 80, 13-17.

[131] Wolozin, B., Kellman, W., Ruosseau, P., Celesia, G.G., & Siegel, G. (2000). Decreased prevalence of Alzheimer disease associated with 3-hydroxy-3-methyglutaryl coenzyme A reductase inhibitors. *Arch Neurol*. 57, 1439-1443.

[132] Rosenberg, P.B., Mielke, M.M., Tschanz, J., Cook, L., Corcoran, C., Hayden, K.M., Norton, M., Rabins, P.V., Green, R.C., Welsh-Bohmer, K.A., Breitner, J.C., Munger, R., & Lyketsos, C.G. (2008). Effects of cardiovascular medications on rate of functional decline in Alzheimer disease. *Am J Geriatr Psychiatry*. 16, 883-892.

[133] Jick, H., Zornberg, G.L., Jick, S.S., Seshadri, S., & Drachman, D.A. (2000). Statins and the risk of dementia. *Lancet*. 356, 1627-1631.

[134] Yaffe, K., Barrett-Connor, E., Lin, F., & Grady, D. (2002). Serum lipoprotein levels, statin use, and cognitive function in older women. *Arch Neurol*. 59, 378-384.

[135] Sparks, D.L., Sabbagh, M.N., Connor, D.J., Lopez, J., Launer, L.J., Browne, P., Wasser, D., Johnson-Traver, S., Lochhead, J., & Ziolwolski, C. (2005). Atorvastatin for the treatment of mild to moderate Alzheimer disease: preliminary results. *Arch Neurol*. 62, 753-757.

[136] Friedhoff, L.T., Cullen, E.I., Geoghagen, N.S., & Buxbaum, J.D. (2001). Treatment with controlled-release lovastatin decreases serum concentrations of human beta-amyloid (A beta) peptide. *Int J Neuropsychopharmacol*. 4, 127-130.

[137] Simons, M., Schwärzler, F., Lütjohann, D., von Bergmann, K., Beyreuther, K., Dichgans, J., Wormstall, H., Hartmann, T., & Schulz, J.B. (2002). Treatment with simvastatin in normocholesterolemic patients with Alzheimer's disease: A 26-week randomized, placebo-controlled, double-blind trial. *Ann Neurol*. 52, 346-350.

[138] Heart Protection Study Collaborative Group. (2002). MRC/BHF Heart Protection Study of cholesterol lowering with simvastatin in 20,536 high-risk individuals: a randomised placebo-controlled trial. *Lancet*. 360, 7-22.

[139] Shepherd, J., Blauw, G.J., Murphy, M.B., Bollen, E.L., Buckley, B.M., Cobbe, S.M., Ford, I., Gaw, A., Hyland, M., Jukema, J.W., Kamper, A.M., Macfarlane, P.W., Meinders, A.E., Norrie, J., Packard, C.J., Perry, I.J., Stott, D.J., Sweeney, B.J., Twomey, C., Westendorp, R.G. & PROSPER study group. (2002). PROspective Study of Pravastatin in the Elderly at Risk. Pravastatin in elderly individuals at risk of vascular disease (PROSPER): a randomised controlled trial. *Lancet*. 360, 1623-1630.

[140] Trompet, S., van Vliet, P., de Craen ,A.J., Jolles, J., Buckley, B.M., Murphy, M.B., Ford, I., Macfarlane, P.W., Sattar, N., Packard, C.J., Stott, D.J., Shepherd, J., Bollen,

E.L., Blauw, G.J., Jukema, J.W., & Westendorp, R.G. (2010). Pravastatin and cognitive function in the elderly. Results of the PROSPER study. *J Neurol.* 257, 85-90.

[141] Feldman, H.H., Doody, R.S., Kivipelto, M., Sparks, D.L., Waters, D.D., Jones, R.W., Schwam, E., Schindler, R., Hey-Hadavi, J., DeMicco, D.A., Breazna, A., & LEADe Investigators. (2010). Randomized controlled trial of atorvastatin in mild to moderate Alzheimer disease: LEADe. *Neurology.* 74, 956-964.

[142] Sano, M., Bell, K.L., Galasko, D., Galvin, J.E., Thomas, R.G., van Dyck, C.H., & Aisen, P.S. (2011). A randomized, double-blind, placebo-controlled trial of simvastatin to treat Alzheimer disease. *Neurology.* 77, 556-563.

[143] Zhou, B., Teramukai, S., & Fukushima, M. (2007). Prevention and treatment of dementia or Alzheimer's disease by statins: a meta-analysis. *Dement Geriatr Cogn Disord.* 23, 194-201.

[144] McGuinness, B., O'Hare, J., Craig, D., Bullock, R., Malouf, R., & Passmore, P. (2010). Statins for the treatment of dementia. *Cochrane Database Syst Rev.* 4, CD007514.

[145] McGuinness, B., Craig, D., Bullock, R., & Passmore, P. (2009). Statins for the prevention of dementia. *Cochrane Database Syst Rev.* 2, CD003160.

[146] Vuletic, S., Riekse, R.G., Marcovina, S.M., Peskind, E.R., Hazzard, W.R., & Albers, J.J. (2006). Statins of different brain penetrability differentially affect CSF PLTP activity. *Dement Geriatr Cogn Disord.* 22, 392-398.

[147] Saheki, A., Terasaki, T., Tamai, I., & Tsuji, A. (1994). In vivo and in vitro blood-brain barrier transport of 3-hydroxy-3-methylglutaryl coenzyme A (HMG-CoA) reductase inhibitors. *Pharm Res.* 11, 305-311.

[148] Dietschy, J.M., & Turley, S.D. (2001). Cholesterol metabolism in the brain. *Curr Opin Lipidol.* 12, 105-112.

[149] Thompson, J.F., Man, M., Johnson, K.J., Wood, L.S., Lira, M.E., Lloyd, D.B., Banerjee, P., Milos, P.M., Myrand, S.P., Paulauskis, J., Milad, M.A., & Sasiela, W.J. (2005). An association study of 43 SNPs in 16 candidate genes with atorvastatin response. *Pharmacogenomics J.* 5, 352-358.

[150] Butterfield, D.A., Barone, E., & Mancuso, C. (2011). Cholesterol-independent neuroprotective and neurotoxic activities of statins: perspectives for statin use in Alzheimer disease and other age-related neurodegenerative disorders. *Pharmacol Res.* 64, 180-186.

[151] Selley, M.L. (2005). Simvastatin prevents 1-methyl-4-phenyl-1,2,3,6-tetrahydropyridine-induced striatal dopamine depletion and protein tyrosine nitration in mice. *Brain Res.* 1037, 1-6.

[152] Mogi, M., Kondo, T., Mizuno, Y., & Nagatsu, T. (2007). p53 protein, interferon-gamma, and NF-kappaB levels are elevated in the parkinsonian brain. *Neurosci Lett.* 414, 94-97.

[153] Levecque, C., Elbaz, A., Clavel, J., Richard, F., Vidal, J.S., Amouyel, P., Tzourio, C., Alpérovitch, A., & Chartier-Harlin, M.C. (2003). Association between Parkinson's disease and polymorphisms in the nNOS and iNOS genes in a community-based case-control study. *Hum Mol Genet.* 12, 79-86.

[154] Huang, X., Chen, P.C., & Poole, C. (2004). APOE-[epsilon]2 allele associated with higher prevalence of sporadic Parkinson disease. *Neurology.* 62, 2198-2202.

[155] Wang, Q., Ting, W.L., Yang, H., & Wong, P.T. (2005). High doses of simvastatin upregulate dopamine D1 and D2 receptor expression in the rat prefrontal cortex:

possible involvement of endothelial nitric oxide synthase. *Br J Pharmacol.* 144, 933-939.

[156] Wang, Q., Wang, P.H., McLachlan, C., & Wong, P.T. (2005). Simvastatin reverses the downregulation of dopamine D1 and D2 receptor expression in the prefrontal cortex of 6-hydroxydopamine-induced Parkinsonian rats. *Brain Res.* 1045, 229-233.

[157] Wolozin, B., Wang, S.W., Li, N.C., Lee, A., Lee, T.A., & Kazis, L.E. (2007). Simvastatin is associated with a reduced incidence of dementia and Parkinson's disease. *BMC Med.* 5, 20.

[158] Mutez, E., Duhamel, A., Defebvre, L., Bordet, R., Destée, A., & Kreisler, A. (2009). Lipid-lowering drugs are associated with delayed onset and slower course of Parkinson's disease. *Pharmacol Res.* 60, 41-45.

[159] Wahner, A.D., Bronstein, J.M., Bordelon, Y.M., & Ritz, B. (2008). Statin use and the risk of Parkinson disease. *Neurology.* 70, 1418-1422.

[160] Huang, X., Chen, H., Miller, W.C., Mailman, R.B., Woodard, J.L., Chen, P.C., Xiang, D., Murrow, R.W., Wang, Y.Z., & Poole, C. (2007). Lower low-density lipoprotein cholesterol levels are associated with Parkinson's disease. *Mov Disord.* 22, 377-381.

[161] de Lau, L.M., Koudstaal, P.J., Hofman, A., & Breteler, M.M. (2006). Serum cholesterol levels and the risk of Parkinson's disease. *Am J Epidemiol.* 164, 998-1002.

[162] Fried, L.F., Orchard, T.J., & Kasiske, B.L. (2001). Effect of lipid reduction on the progression of renal disease: a meta-analysis. *Kidney Int.* 59, 260-269.

[163] Bussolati, B., Deregibus, M.C., Fonsato, V., Doublier, S., Spatola, T., Procida, S., Di Carlo, F., & Camussi, G. (2005). Statins prevent oxidized LDL-induced injury of glomerular podocytes by activating the phosphatidylinositol 3-kinase/AKT-signaling pathway. *J Am Soc Nephrol.* 16, 1936-1947.

[164] Chen, H.C., Guh, J.Y., Shin, S.J., & Lai, Y.H. (2002). Pravastatin suppress superoxide and fibronectin production of glomerular mesangial cells induced by oxidized-LDL and high glucose. *Atherosclerosis.* 160, 141-146.

[165] Reisin, E., Ebenezer, P.J., Liao, J., Lee, B.S., Larroque, M., Hu, X., Aguilar, E.A., Morse, S.A., & Francis, J. (2009). Effect of the HMG-CoA reductase inhibitor rosuvastatin on early chronic kidney injury in obese zucker rats fed with an atherogenic diet. *Am J Med Sci.* 338, 301-309.

[166] Sabbatini, M., Pisani, A., Uccello, F., Serio, V., Serù, R., Paternò, R., Cianciaruso, B., Fuiano, G., & Andreucci, M. (2004). Atorvastatin improves the course of ischemic acute renal failure in aging rats. *J Am Soc Nephrol.* 15, 901-909.

[167] Blantz, R.C., & Munger, K. (2002). Role of nitric oxide in inflammatory conditions. *Nephron.* 90, 373-378.

[168] Vázquez-Pérez, S., Aragoncillo, P., de Las Heras, N., Navarro-Cid, J., Cediel, E., Sanz-Rosa, D., Ruilope, L.M., Díaz, C., Hernández, G., Lahera, V., & Cachofeiro, V. (2001). Atorvastatin prevents glomerulosclerosis and renal endothelial dysfunction in hypercholesterolaemic rabbits. *Nephrol Dial Transplant.* 16 Suppl 1:40-44.

[169] Vieira, J.M. Jr, Mantovani, E., Rodrigues, L.T., Dellê, H., Noronha, I.L., Fujihara, C.K., & Zatz, R. (2005). Simvastatin attenuates renal inflammation, tubular transdifferentiation and interstitial fibrosis in rats with unilateral ureteral obstruction. *Nephrol Dial Transplant.* 20, 1582-1591.

[170] Tonelli, M., Moyé, L., Sacks, F.M., Cole, T., Curhan, G.C. & Cholesterol and Recurrent Events Trial Investigators. (2003). Effect of pravastatin on loss of renal

function in people with moderate chronic renal insufficiency and cardiovascular disease. *J Am Soc Nephrol.* 14, 1605-1613.

[171] Bianchi, S., Bigazzi, R., Caiazza, A., & Campese, V.M. (2003). A controlled, prospective study of the effects of atorvastatin on proteinuria and progression of kidney disease. *Am J Kidney Dis.* 41, 565-570.

[172] Di Lullo, L., Addesse, R., Comegna, C., Firmi, G., Galderisi, C., Iannacci, G.R., & Polito, P. (2005). Effects of fluvastatin treatment on lipid profile, C-reactive protein trend, and renal function in dyslipidemic patients with chronic renal failure. *Adv Ther.* 22, 601-612.

[173] Athyros, V.G., Mikhailidis, D.P., Papageorgiou, A.A., Symeonidis, A.N., Pehlivanidis, A.N., Bouloukos, V.I., & Elisaf, M. (2004). The effect of statins versus untreated dyslipidaemia on renal function in patients with coronary heart disease. A subgroup analysis of the Greek atorvastatin and coronary heart disease evaluation (GREACE) study. *J Clin Pathol.* 57, 728-734.

[174] *http://www.theheart.org/article/1095269.do*

[175] Tonelli, M., Isles, C., Craven, T., Tonkin, A., Pfeffer, M.A., Shepherd, J., Sacks, F.M., Furberg, C., Cobbe, S.M., Simes, J., West, M., Packard, C., & Curhan, G.C. (2005). Effect of pravastatin on rate of kidney function loss in people with or at risk for coronary disease. *Circulation.* 112, 171-178.

[176] Kimura, K., Shimano, H., Yokote, K., Urashima, M., & Teramoto, T. (2010). Effects of pitavastatin (LIVALO tablet) on the estimated glomerular filtration rate (eGFR) in hypercholesterolemic patients with chronic kidney disease. Sub-analysis of the LIVALO Effectiveness and Safety (LIVES) Study. *J Atheroscler Thromb.* 17, 601-609.

[177] Vidt, D.G., Harris, S., McTaggart, F., Ditmarsch, M., Sager, P.T., & Sorof, J.M. (2006). Effect of short-term rosuvastatin treatment on estimated glomerular filtration rate. *Am J Cardiol.* 97, 1602-1606.

[178] Asselbergs, F.W., Diercks, G.F., Hillege, H.L., van Boven, A.J., Janssen, W.M., Voors, A.A., de Zeeuw, D., de Jong, P.E., van Veldhuisen, D.J., van Gilst, W.H., & Prevention of Renal and Vascular Endstage Disease Intervention Trial (PREVEND IT) Investigators. (2004). Effects of fosinopril and pravastatin on cardiovascular events in subjects with microalbuminuria. *Circulation.* 110, 2809-2816.

[179] Ridker, P.M., MacFadyen, J., Cressman, M., & Glynn, R.J. (2010). Efficacy of rosuvastatin among men and women with moderate chronic kidney disease and elevated high-sensitivity C-reactive protein: a secondary analysis from the JUPITER (Justification for the Use of Statins in Prevention-an Intervention Trial Evaluating Rosuvastatin) trial. *J Am Coll Cardiol.* 55, 1266-1273.

[180] Baigent, C., Landray, M.J., Reith, C., Emberson, J., Wheeler, D.C., Tomson, C., Wanner, C., Krane, V., Cass, A., Craig, J., Neal, B., Jiang, L., Hooi, L.S., Levin, A., Agodoa, L., Gaziano, M., Kasiske, B., Walker, R., Massy, Z.A., Feldt-Rasmussen ,B., Krairittichai, U., Ophascharoensuk, V., Fellström, B., Holdaas, H., Tesar, V., Wiecek, A., Grobbee, D., de Zeeuw, D., Grönhagen-Riska, C., Dasgupta, T., Lewis, D., Herrington, W., Mafham, M., Majoni, W., Wallendszus, K., Grimm, R., Pedersen, T., Tobert, J., Armitage, J., Baxter, A., Bray, C., Chen, Y., Chen, Z., Hill, M., Knott, C., Parish, S., Simpson, D., Sleight, P., Young, A,, Collins, R. & SHARP Investigators. (2011). The effects of lowering LDL cholesterol with simvastatin plus ezetimibe in

patients with chronic kidney disease (Study of Heart and Renal Protection): a randomised placebo-controlled trial. *Lancet.* 2011 377, 2181-2192.

[181] Kendrick, J., Shlipak, M.G., Targher, G., Cook, T., Lindenfeld, J., & Chonchol, M. (2010). Effect of lovastatin on primary prevention of cardiovascular events in mild CKD and kidney function loss: a post hoc analysis of the Air Force/Texas Coronary Atherosclerosis Prevention Study. *Am J Kidney Dis.* 55, 42-49.

[182] Navaneethan, S.D., Pansini, F., Perkovic, V., Manno, C., Pellegrini, F., Johnson, D.W., Craig, J.C., & Strippoli, G.F. (2009). HMG CoA reductase inhibitors (statins) for people with chronic kidney disease not requiring dialysis. *Cochrane Database Syst Rev.* 2, CD007784.

[183] Strippoli, G.F., Navaneethan, S.D., Johnson, D.W., Perkovic, V., Pellegrini, F., Nicolucci, A., & Craig, J.C. (2008). Effects of statins in patients with chronic kidney disease: meta-analysis and meta-regression of randomised controlled trials. *BMJ.* 336, 645-651.

[184] Sandhu, S., Wiebe, N., Fried, L.F., & Tonelli, M. (2006). Statins for improving renal outcomes: a meta-analysis. *J Am Soc Nephrol.* 17, 2006-2016.

[185] Douglas, K., O'Malley, P.G., & Jackson, J.L. (2006). Meta-analysis: the effect of statins on albuminuria. *Ann Intern Med.* 145, 117-124.

[186] Del Castillo, D., Cruzado, J.M., Manel Díaz, J., Beneyto Castelló, I., Lauzurica Valdemoros, R., Gómez Huertas, E., & Checa Andrés, M.D. (2004). The effects of hyperlipidaemia on graft and patient outcome in renal transplantation. *Nephrol Dial Transplant.* 19 Suppl 3, iii 67-71.

[187] Masterson, R., Hewitson, T., Leikis, M., Walker, R., Cohney, S., & Becker, G. (2005). Impact of statin treatment on 1-year functional and histologic renal allograft outcome. *Transplantation.* 80, 332-338.

[188] Lisik, W., Schoenberg, L., Lasky, R.E., & Kahan, B.D. (2007). Statins benefit outcomes of renal transplant recipients on a sirolimus-cyclosporine regimen. *Transplant Proc.* 39, 3086-3092.

[189] Fellström, B., Holdaas, H., Jardine, A.G., Holme, I., Nyberg, G., Fauchald, P., Grönhagen-Riska, C., Madsen, S., Neumayer, H.H., Cole, E., Maes, B., Ambühl, P., Olsson, A.G., Hartmann, A., Logan, J.O., Pedersen, T.R., & Assessment of Lescol in Renal Transplantation Study Investigators. (2004). Effect of fluvastatin on renal end points in the Assessment of Lescol in Renal Transplant (ALERT) trial. *Kidney Int.* 66, 1549-1555.

[190] Kasiske, B.L., Heim-Duthoy, K.L., Singer, G.G., Watschinger, B., Germain, M.J., & Bastani, B. (2001). The effects of lipid-lowering agents on acute renal allograft rejection. *Transplantation.* 72, 223-227.

[191] Navaneethan, S.D., Perkovic, V., Johnson, D.W., Nigwekar, S.U., Craig, J.C., & Strippoli, G.F. (2009). HMG CoA reductase inhibitors (statins) for kidney transplant recipients. *Cochrane Database Syst Rev.* 2, CD005019.

[192] Mundy, G., Garrett, R., Harris, S., Chan, J., Chen, D., Rossini, G., Boyce, B., Zhao, M., & Gutierrez, G. (1999). Stimulation of bone formation in vitro and in rodents by statins. *Science.* 286, 1946-1949.

[193] Bauer, D.C. (2003). HMG CoA reductase inhibitors and the skeleton: a comprehensive review. *Osteoporos Int.* 14, 273-282.

[194] Wang, P.S., Solomon, D.H., Mogun, H., & Avorn, J. (2000). HMG-CoA reductase inhibitors and the risk of hip fractures in elderly patients. *JAMA*. 283, 3211-3216.
[195] Meier, C.R., Schlienger, R.G., Kraenzlin, M.E., Schlegel, B., & Jick, H. (2000). HMG-CoA reductase inhibitors and the risk of fractures. *JAMA*. 283, 3205-3210.
[196] Solomon, D.H., Finkelstein, J.S., Wang, P.S., & Avorn, J. (2005). Statin lipid-lowering drugs and bone mineral density. *Pharmacoepidemiol Drug Saf*. 14, 219-226.
[197] van Staa, T.P., Wegman, S., de Vries, F., Leufkens, B., & Cooper, C. (2001). Use of statins and risk of fractures. *JAMA*. 285, 1850-1855.
[198] LaCroix, A.Z., Cauley, J.A., Pettinger, M., Hsia, J., Bauer, D.C., McGowan, J., Chen, Z., Lewis, C.E., McNeeley, S.G., Passaro, M.D., & Jackson, R.D. (2003). Statin use, clinical fracture, and bone density in postmenopausal women: results from the Women's Health Initiative Observational Study. *Ann Intern Med*. 139, 97-104.
[199] Bjarnason, N.H., Riis, B.J., & Christiansen, C. (2001). The effect of fluvastatin on parameters of bone remodeling. *Osteoporos Int*. 12, 380-384.
[200] Berthold, H.K., Unverdorben, S., Zittermann, A., Degenhardt, R., Baumeister, B., Unverdorben, M., Krone, W., Vetter, H., & Gouni-Berthold, I. (2004). Age-dependent effects of atorvastatin on biochemical bone turnover markers: a randomized controlled trial in postmenopausal women. *Osteoporos Int*. 15, 459-467.
[201] Uzzan, B., Cohen, R., Nicolas, P., Cucherat, M., & Perret, G.Y. (2007). Effects of statins on bone mineral density: a meta-analysis of clinical studies. *Bone*. 40, 1581-1587.
[202] Toh, S., & Hernández-Díaz, S. (2007). Statins and fracture risk. A systematic review. *Pharmacoepidemiol Drug Saf*. 16, 627-640.
[203] Hatzigeorgiou, C., & Jackson, J.L. (2005). Hydroxymethylglutaryl-coenzyme A reductase inhibitors and osteoporosis: a meta-analysis. *Osteoporos Int*. 16, 990-998.
[204] Bauer, D.C., Mundy, G.R., Jamal, S.A., Black, D.M., Cauley, J.A., Ensrud, K.E., van der Klift, M., & Pols, H.A. (2004). Use of statins and fracture: results of 4 prospective studies and cumulative meta-analysis of observational studies and controlled trials. *Arch Intern Med*. 164, 146-152.
[205] Yue, J., Zhang, X., Dong, B., & Yang, M. (2010). Statins and bone health in postmenopausal women: a systematic review of randomized controlled trials. *Menopause*. 17, 1071-1079.
[206] Rejnmark, L., Buus, N.H., Vestergaard, P., Heickendorff, L., Andreasen, F., Larsen, M.L., & Mosekilde, L. (2004). Effects of simvastatin on bone turnover and BMD: a 1-year randomized controlled trial in postmenopausal osteopenic women. *J Bone Miner Res*. 19, 737-744.
[207] Mundy, G.R. (2001). Statins and their potential for osteoporosis. *Bone*. 29, 495-497.
[208] Hamelin, B.A., & Turgeon, J. (1998). Hydrophilicity/lipophilicity: relevance for the pharmacology and clinical effects of HMG-CoA reductase inhibitors. *Trends Pharmacol Sci*. 19, 26-37.
[209] Ohnaka, K., Shimoda, S., Nawata, H., Shimokawa, H., Kaibuchi, K., Iwamoto, Y., & Takayanagi, R. (2001). Pitavastatin enhanced BMP-2 and osteocalcin expression by inhibition of Rho-associated kinase in human osteoblasts. *Biochem Biophys Res Commun*. 287, 337-342.
[210] Matthews, S.J. (2005). Biological activity of bone morphogenetic proteins (BMP's). *Injury*. 36 Suppl 3, S34-S37.

[211] Maeda, T., Kawane, T., & Horiuchi, N. (2003). Statins augment vascular endothelial growth factor expression in osteoblastic cells via inhibition of protein prenylation. *Endocrinology*. 144, 681-692.

[212] Bouletreau, P.J., Warren, S.M., Spector, J.A., Peled, Z.M., Gerrets, R.P., Greenwald, J.A., & Longaker, M.T. (2002). Hypoxia and VEGF up-regulate BMP-2 mRNA and protein expression in microvascular endothelial cells: implications for fracture healing. *Plast Reconstr Surg*. 109, 2384-2397.

[213] Deckers, M.M., van Bezooijen, R.L., van der Horst, G., Hoogendam, J., van Der Bent, C., Papapoulos, S.E., & Löwik, C.W. (2002). Bone morphogenetic proteins stimulate angiogenesis through osteoblast-derived vascular endothelial growth factor A. *Endocrinology*. 143, 1545-1553.

[214] Eghbali-Fatourechi, G.Z., Mödder, U.I., Charatcharoenwitthaya, N., Sanyal, A., Undale, A.H., Clowes, J.A., Tarara, J.E., & Khosla, S. (2007). Characterization of circulating osteoblast lineage cells in humans. *Bone*. 40, 1370-1377.

[215] Russell, R.G., & Rogers, M.J. (1999). Bisphosphonates: from the laboratory to the clinic and back again. *Bone*. 25, 97-106.

[216] Coxon, F.P., Helfrich, M.H., Van't Hof, R., Sebti, S., Ralston, S.H., Hamilton, A., & Rogers, M.J. (2000). Protein geranylgeranylation is required for osteoclast formation, function, and survival: inhibition by bisphosphonates and GGTI-298. *J Bone Miner Res*. 15, 1467-1476.

[217] Bergstrom, J.D., Bostedor, R.G., Masarachia, P.J., Reszka, A.A., & Rodan, G. (2000). Alendronate is a specific, nanomolar inhibitor of farnesyl diphosphate synthase. *Arch Biochem Biophys*. 373, 231-241.

[218] Newman, T.B., & Hulley, S.B. (1996). Carcinogenicity of lipid-lowering drugs. *JAMA*. 275,55-60.

[219] Duncan, R.E., El-Sohemy, A., & Archer, M.C. (2004). Mevalonate promotes the growth of tumors derived from human cancer cells in vivo and stimulates proliferation in vitro with enhanced cyclin-dependent kinase-2 activity. *J Biol Chem*. 279, 33079-33084.

[220] Blais, L., Desgagné ,A., & LeLorier, J. (2000). 3-Hydroxy-3-methylglutaryl coenzyme A reductase inhibitors and the risk of cancer: a nested case-control study. *Arch Intern Med*. 160, 2363-2368.

[221] Poynter, J.N., Gruber, S.B., Higgins, P.D., Almog, R., Bonner, J.D., Rennert, H.S., Low, M., Greenson, J.K., & Rennert, G. (2005). Statins and the risk of colorectal cancer. *N Engl J Med*. 352, 2184-2192.

[222] Khurana, V., Bejjanki, H.R., Caldito, G., & Owens, M.W. (2007). Statins reduce the risk of lung cancer in humans: a large case-control study of US veterans. *Chest*. 131, 1282-1288.

[223] Gutt, R., Tonlaar, N., Kunnavakkam, R., Karrison, T., Weichselbaum, R.R., & Liauw, S.L. (2010). Statin use and risk of prostate cancer recurrence in men treated with radiation therapy. *J Clin Oncol*. 28, 2653-2659.

[224] Khurana, V., Sheth, A., Caldito, G., & Barkin, J.S. (2007). Statins reduce the risk of pancreatic cancer in humans: a case-control study of half a million veterans. *Pancreas*. 34, 260-265.

[225] Khurana, V., Caldito, G., & Ankem, M. (2008). Statins might reduce risk of renal cell carcinoma in humans: case-control study of 500,000 veterans. *Urology*. 71, 118-122.

[226] Coogan, P.F., Rosenberg, L., Palmer, J.R., Strom, B.L., Zauber, A.G., & Shapiro, S. (2002). Statin use and the risk of breast and prostate cancer. *Epidemiology*. 13, 262-267.

[227] Kaye, J.A., & Jick, H. (2004). Statin use and cancer risk in the General Practice Research Database. *Br J Cancer*. 90, 635-637.

[228] Jacobs, E.J., Rodriguez, C., Brady, K.A., Connell, C.J., Thun, M.J., & Calle, E.E. (2006). Cholesterol-lowering drugs and colorectal cancer incidence in a large United States cohort. *J Natl Cancer Inst*. 98, 69-72.

[229] Matsushita, Y., Sugihara, M., Kaburagi, J., Ozawa, M., Iwashita, M., Yoshida, S., Saito, H., & Hattori,Y. (2010). Pravastatin use and cancer risk: a meta-analysis of individual patient data from long-term prospective controlled trials in Japan. *Pharmacoepidemiol Drug Saf*. 19, 196-202.

[230] Browning, D.R., & Martin, R.M. (2007). Statins and risk of cancer: a systematic review and metaanalysis. *Int J Cancer*. 120, 833-843.

[231] Kuoppala, J., Lamminpää, A., & Pukkala, E. (2008). Statins and cancer: A systematic review and meta-analysis. *Eur J Cancer*. 44, 2122-2132.

[232] Dale, K.M., Coleman, C.I., Henyan, N.N., Kluger, J., & White, C.M. (2006). Statins and cancer risk: a meta-analysis. *JAMA*. 295, 74-80.

[233] Cholesterol Treatment Trialists' (CTT) Collaboration, Baigent, C., Blackwell, L., Emberson, J., Holland, L.E., Reith, C., Bhala, N., Peto, R., Barnes, E.H., Keech, A., Simes, J., & Collins, R. (2010). Efficacy and safety of more intensive lowering of LDL cholesterol: a meta-analysis of data from 170,000 participants in 26 randomised trials. *Lancet*. 376, 1670-1681.

[235] Brugts, J.J., Yetgin, T., Hoeks, S.E., Gotto, A.M., Shepherd, J., Westendorp, R.G., de Craen, A.J., Knopp, R.H., Nakamura, H., Ridker, P., van Domburg, R., & Deckers, J.W. (2009). The benefits of statins in people without established cardiovascular disease but with cardiovascular risk factors: meta-analysis of randomised controlled trials. *BMJ*. 2009 338, b2376.

[236] Mills, E.J., Rachlis, B., Wu, P., Devereaux, P.J., Arora, P., & Perri, D. (2008). Primary prevention of cardiovascular mortality and events with statin treatments: a network meta-analysis involving more than 65,000 patients. *J Am Coll Cardiol*. 52, 1769-1781.

[237] Alsheikh-Ali, A.A., Trikalinos, T.A., Kent, D.M., & Karas, R.H. (2008). Statins, low-density lipoprotein cholesterol, and risk of cancer. *J Am Coll Cardiol*. 52, 1141-1147.

[238] Bonovas, S., & Sitaras, N.M. (2007). Does pravastatin promote cancer in elderly patients? A meta-analysis. *CMAJ*. 176, 649-654.

[239] Bonovas, S., Filioussi, K., Tsavaris, N., & Sitaras, N.M. (2006). Statins and cancer risk: a literature-based meta-analysis and meta-regression analysis of 35 randomized controlled trials. *J Clin Oncol*. 24, 4808-4817.

[240] Bjerre, L.M., & LeLorier, J. (2001). Do statins cause cancer? A meta-analysis of large randomized clinical trials. *Am J Med*. 110, 716-723.

[241] Shimoyama, S. (2011). Statins and gastric cancer risk. *Hepatogastroenterology*. 58, 1057-1061.

[242] Bonovas, S., Filioussi, K., Flordellis, C.S., & Sitaras, N.M. (2007). Statins and the risk of colorectal cancer: a meta-analysis of 18 studies involving more than 1.5 million patients. *J Clin Oncol*. 25, 3462-3468.

[243] Stein, E.A., Corsini ,A., Gimpelewicz, C.R., Bortolini, M., & Gil, M. (2006). Fluvastatin treatment is not associated with an increased incidence of cancer. *Int J Clin Pract.* 60, 1028-1034.

[244] Baigent, C., Keech, A., Kearney, P.M., Blackwell, L., Buck, G., Pollicino, C., Kirby, A., Sourjina, T., Peto, R., Collins, R., Simes, R., & Cholesterol Treatment Trialists' (CTT) Collaborators. (2005). Efficacy and safety of cholesterol-lowering treatment: prospective meta-analysis of data from 90,056 participants in 14 randomised trials of statins. *Lancet.* 366, 1267-1278.

[245] Bonovas, S., Filioussi, K., & Sitaras, N.M. (2008). Statins are not associated with a reduced risk of pancreatic cancer at the population level, when taken at low doses for managing hypercholesterolemia: evidence from a meta-analysis of 12 studies. *Am J Gastroenterol.* 103, 2646-2651.

[246] Bonovas, S., Filioussi, K., Tsavaris, N., & Sitaras, N.M. (2005). Use of statins and breast cancer: a meta-analysis of seven randomized clinical trials and nine observational studies. *J Clin Oncol.* 23, 8606-8612.

[247] Freeman, S.R., Drake, A.L., Heilig, L.F., Graber, M., McNealy, K., Schilling, L.M., & Dellavalle, R.P. (2006). Statins, fibrates, and melanoma risk: a systematic review and meta-analysis. *J Natl Cancer Inst.* 98, 1538-1246.

[248] Bonovas, S., Filioussi, K., & Sitaras, N.M. (2008). Statin use and the risk of prostate cancer: A metaanalysis of 6 randomized clinical trials and 13 observational studies. *Int J Cancer.* 123, 899-904.

[249] Bonovas, S., Nikolopoulos, G., Filioussi, K., Peponi, E., Bagos ,P., & Sitaras, N.M. (2010). Can statin therapy reduce the risk of melanoma? A meta-analysis of randomized controlled trials. *Eur J Epidemiol.* 25, 29-35.

[250] Dellavalle, R.P., Drake, A., Graber, M., Heilig, L.F., Hester, E.J., Johnson, K.R., McNealy, K., & Schilling, L. (2005). Statins and fibrates for preventing melanoma. *Cochrane Database Syst Rev.* 4, CD003697.

[251] Bonovas, S., Filioussi, K., Tsantes, A., & Sitaras, N.M. (2007). Use of statins and risk of haematological malignancies: a meta-analysis of six randomized clinical trials and eight observational studies. *Br J Clin Pharmacol.* 64, 255-262.

[252] Demierre, M.F., Higgins, P.D., Gruber, S.B., Hawk, E., & Lippman, S.M. (2005). Statins and cancer prevention. *Nat Rev Cancer.* 5, 930-942.

[253] Kato, S., Smalley, S., Sadarangani ,A., Chen-Lin, K., Oliva, B., Brañes, J., Carvajal, J., Gejman, R., Owen, G.I., & Cuello, M. (2010). Lipophilic but not hydrophilic statins selectively induce cell death in gynaecological cancers expressing high levels of HMGCoA reductase. *J Cell Mol Med.* 14, 1180-1193.

[254] Agarwal, B., Bhendwal, S., Halmos, B., Moss, S.F., Ramey, W.G., & Holt, P.R. (1999). Lovastatin augments apoptosis induced by chemotherapeutic agents in colon cancer cells. *Clin Cancer Res.* 5, 2223-2229.

[255] Cho, S.J., Kim, J.S., Kim, J.M., Lee, J.Y., Jung, H.C., & Song, I.S. (2008). Simvastatin induces apoptosis in human colon cancer cells and in tumor xenografts, and attenuates colitis-associated colon cancer in mice. *Int J Cancer.* 123, 951-957.

[256] Narisawa, T., Fukaura, Y., Terada, K., Umezawa, A., Tanida, N., Yazawa, K., & Ishikawa, C. (1994). Prevention of 1,2-dimethylhydrazine-induced colon tumorigenesis by HMG-CoA reductase inhibitors, pravastatin and simvastatin, in ICR mice. *Carcinogenesis.* 15, 2045-2048.

[257] Kaneko, R., Tsuji, N., Asanuma, K., Tanabe, H., Kobayashi, D., & Watanabe, N. (2007). Survivin down-regulation plays a crucial role in 3-hydroxy-3-methylglutaryl coenzyme A reductase inhibitor-induced apoptosis in cancer. *J Biol Chem.* 282, 19273-19281.

[258] Thibault, A., Samid, D., Tompkins, A.C., Figg, W.D., Cooper, M.R., Hohl, R.J., Trepel, J., Liang, B., Patronas, N., Venzon, D.J., Reed, E., & Myers, C.E. (1996). Phase I study of lovastatin, an inhibitor of the mevalonate pathway, in patients with cancer. *Clin Cancer Res.* 2, 483-491.

[259] Knox, J.J., Siu, L.L., Chen, E., Dimitroulakos, J., Kamel-Reid, S., Moore, M.J., Chin, S., Irish, J., LaFramboise, S., & Oza, A.M. (2005). A Phase I trial of prolonged administration of lovastatin in patients with recurrent or metastatic squamous cell carcinoma of the head and neck or of the cervix. *Eur J Cancer.* 41, 523-530.

[260] Larner, J., Jane, J., Laws, E., Packer, R., Myers, C., & Shaffrey, M. (1998). A phase I-II trial of lovastatin for anaplastic astrocytoma and glioblastoma multiforme. *Am J Clin Oncol.* 21, 579-583.

[261] Kim, W.S., Kim, M.M., Choi, H.J., Yoon, S.S., Lee, M.H., Park, K., Park, C.H., & Kang, W.K. (2001). Phase II study of high-dose lovastatin in patients with advanced gastric adenocarcinoma. *Invest New Drugs.* 19, 81-83.

[262] Kawata, S., Yamasaki, E., Nagase, T., Inui, Y., Ito, N., Matsuda, Y., Inada, M., Tamura, S., Noda, S., Imai, Y., & Matsuzawa, Y. (2001). Effect of pravastatin on survival in patients with advanced hepatocellular carcinoma. A randomized controlled trial. *Br J Cancer.* 84, 886-891.

[263] *http://www.ClinicalTrial.gov.* accessed November 2011.

[264] Lersch, C., Schmelz, R., Erdmann, J., Hollweck, R., Schulte-Frohlinde, E., Eckel, F., Nader, M., & Schusdziarra, V. (2004). Treatment of HCC with pravastatin, octreotide, or gemcitabine--a critical evaluation. *Hepatogastroenterology.* 51, 1099-1103.

[265] Shimoyama, S. (2011). Statins are logical candidates for overcoming limitations of targeting therapies on malignancy: their potential application to gastrointestinal cancers. *Cancer Chemother Pharmacol.* 67, 729-739.

[266] Rockwood, K., Kirkland, S., Hogan, D.B., MacKnight, C., Merry, H., Verreault, R., Wolfson, C., & McDowell, I. (2002). Use of lipid-lowering agents, indication bias, and the risk of dementia in community-dwelling elderly people. *Arch Neurol.* 59, 223-227.

[267] Meske, V., Albert, F., Richter, D., Schwarze, J., & Ohm, T.G. (2003). Blockade of HMG-CoA reductase activity causes changes in microtubule-stabilizing protein tau via suppression of geranylgeranylpyrophosphate formation: implications for Alzheimer's disease. *Eur J Neurosci.* 17, 93-102.

In: Statins
Editors: Benedetta La Grua and Alessandro Molinelli
ISBN: 978-1-62081-367-6

Chapter III

Anti-inflammatory Activity of Statins in Asthma and COPD

Kittipong Maneechotesuwan and Adisak Wongkajornsilp
Faculty of Medicine Siriraj Hospital, Mahidol University, Thailand

Abstract

Statins are conventionally known as 3-hydroxy-3-methylglutaryl coenzyme A (HMG-CoA) reductase inhibitors that deplete mevalonic acid. Statins possess pleiotropic effects on the inhibition of multiple inflammatory signals independent of their cholesterol-lowering capacity. Statins suppress mevalonic acid-induced smooth muscle proliferation. In animal studies, statins could inhibit eosinophilic and neutrophilic airway inflammation, a key pathology of asthma and COPD respectively, by modulating a variety of signal transductions. These include the inhibition of guanosine triphosphatase, nuclear factor-κB mediated activation of inflammatory / matrix remodelling pathways, and p38 MAPK mediated eosinophilic inflammation. In addition, statins attenuate airway remodeling, particularly the suppression of airway smooth muscle hyperplasia, and therefore improve airway hyperresponsiveness in asthma. Clinical studies suggested that statins enhance anti-inflammatory effects of corticosteroids on eosinophilic airway inflammation in asthma through the induction of the immunosuppressive indoleamine 2, 3-dioxygenase activity and the release of an anti-inflammatory cytokine, IL-10. Statins also mediate their effective anti-inflammatory effects through the suppression of the mevalonic acid cascade in alveolar macrophages that have emerged as critical modulators in the COPD pathophysiology. This chapter provides the proposed molecular mechanisms underlying the anti-inflammatory / anti-airway remodeling actions and the clinical effectiveness of statins in both asthma and COPD.

Affected Signaling Pathways

Statins have been conventionally known to competitively bind HMG-CoA reductase at nanomolar concentrations. This binding impedes the conversion of HMG-CoA to L-mevalonate, resulting in the reduction of the intermediates of the cholesterol biosynthetic pathway, in particular the 15-carbon farnesyl pyrophosphate (FPP) and the 20-carbon geranylgeranyl pyrophosphate (GGPP). These intermediates not only are precursors for cholesterol synthesis, but also peptide prenylation, a crucial regulator of intracellular signaling.

Peptide prenylation regulates the reorganization of the cytoskeleton, the intracellular membrane trafficking, and the protein-protein interactions. The regulation of the cytoskeletons is mediated by the prenylation of a motif on the carboxy-terminal of over 40 members of the small GTPase family of molecular switch proteins. These include cell-division cycle 42 (CDC42), RAC and RAS homologue (RHO).

These proteins control multiple signaling pathways involving reorganization of cytoskeleton. [1] The intracellular membrane trafficking is also controlled by the prenylation of the members of the RAB family of RAS-related G proteins containing a CC or CXC C-terminal sequence. The inhibition of HMG-CoA reductase by statins depletes the availability of these prenylated proteins.

Statins possess pleiotropic immunomodulatory effects toward diverse immune cells, including T cells, regulatory T cells, B cells, macrophages, dendritic cells (DCs) and endothelial cells. [2]

The immunomodulatory effects of statins are mainly mediated by depleting prenylated proteins that regulate motility, activation, proliferation, transendothelial migration of leukocytes; the antigen uptake, processing and presentation of DCs; the phagocytic function of macrophages; and the endothelial cell function. [1]

Tissue and Cellular Targets

Conventionally Targeted Tissues

Biochemical Intervention

Statins inhibit 3-hydroxy-3-methylglutaryl coenzyme A (HMG-CoA) reductase, the rate-limiting step in hepatic cholesterol synthesis. This results in decreasing synthesis and secretion of lipoproteins from the liver, upregulating LDL receptors on hepatocytes, and increasing clearance of circulating apolipoprotein E- and B-containing lipoproteins. Statins effectively reduce LDL levels and other remnant particles, including very low-density lipoprotein remnants and intermediate-density lipoprotein. [3] Statin therapy effectively lowers plasma concentrations of non-high-density lipoprotein (HDL) cholesterol, including LDL-C. Statins also decrease the underlying biological mechanisms of the atherosclerotic process by their non-LDL-mediated effects.

These include 1) increasing expression of endothelial nitric oxide (NO) synthase, 2) decreasing the production of endothelin-1 and reactive oxygen species, 3) improving the thrombogenic profiles, 4) attenuating inflammation through decreasing the expression of cytokines, chemokines, adhesion molecules, and lowering C-reactive protein (CRP) levels, 5) suppressing macrophage growth and smooth muscle cell (SMC) migration and proliferation.

Endothelium

Lipid-mediated Effects

Endothelial cells benefit from simvastatin mainly through the reduction of LDL-C. LDL-C is a potent inducer of endothelial dysfunction, inflammation, and atherogenesis. The arterial wall was adversely affected by LDL-C through 1) recruiting monocytes and T lymphocytes; 2) expressing growth factors and adhesion molecules; 3) inducing proliferative activity in macrophages and SMCs; 4) attracting complement and CRP that leads to free radical production; and 5) enhancing thrombogenic potential. The etiologic role for cholesterol in atherosclerosis is well established. The large-scale lipid-lowering trials consistently showed the reduction in cardiovascular morbidity and mortality. [4-10]

Non-lipid Mediated Effects

There are two lines of evidence suggesting the role of non-lipid-mediated effects in clinical effects of statins: 1) only a temporal relationship between LDL lowering and clinical benefit after statin initiation; 2) the observed clinical benefit from statins are not sufficiently explained solely by their effect on lipid levels. The clearest evidence of non-lipid-mediated effects of statins came from the prospective clinical trials, especially the Justification for the Use of Statins in Primary Prevention: an Intervention Trial Evaluating Rosuvastatin (JUPITER). [11] This study addressed primary prevention of statin therapy in enrolled 17,802 subjects who had no cardiovascular disease but had LDL levels < 130 mg/dL and hsCRP levels ≥ 2 mg/L. All study participants were randomized to receive treatment with 20 mg rosuvastatin daily or placebo and monitored for vascular events. The JUPITER trial was stopped early due to a 445 reduction in the primary end point of all vascular events, a 54% reduction in myocardial infarction, a 48% reduction in stroke, a 46% reduction in the need for arterial revascularization, and a 20% reduction in all-cause mortality. [11] The protective effect of statins toward cardiovascular system could be independent upon the lipid lowering effect. The non-lipid-mediated effects of statins were demonstrated in a clinical trial. Statins benefited healthy persons with elevated CRP, but no hyperlipidemia by decreasing the incidence of major cardiovascular events. [11]

One of the non-lipid mediated effects of statins is mediated through the upregulation of regulatory pathways of endothelial NO synthase. [12-14] Statins increase the stability of eNOS mRNA, leading to increased eNOS expression possibly by suppressing Rho/ROCK signaling, a negative regulatory pathway for eNOS. [15, 16] Statins activate eNOS phosphorylation by rapidly enhancing the activation of Akt through the upregulation of phosphatidylinositol-3 kinase (PI3K) signaling. [17] In addition, the inhibition of the Rho/ROCK pathway also rapidly enhances the activation of PI3K/Akt pathway resulting in cardioprotection. This indicates that statins upregulate eNOS expression through the cross-talk of these two signaling pathways. [18] Statins can restore eNOS activity in endothelial cells by decreasing the expression of caveolin-1 [19], a membrane protein that binds to eNOS in caveolae. [20] This effect is completely reversed by the addition of mevalonate. [19] The increasing expression of eNOS by statins can be mediated through the modulation of the Lung-Kruppel-like factor (LKLF/KLF2). Statins induce angiogenesis by enhancing the mobilization, proliferation, migration and survival of circulating endothelial progenitor cells

(EPCs). [21-24] Interestingly, this effect is mediated at lower concentrations of statins only, while higher concentrations of statins induce anti-angiogenic effects. [25]

Vascular Smooth Muscle

Statins have been reported to alleviate pathologic conditions of vascular smooth muscle cells (VSMC) in vascular proliferative diseases. Statins can attenuate cytokine-mediated VSMC proliferation in coronary artery disease and in transplant-related arteriopathy. [26, 27] This anti-proliferative effect of statins is mediated through isoprenoid-dependent pathway since 1) the statin-induced G1 cell cycle arrest can be reversed by the addition of mevalonate or GGPP [28] and 2) DNA synthesis in VSMC can be restored by isoprenoid, but not cholesterol. [29] The anti-proliferative effect of statins on VSMC proliferation may be mediated through the inhibition of Rho. [30] Statins inhibit serotonin-induced mitogenesis and migration through the inhibition of GTP-RhoA formation in pulmonary artery smooth muscle cells. [31] These data indicate that the Rho/ROCK pathway mediates SMC proliferation and inhibition of Rho isoprenylation may be the main mechanism by which statins inhibit vascular SMC proliferation.

Cardiac Myocyte

Beneficial effect of statins toward cardiac myocytes has been agreed upon. Cardiac hypertrophy can be mediated by oxidative stress molecules including Rac1. Rac1, a critical component for NADPH oxidase activity, can be inhibited by statins through the inhibition of Rac1 geranylgeranylation. Statins have protective action against ischemic myocardial injury [32, 33] as demonstrated by the studies in normocholesterolemic and hypercholesterolemic animal models. [34, 35] The mechanism responsible for myocardial protection is the replenishment of NO, resulting in vasodilation and increasing regional myocardial blood flow under hypoxic conditions. [36, 37]

Cardiovascular System

Beneficial effects of statins have been well established. In animal models with experimental pulmonary arterial hypertension (PAH), statins improved mean pulmonary arterial pressure [38-42], right ventricular pressure [43] and hypertrophy [40, 41, 44], pulmonary vascular remodeling (neointimal formation) [44], endothelial dysfunction, oxidative stress and inflammation. Statins improved muscularization and medial thickening [38, 39, 42] by suppressing the proliferation and enhancing apoptosis of smooth muscle cells, endothelial cells [40, 44] and adventitial fibroblasts. [45] Oxidative stress also was lessened by statin-induced upregulation of endothelial nitric oxide synthase [44, 46, 47] and the decrease in reactive oxygen species production. [41] The peribronchial and perivascular inflammation was suppressed by statin-downregulated inflammatory gene expression (i.e. Fos, Jun and TNF-α). [46, 47] Statins can attenuate the binding of serotonin to its receptors [48] and the serotonin-induced contractions of coronary arteries. [49] This raises the possibility that statins may reverse serotonin-induced pulmonary arterial contractions. However, the distribution of serotonin receptors in the pulmonary circulation differs from those of other arterial beds [50] that might not yield the predicted outcome. In contrast to experimental studies, human studies are limited. Simvastatin at 20-80 mg/day improved the 6-min walk test, cardiac output and right ventricular systolic pressures with slow rate of disease progression. [51] The 6-month RCT called SiPHT (Simvastatin as a Treatment for Pulmonary hypertension Trial) demonstrated that simvastatin (80 mg/day) in addition to standard treatment with sildenafil and/or endothelin-1 antagonist significantly reduced right ventricular mass, whereas it was increased in the placebo group. [52] However, there were no significant changes in 6-min walk test, cardiac output, plasma nitric oxide metabolites or cytokines. The effect of pravastatin on the improvement of PAH and exercise capacity was also studied in a RCT. Pravastatin (40 mg/day) could significantly increase exercise time and reduced systolic pulmonary arterial pressure in COPD patients with PAH. [53]

Airway Epithelial Cells

Airway epithelial cell is the primary afflicted site in asthma and plays a central role in airway inflammation. [54, 55] A compromise in epithelial barrier makes the airway susceptible to virus infection in children. [55] The viral invasion primes immature dendritic cells toward a T_H2 maturation with local allergen sensitization. [55] The barrier impairment of airway epithelium lessens its antioxidant capacity, leading to the unusual susceptibility to oxidative stress. The ongoing malfunction includes aberrant innate immune response in ozone and endotoxin-induced allergic airway disease and pollutant-induced asthma exacerbation. [56, 57]

The lessening nitric oxide (NO) production, primarily resulting from nitric oxide synthase (NOS) 2 inhibition, plays a role in certain airway diseases (i.e. cystic fibrosis and diffuse panbronchiolitis). NOS2 is regulated by a wide variety of signal transduction pathways in airway epithelial cells. The Rho GTPase cascade is one of the signaling pathways necessary for balancing inflammatory response and NO production. Rho signaling suppresses NO production through the inhibition at NOS2 promoter, possibly as a feedback mechanism. Since the activation of Rho requires posttranslational prenylation, the inhibition of HMG-CoA reductase recovers NOS2 promoter activity and expression. [58] However, an earlier study indicated that mevastatin-induced NOS2 promoter activity is dependent of neither the Rho GTPase pathway nor the activation of NF-κB / AP-1. [58] This is evidenced through the inhibition of ROCK, a downstream effector of the Rho GTPase pathway, by Y-27632. The ROCK inhibition resulted in the suppression of NF-κB and AP-1-dependent NOS2 promoter with a paradoxical increase in NOS2 mRNA and protein. Therefore ROCK is another key regulator in balancing NO production in response to inflammatory stimuli. The limitation of NO production may lead to the overzealous production of reactive oxygen species with subsequent airway damage.

Airway Smooth Muscle (ASM)

Statin can lessen the contribution of ASM cells to airway remodeling. These include the suppression of extracellular matrix (ECM) protein synthesis and secretion from human airway smooth muscles [59]; autophagy and apoptosis of human airway smooth muscles and fibroblast through the inhibition of mevalonate cascade [60]; inhibition of Rho A, a critical inducer for the proliferation of human airway smooth muscle. [61] All aforementioned mechanisms lead to the alleviation of ASM hyperplasia, attenuation of airway remodeling and airway hyperresponsiveness in asthma. This possibly explains the observation of lessening airway hyperactivity in the mice model of asthma. [62]

Airway Remodeling

Statins could inhibit TGF-β-induced airway remodeling in a mouse model of allergic asthma by suppressing TGF-β signaling. [63, 64] The induction of WNT/β-catenin pathway expression and activation in pulmonary fibroblasts by TGF-β is required for ECM production and myofibroblasts differentiation in COPD. [65] However, the clinical study of simvastatin showed the reversal of smoke-induced pulmonary hypertension and the prevention of emphysema, but no effect on airway remodeling. [66]

Platelet

Hypercholesterolemia is associated with increasing platelet reactivity. [67] Statins could decrease platelet reactivity through both cholesterol-dependent and independent mechanisms. A cholesterol-independent mechanism involves the statin-upregulated eNOS expression in platelets, resulting in decreasing platelet activation. [68] This effect was demonstrated for atorvastatin in an animal model [68] and fluvastatin in a clinical study with hypercholesterolemia. [69] In addition, statins inhibit tissue factor expression in macrophages and thereby reducing the thrombotic potential of the vascular wall. [70]

Immunomodulatory Activity, an Unanticipated Action of Statins

Evidences of Immunological Action

Statins can reduce the transendothelial migration of neutrophils [71], the reactive oxygen species production [72], the release of neutrophil chemoattractants and proteases from activated epithelial cells. [73] Statins also dampen innate immune response by suppressing TLR2 and TLR4 expression [74] and MHC class II molecules [75] on monocytes, and impeding the maturation of dendritic cells. [75] In addition, statins induce the unfolded protein response (UPR) in macrophages [76], leading to the inhibition of innate immunity and protection against excessive inflammatory responses. [77, 78] Interestingly, statins suppress the activation of IFN regulatory factor 7, a key transcription factor for type I IFN expression in plasmacytoid DCs through the inhibition of Rho generylgenerylation. [79]

Statins Regulate Both Innate and Adaptive Immune Responses

The inflammatory response in atherosclerosis involves both innate and adaptive immunity. In human, hyperlipidemia actively recruits proinflammatory monocytes that express P-selectin glycoprotein ligand. [80] These proinflammatory monocytes provoke the innate immune response through the release of proinflammatory cytokines and other mediators including matrix metalloproteases. [81] Lipoproteins have been associated with innate immune response. The binding of oxidized LDL to scavenger receptors can induce proinflammatory signals in endothelial cells. [81] Likewise, apolipoprotein CIII (a component of certain triglyceride-rich lipoproteins) initiates inflammation through the binding with an innate immune cell receptor, TLR2. [82] The innate immunity-inducing inflammatory signals in atherosclerosis produce considerable crosstalk with thrombotic pathways that put atherosclerotic patients at high thrombotic risk. [83] In reverse, thrombin can induce the expression of proinflammatory cytokines from vascular endothelial and smooth muscle cells. In addition, activated platelets can shed the potent proinflammatory stimulus CD40-ligand (CD154) and release preformed proinflammatory mediators including the myeloid-related protein (MRP)-8/14. MRP-8/14 serves as a biomarker for adverse cardiovascular events in survivors of acute coronary syndromes. [84, 85] MRP-8/14 exerts its inflammatory actions by activating innate immune response through the binding to TLR4. [86] MRP-8/14 can also promote endothelial cell apoptosis, a molecular mechanism involved in plaque thrombosis. [87]

Innate Immune Response

Statins Reduced Leukocyte-endothelial Adhesion

Statins reduced leukocyte adhesion, attenuated macromolecular leak and restored endothelial-dependent NO-mediated relaxation in the rat mesentery during sepsis. [88] Pravastatin, simvastatin, and atorvastatin suppressed neutrophil transendothelial migration toward the chemoattractant fMLP. This effect depended on the ability of statins to reduce fMLP-induced Rho activity in neutrophils, but not the induction of neutrophil adhesion or adhesion molecule expression. This action was substantiated by the reversal of the statin-mediated reduction in neutrophil transendothelial migration after the addition of Rho precursor geranylgeranyl pyrophosphate. In addition, statins could suppress histamine-induced tethering interactions and TNF-α-stimulated rolling of neutrophils on endothelial cells that was consistent with the downregulation of P-selectin and E-selectin, respectively. This action of statins was mediated through mevalonate blockade since the pre-treatment of endothelial cells with mevalonate dramatically reversed both tethering and rolling actions of statins.

Increased Endoplasmic Reticulum Stress/Unfolded Protein Response

Macrophage apoptosis can be induced by the stress to the endoplasmic reticulum (ER) as reflected by the accumulation of unfolded protein response (UPR). The UPR is considered as a cytoprotective and survival mechanism. The UPR is regulated by three ER intermembrane transducers: PKR-like ER kinase (PERK), inositol requiring 1 (IRE1), and activating transcription factor 6 (ATF6). The activation of the UPR leads to the triggering of several molecular events: 1) IRE1-mediated expression of X box protein-1 (XBP1) transcription factor; 2) PERK-induced ATF4-activated transcription of CHOP (CCAAT/enhancer binding protein-homologous protein), an apoptotic mediator under ER stress; 3) the ATF6 cleavage-induced nuclear translocation of cytosolic domain of ATF6 to activate the UPR genes. ER stress and CHOP expression can be induced by trafficking of free cholesterol to the ER, that eventually lead to macrophage apoptosis. Statins can regulate sensor proteins of the UPR by enhancing ATF6 and XBP1 activation without affecting CHOP and ATF4 expression, by inducing the expression of the GRP78 (78kDa glucose-regulated protein) stress protein.

Statins Decreased Type I IFN Production in Plasmacytoid DCs (pDCs)

Statins were shown to heavily suppress IFN-α production in human pDCs. [79] The suppression of IFN-α production is mediated through the inactivation of geranylgeranylated Rho since 1) the suppression could be was reversed by geranylgeranyl pyrophosphate and 2) the suppression was intensified by either geranylgeranyl transferase inhibitor or Rho kinase inhibitor. In addition to the inactivation of geranylgeranylated Rho, statins also suppressed the expression of phosphorylated p38 MAPK, PI 3-kinase/Akt, and nuclear translocation of IRF-7 that otherwise transduce the intracellular signal toward type I IFN synthesis in pDCs.

Statins Promote the Resolution of Inflammation through the Production of 15-epi-lipoxins that Might Alleviate Severe Asthma

Statins have been reported to induce the production of 15-epi-lipoxins. [89-91] The 15-epi-lipoxins have been proposed as mediators for anti-inflammatory action of ASA. Lipoxins are eicosanoids generated from arachidonic acid (AA) via lipoxygenase. Lipoxins comprise 2 distinct isomers, lipoxin (LX)A_4 and LXB_4. The biosynthesis of lipoxins is initiated by the conversion of AA to 15- hypdroxyeicosatetraenoic acid (HETE) during cell-cell interactions (e.g. epithelial cell-leukocyte, leukocyte-leukocyte) [92] or platelet-leukocyte interactions. Lipoxygenase-initiated lipoxin biosynthesis also involves cyclooxygenase-2 (COX-2). The acetylation of COX-2 by ASA hampered the production of PGH_2 but not the production of 15R-HETE from arachidonate. This intermediate is therefore readily transformed to epimeric lipoxins (15-epi-lipoxins). [93] The 15-epi-lipoxin biosynthesis can also be initiated by cytochrome P450 in the absence of ASA. [94]

LXA_4 and 15-epi-LXA_4 play a protective role against allergic inflammation in asthma. LXA_4 mediates its anti-inflammatory action through the interaction with its specific receptors (lipoxin A_4 receptor, ALX) on both leukocytes [95] and airway epithelial cells. [96] LXA_4 and 15-epi-LXA_4 suppress both airway hyperresponsiveness and eosinophilic airway inflammation [97, 98] with dwindling levels of IL-5, IL-13, eotaxin, IgE prostanoids and CysLTs. [99] The decrease in lipoxin production with downregulation of lipoxin biosynthetic enzymes and LXA_4 receptors in bronchial biopsy are associated with severe asthma. [100] The basal LXA_4 biosynthesis in alveolar macrophages from severe asthma was decreased and impaired upon LPS stimulation. [101] The low urinary concentrations of 15-epi-LXA_4 in patients with aspirin-intolerant asthma implicated the suppression of lipoxin biosynthesis. [102] In contrast, the increasing 15-epi-LXA_4 production through the interaction of leukocytes and airway epithelial cells after lovastatin administration attenuates mucosal inflammation. [89] Statins might improve the resolution of airway inflammation in severe asthmatics possessing low 15-epi- LXA_4. However more data are needed to bolster this paradigm.

Statins Exert its Anti-inflammatory Effects on Pulmonary and Systemic Inflammation in COPD

Statins inhibit key inflammatory and remodeling pathways in COPD through their pleiotropic pharmacologic actions: [103] 1) suppressing the production of TNF-α, IL-6, IL-8 with decreasing neutrophil infiltration into the lungs; 2) alleviating small airway fibrosis and irreversible airflow obstruction; 3) exerting antioxidant and anti-inflammatory effects on skeletal muscle; 4) attenuating inflammatory response to pulmonary infection; 5) interfering the development of epithelial-mesenchymal transition, an initiating process to lung cancer.

Adaptive Immune Response

Statins Perturb the Balance of T Cell Subsets (T_H1, T_H2, T_H0, Treg and T_H17)

The statin-mediated disease alleviation could be mediated through the shift in the balance of T cell subsets. Statins prevent the development and progression of experimental T_H1-cell mediated autoimmune disease. [1] Statin administered after the onset of the acute phase of chronic-relapsing model of multiple sclerosis (i.e. EAE) could reverse the disease [104] while the administration during disease remission could prevent the relapse. [104-106] The treatment for EAE with atorvastatin suppressed T cell proliferation with a concomitant shift in T cell cytokine profiles. The profiles shifted toward T_H2 cytokines (IL-4, IL-5 and IL-10) possibly through the phosphorylation of signal transducer and activator of transcription 6 (STAT6) that induced IL-4-dependent T_H2 differentiation. [104] The phosphorylation of STAT4 and IL-12-dependent T_H1 differentiation was suppressed with diminishing secretion of IL-2, IL-12, TNF and IFN-γ [104]. The suppression of T_H1 cytokines resulted from statins-induced upregulation of T_H2 transcription factor GATA-3 and downregulation of NF-κB and T-bet (T-box transcription factor). [107] The ability of statins to shift T cell phenotype from T_H1 to T_H2 has also been documented in an experimental autoimmune myocarditis. [108] However, not all studies have demonstrated a statin-induced bias towards T_H2 cytokine profile. In experimental autoimmune uveitis, lovastatin, but not atorvastatin, attenuated the disease and inhibited IFN-γ production with trivial effect on T_H2 cytokine production. [109, 110] High dose simvastatin suppressed collagen-specific T_H1 humoral and cellular immune responses in an animal model of collagen-induced arthritis with no upregulation of T_H2 cytokine production. [111] Simvastatin, lovastatin and mevastatin failed to stimulate either a T_H1 or T_H2 bias in PBMCs from patients with multiple sclerosis, but the IFN-γ and IL-12 productions were increased. [112] This observation was recited with $CD3^+$ T cells from simvastatin–treated multiple sclerosis possessing clinical improvement without cytokine alteration. [113] Despite these discrepancies, the most robust observation is the beneficial suppression of the T_H1 immune response by statins. The precise mechanisms underlying the shift on the T_H1/T_H2 balance remain to be dissected. Either mevalonate or its metabolites might promote T_H1 differentiation since mevalonate could reverse atorvastatin-mediated T_H2 differentiation. [104] In addition, the specific isoprenoid intermediates modulate T_H2 differentiation through differential farnesylation and prenylation of RAS and RHO. [114] In contrast, statins suppress T_H2 cytokine production in a murine model of allergic asthma [115, 116] through the inhibition of NF-κB and p38 MAPK [117] that controls GATA-3 nuclear import for the activation of T_H2 cytokine expression. [118]

Simvastatin could suppress T_H17 cell differentiation and the release of IL-17A, IL-17F, IL-21 and IL-22 from $CD4^+$ T cells of multiple sclerosis through the down-regulation of IFN regulatory factor 4. [119] Pravastatin also attenuated allergic airway inflammation through the suppression of IL-17 production. [115]

Polarization toward Regulatory T Cells

Regulatory T cells (Tregs) are $CD4^+$ T cells that possess suppressive activity toward other effector T helper cells (e.g., T_H1, T_H2 and T_H17). They can develop in native immune system (naturally occurring Tregs) or in response to antigenic exposure (adaptive Tregs). [120] Tregs are characterized by the high constitutive expression of surface CD25 [121] and forkhead-winged helix family protein of transcription regulators (Foxp3). Tregs do not proliferate when stimulated with antigen *in vitro*, but actively suppress proliferation and cytokine production from other T cells. The high expression of Foxp3 contributed to the suppressive activity of Tregs since the removal of Foxp3 reversed the suppressive activity in Tregs while the transfer of Foxp3 to other effector T cells gave rise to the suppressive activity. [122-125] The suppressive mechanisms of Tregs are mediated through the action of released cytokines (e.g. IL-10 and TGF-β), surface molecules (e.g. CTLA4, PD-1 and BTLA). [121, 126] Tregs can reduce the ability of antigen presenting cells such as DCs to activate effector T cell response through the downregulation of the co-stimulatory molecules (i.e. CD80 and CD86) [127]. Tregs also compete with naïve T cells for the access to DCs.

The differentiation of Tregs is induced by a variety of immunosuppressive cytokines and enzymes such as TGF-β and IL-10, indoleamine 2, 3-dioxygenase. [128] The fetus is persistently exposed to non-inherited maternal antigens that pass through placenta and induce the development of Tregs in the fetal lymph nodes. Tregs constitute a high percentage of total lymphocytes in the fetal lymph nodes. This pool of Tregs prevents fetal immune responses against maternal antigens. During or after pregnancy, the transfer of antigen and TGF-β across placenta or via breast milk induces antigen-specific Tregs [129, 130] whose generation depends on a functional TGF-β receptor. [129, 131] The induced allergen-specific Tregs in early life may warrant subsequent asthma-free life. [131] Foxp3 is the master transcription factor mediating immunosuppressive function of Tregs. [122, 123] TGF-β induces Foxp3 expression in Tregs by activating the enhancer and the promoter regions of Foxp3. These actions involve histone acetylation and demethylation of the Foxp3 gene. [132, 133] Simvastatin can induce Foxp3 expressing inducible Tregs (iTregs) by itself and synergistically with low concentrations of TGF-β to convert $Foxp3^-$ to $Foxp3^+$T cells. [134] The synergistic effects of simvastatin on the induction of Foxp3 expression are mediated primarily through the blockade of protein geranylgeranylation. [134] In addition, the synergistic action of simvastatin on TGF-β-mediated induction of Foxp3 may be mediated by methylation of the Foxp3 promoter. One of the primary mechanisms underlying the synergistic effects of simvastatin on TGF-β-mediated induction of Foxp3 is the blockade of the negative regulatory Smad (Smad6/7) toward TGF-β signaling. [134]

Tregs might bring beneficial role in suppressing pathogenic T_H2 cells in patients with allergic disease. Allergic conditions usually contain defective Tregs through their pathophysiological ontology. The number of $CD4^+CD25^+$ T cells and the levels of Foxp3 mRNA in bronchoalveolar lavage fluid (BAL) from asthmatic children were lower than those from healthy controls. [135] Isolated $CD4^+CD25^+$ T cells from asthmatics possess low suppressive activity to effector T cell proliferation and cytokine production. In contrast, the number of $CD4^+CD25^+$ T cells and the levels of Foxp3 mRNA in BAL were reversed after the treatment with inhaled corticosteroids. [135] The addition of a statin to corticosteroid further improved the numbers and function of Tregs.

Up-regulation of KLF2 in T Cells

The transcription factor Kruppel-like factor 2 (KLF2) plays several roles in the regulation of T cell function. These include the inhibition of T cell proliferation, the modulation of the expression of molecules that both control naïve T-cell recirculation and maintain T cell quiescence. [2] Ectopic expression of the KLF2 gene in the actively proliferative Jurkat, a human T cell line, resulted in decreasing mitotic activity. [136, 137] KLF2-deficient mouse T cells became hyper-proliferative. [136, 137] KLF2 transcript is expressed in naïve and memory T cells and is rapidly downregulated following TCR stimulation. [138, 139] KLF2 also promotes the very early stages of T cell activation where its expression is transiently upregulated in Jurkat cells to activate IL-2 promoter. [140] In mouse $CD8^+$ T cells, the expression of KLF2 is required for the transition from effector to memory stages. [139] KLF2 deficiency leads to the downregulation of sphingosine-1-phosphate (S1P) receptor 1 and the subsequent defect in SIP-mediated egress of T cells from the thymus and peripheral lymphoid organs. KLF2 drives naïve T cell migration into lymph nodes through CD62L. The suppression of KLF2 and S1P (1) drove T_H2 egress from lymph node resulting from the action of extracellular matrix protein-1 (ECM1). [141] This egress might explain the association of KLF2 with asthma. Taken together, KLF2 modulates normal peripheral T cell recirculation but the effect on T cell function remains unclear. Statins could upregulate KLF2 expression in effector T cells in a mevalonate-dependent manner, that in turn inhibited T cell proliferation and IFN-γ expression. [142] The relationship of statins with KLF2 to suppress T_H2 egress from lymph nodes in asthma has yet been established. The possible mechanism might be the inhibition of the mammalian target of rapamycin complex 1 (MTORC1), a well-known inhibitor of KLF2 expression in activated T cells, by statins. [143] This hypothesis was formulated based on the observation that statins-inhibited activation of Ras homolog enriched in brain (Rheb) could suppress MTORC1 activation in vascular smooth muscle cells. [144] However, the possibility that the inhibition of MTORC1 by statins is mediated through the inhibition of Rheb has yet been investigated.

Suppression of T Cell Cytotoxic Activity

The development of allergic eosinophilic airway disease is controlled by NK cells. [145] Simvastatin could suppress the cytotoxicity of natural killer cells isolated from patients with cardiovascular disease that could alleviate atherosclerosis. [146] Pravastatin and cyclosporine could synergistically reduce NK cell cytotoxicity in heart transplant recipients leading to the reduction in solid organ graft rejection in both acute and chronic stages. [147, 148] The suppressive effects of statins on T cell cytotoxicity encompassed other cell types such as Jurkat cells. [149] Atorvastatin also inhibited cytotoxic activity of phorbol ester/ionomycin-activated Jurkat cells with Fas ligand (FasL) sensitivity. [149] In addition, atorvastatin or simvastatin antagonized the upregulation of FasL expression in activated Jurkat cells involving RhoA and is mediated through mevalonate and geranylgeranylpyrophosphate. A suppression of sterol synthesis greater than 90% by statins in NK cells was required to observe the inhibition of NK cell cytotoxicity. This effect could be achieved with a minimal concentration of simvastatin or simvastatin sodium salt of 2 μM. [150] This suppression was similar to those observed with theophylline at therapeutic level. [151] The suppression of NK cells may benefit both asthma and COPD. The enhancement of NK cell activity was observed in patients with asthma [152-154] and COPD. [155, 156] This implied that the suppression of the MHC-unrestricted cytotoxicity (i.e. NK cell activity) by statins might alleviate airway inflammation in asthma and COPD.

Decreasing Antigen Presenting Function of DCs

The prerequisite for antigen presentation by DCs involves endocytosis of antigen, internal processing, and presentation by MHC class II molecules on the cell surface. [1] The antigen presentation is controlled in part by the remodeling of the cytoskeleton and the action of small GTPases. [1] Decreasing small GTPases activity may lead to the modification of the actin cytoskeleton. [1] The constitutively active CDC42 and RHO enhance the antigen presentation function of DCs to T cells due to the maintenance of endocytosis through the activation of RAC and CDC42. [1, 157] CDC42 and RAC contribute to the formation of the T-cell receptor complex as it binds to the MHC class II complex, whereas CDC42, RAS, RHO and RAC1 are all involved in cell-cycle progression and proliferation. [1] Statin-mediated inhibition of antigen-induced T-cell proliferation is mediated through the negative regulation of cell-cycle progression and the inhibition of GTPases-mediated cell proliferation. [105] Lovastatin, simvastatin and mevastatin could inhibit the proliferation of peripheral blood mononuclear cells (PBMCs) in a dose-dependent manner. [112] Statins also interfered the expression of MHC class II by disrupting the integrity of cell-membrane lipid rafts, the important microdomains for the assembly of signaling complexes, leading to a loss of association of MHC class II molecules. [158]

Other Immunological Targets in Asthma and COPD

Eosinophils

Statins suppress airway eosinophilia in a mouse model of asthma. [62, 117] Simvastatin (40 mg/kg) attenuated airway eosinophil influx by 67% in mice and this effect was reversed by the addition of mevalonate. [62] The suppressive effects of statins on eosinophilic influx were mediated through the downregulation of VCAM-1 and the inhibition of IL-5. [117] There has yet been any study that investigates the direct effects of statins on eosinophil functions.

Macrophages

Since macrophages have been known to play critical roles in innate and adaptive immune responses, they are postulated to commence the development of inflammatory airway diseases such as asthma and COPD. Macrophages are conspicuously activated as classically (M1) and alternatively (M2) macrophages consecutively during asthmatic response in the alveolar tissue of asthmatic lungs. [159] M2 subset is activated by IL-4 and IL-13 whereas M1 subset is driven by interferon-γ. [160] The localizations of macrophages determine their fates of polarization. Macrophages localized in the lung interstitium (immunoregulatory macrophages) with less exposure to airway stimuli are less prone to polarization towards either M1 or M2 phenotype as these cells predominantly express IL-10 with immunoregulatory activity. [159] The manifestation of asthma might depend upon the balance between M1, M2 and immunoregulatory macrophages in the lungs. [159] Alternatively-activated macrophages (AAM) are a major source of IL-13 that induces mucus production and airway hyperresponsiveness in asthma. [160] The M2 subtype could be induced by respiratory viruses. Sendai virus could induce the M2 polarization in mice as characterized by the enhancing expression of chitinase-like proteins *(Chi3l3/4),* resistin-like molecules *(Rtnla or Fizz1)*, arginase 1 (*Arg1*), matrix metalloproteinases (*Mmp12*), and arachidonate 12-lipoxygenase (*Alox12e*). [161] The expression of Chi3l3/4 proteins is principally restricted to $CD68^+$ macrophages. [161] The expression of a chitinase-like protein is anticipated in human since YKL-40, also a chitinase-like protein, plays a critical role in the development and progression of allergic inflammation and airway remodeling. The serum and airway levels of YKL-40 were correlated with the severity of asthma. [162] The chitin secreted from AAM is critical for the subsequent inflammatory response [163] and wound healing. [164] Chitin directly activates macrophage to express TNF-α and IL-17 via TLR-2 and MyD-88-dependent but TLR-4-independent pathways. [165] Chitin can interact with macrophages via mannose receptors, TLR2 [165, 166] and C-type lectin receptor dectin-1. The expression of pro-inflammatory mediators such as LTB_4 [163] by macrophages after the stimulation with chitin recruits eosinophils and other innate immune cells secreting type II cytokines. Simvastatin attenuated allergic immune response with decreasing alveolar macrophages infiltration in the lungs of ovalbumin-challenged mice through the suppression of small G proteins/MAP kinases/NF-κB. [117] Atorvastatin suppressed pro-inflammatory (M1) macrophage infiltration while augmented anti-inflammatory (M2) macrophages with accompanying M2 chemokines and cytokines. [167]

The immunomodulating factors secreted from alveolar macrophages include prostaglandin E_2 (PGE_2), IL-10 and TGF-β. PGE_2 enhances IL-10 expression and release from peripheral blood T cells. IL-10 and TGF-β suppress the secretion of pro-inflammatory cytokines and T cell proliferation. These immunomodulatory cytokines decrease the apoptosis of alveolar macrophages and therefore enhance macrophage-mediated inhibition of T cell proliferation. Statins heighten the immunoregulatory activity of macrophages. Simvastatin enhanced the upregulatory effects of corticosteroids on IL-10 expression and release from alveolar macrophages. [168] Statins also potentiate corticosteroids on the upregulation of the immunosuppressive indoleamine 2, 3-dioxygenase (IDO) by increasing GITRL-activated and type I IFN-mediated IDO expression. [168] IDO, mainly expressed in antigen presenting cells (macrophages and dendritic cells), could inhibit T and natural killer cell proliferation, [128, 169-171] but upregulate regulatory T cells. [128] In addition, IDO could prevent the development of T_H2-mediated eosinophilic airway inflammation in animal model of asthma [172] and reduce sputum eosinophils in human asthma. [173]

Neutrophils

Statins reduce the expression of chemokines (e.g., CXCL8 and CCL2, and MMPs especially MMP-9) that has been upregulated in COPD. [174] Statins also suppress the expression of adhesion molecules (e.g., inter-cellular adhesion molecule 1, vascular cell adhesion molecule 1 and E-selectin) involving the recruitment of inflammatory cells (neutrophils, monocytes and lymphocytes) from the circulation into the lungs. Statins activate the uptake of apoptotic neutrophils by alveolar macrophages through efferocytosis. This effect is mediated through the inhibition of the prenylation and the suppression of RhoA activation, the known suppressors in the phagocytosis of apoptotic cells. [175] Therefore statins may accelerate the resolution of neutrophilic inflammation in COPD since the impairment of phagocytosis is well-established in COPD. [176] In mice, statins can inhibit

T_H17 cells through the suppression of retinoic acid-related orphan receptor γt. [177] T_H17 cells orchestrate neutrophilic inflammation in mice COPD through the release of IL-17 that triggers epithelial cells to release CXCL1 and CXCL18. [178] Taken together, statins may alleviate COPD through the control of neutrophilic airway inflammation.

Molecular Targets

Mevalonate Pathway

Immunomodulation of statins is mediated through the inhibition of L-mevalonate pathway that results in the depletion of farnesylated and geranylgeranylated downstream proteins. [179] Geranylgeranyl-PP attachment to small G-proteins including Rho, allows the adhesion and intracellular trafficking of membrane-associated signaling proteins, [180, 181] and involves in post-translational prenylation of cell signaling proteins. [1] For instance, the blockade of mevalonate pathway in T cells diminishes the prenylation to GTPases, Ras, Rho-B and Rap-1. These proteins become inactive and could not translocate to the T cell membrane. This retards the activation and proliferation of T cells, resulting in the inhibition of T_H1 cytokine production. [179]

Mevalonate-regulated Cell Signaling

NF-κB Signaling

Statins (atorvastatin and lovastatin) can suppress proinflammatory cytokine and chemokine expression in mononuclear cells and smooth muscle cells through the inhibition of the classical nuclear factor kappa B (NF-κB) signaling pathway. [182] NF-κB mediates signaling events in several cell types underlying airway inflammation in stable and exacerbation phases of both asthma and COPD. [183] NF-κB regulates proinflammatory molecules (adhesion molecules, enzymes, cytokines and chemokines), cell adhesion, differentiation, proliferation and apoptosis. [184] Activators of NF-κB include inflammatory stimuli, such as IL-1β and TNF-α. Upon stimulation, NF-κB translocates into the nucleus where it induces inflammatory genes. [185] Increased NF-κB activity has been identified in alveolar macrophages and airway epithelial cells from asthmatic patients. [186]

The activation of NF-κB in airway epithelium with allergen or viral infection results in asthma exacerbations through the induction of inducible nitric oxide synthase [187], ICAM-1 [188], IL-8 [189, 190] and IL-11. [191-193] Corticosteroids effectively suppress classical NF-κB activation in asthmatics [185] but less in COPD. [194] The effectiveness of statins to inhaled corticosteroid treatment for COPD patients to suppress NF-κB activity and subsequent downregulation of airway inflammation requires further study. However, statins enhance the effect of corticosteroids to induce the non-canonical NF-κB-induced IDO expression in mild asthmatics, resulting in the suppression of eosinophilic airway inflammation. [168]

p38 MAPK Signaling

Statins can suppress the hypoxic-induced fibroblast proliferation through the inhibition of p38 MAPK activation in pulmonary artery fibroblasts. [45] The activation of p38 MAPK signaling is involved in inflammatory response to oxidative stress, endotoxin and cigarette smoking exposure. The p38 MAPK drives allergen-induced airway eosinophilia, mucus hypersecretion, and airway hyperresponsiveness by inhibiting eosinophil apoptosis and promoting production of cytokines and chemokines from airway smooth muscle. [195] The activation of p38 MAPK in alveolar macrophages and airway epithelial cells may contribute to corticosteroid insensitivity of severe asthma and COPD. Therefore, statins might reverse refractory airway inflammation in severe asthmatics and COPD patients after the treatment with corticosteroids.

Smad6/7

Statins enhance TGF-β signaling through the suppression of the inhibitory Smad (Smad 6 and Smad 7). [134] This disinhibition resulted in the induction of $Foxp3^+$ T regulatory cells that may aid in the control of T_H2-mediated airway inflammation in asthma. In contrast, statins may ignite the progression of peribronchial fibrosis of COPD since TGF-β signaling could induce airway fibrosis. The exposure to cigarette smoke further down-regulates Smad6/7 [196] that could exacerbate the disability. However, this postulation may not be implicated in the clinical manifestation of COPD since statins already impede the decline in lung function. [197, 198]

PI3K/Akt

Statins inhibited cigarette smoking-induced pulmonary emphysema in mice model [47] through several mechanisms. In alveolar macrophages, PI3K/Akt induces MMP-9 that damages surrounding matrices during the development of emphysema in COPD. Statins can suppress cigarette smoke extract (CSE)-mediated MMP-9 induction in alveolar macrophages through the suppression of CSE-induced phosphorylation of PI3K and Akt. [199] Statins can also provide other beneficial actions. They promote alveolar epithelial cell proliferation and reverse elastase-induced pulmonary emphysema. [200] However, the beneficial effect of statins in pulmonary emphysema requires further clinical trials.

Indoleamine 2, 3-dioxygenase

Statins heightened the upregulatory effects of inhaled corticosteroids (ICS) on the expression and activity of indoleamine 2, 3-dioxygenase (IDO) through the induction of glucocorticoid- inducible tumor necrosis factor receptor related ligand (GITRL)-activated noncanonical nuclear factor-κB and IL-10 release. [168] This effect of statins resulted in the enhancement of anti-inflammatory effects of ICS on eosinophilic airway inflammation in asthmatics. [168] However, it remains unknown whether this effect of statins is mevalonate-dependent.

Asymmetric Dimethyl-arginine and Inducible Nitric Oxide Synthase

Simvastatin can suppress airway inflammation, airway hyperrespon-siveness and airway remodeling in OVA-sensitized mice. [201] The restoring effects of simvastatin on epithelial dysfunction and airway hyperrespon-siveness are mediated through the suppression of asymmetrical dimethyl-arginine (ADMA) and inducible nitric oxide synthase (NOS), but the enhancement of endothelial NOS. [201] This resulted in the dwindling of NOS – ADMA complex that in turn prevented airway epithelial cell injury through the suppression of oxo-nitrosative stress. [201] Alteration in arginine metabolism underlies the link between asthma and metabolic syndrome. [202] From this perspective point of view, statins may restore the altered L-arginine metabolism in metabolic syndrome-risked asthma.

Clinical Efficacy of Statins in Asthma and COPD

Asthma

Statins could not be used as a single therapy for asthma due to their inadequate anti-inflammatory effects. A randomized double-blind placebo control study [203] investigated certain anti-inflammatory activity of simvastatin (20 mg/d for 2 weeks, then 40 mg/d for 2 weeks). These parameters included exhaled tidal nitric oxide, sputum eosinophils, methacholine hyperresponsiveness, saliva eosinophilic cationic protein and C-reactive protein. They observed the decrease in exhaled nitric oxide and some improvement of methacholine hyperresponsiveness albeit statistically insignificant. There was no significant alteration in other inflammatory markers.

The addition of statins to inhaled corticosteroids did not provide short-term improvement in asthma control but decreased sputum macrophages and sputum leukotriene B_4. A double-blinded randomized controlled crossover study [204] demonstrated that there were no clinically important improvements in clinical indices of asthma control after 8 weeks of treatment with atorvastatin (40 mg/day for 8 weeks) added to ICS. They could only observe the decrease in absolute sputum macrophage count and sputum leukotriene B_4.

Statins augmented the anti-inflammatory effects of ICS on eosinophilic airway inflammation in asthma. We demonstrated that the addition of simvastatin to inhaled budesonide markedly reduced the percentage of sputum eosinophils through the activation of IDO in mild asthmatics. [168] The mechanisms underlying the activation of IDO were mediated through two distinct interacting molecular pathways. First, corticosteroids activate IDO by inducing the GITRL-associated noncanonical NF-κB signaling with p52 nuclear translocation and enhance IL-10 production. Second, simvastatin added to budesonide further augments type I IFN- and GITRL-activated noncanonical NF-κB–dependent induction of IDO and enhances IL-10 release. [168]

COPD

Statins may exert beneficial effects on a number of different COPD-specific outcomes. These include lung function and exercise capacity, COPD exacerbation rates, COPD-related hospitalization, intubation, and COPD-related mortality. COPD exacerbations were alleviated in observational studies. [197, 205-207] These beneficial effects could be explained by the pleiotropic effects of statins on neutrophilic airway inflammation. [208] The protection from the retardation in FEV_1 and FVC in COPD patients treated with statins suggested that statins directly mediated a protective effect on lung function. [197, 209] This protective effect was bolstered by the observation of slower decline in lung function in statin users than that in nonusers. [198] Statins prevent the development of emphysema in mice exposed to cigarette smoke with an accompanying reduction in the expression of TNF-α, IFN-γ and MMP-2, -9 and -12 and a reduction in neutrophils in bronchoalveolar lavage fluid. [47] Statins could prevent elastase-mediated emphysema in mice and promote the proliferation and regeneration of alveolar epithelial cells. [200] At a cellular level, statins dampened the effect of IL-17 and TGF-β in stimulating mediator release from primary airway epithelial cells. These indicated the potential of statins to suppress the inflammatory response and small airway fibrosis in COPD [73] and subsequently disease progression. [209]

Statins may decrease mortality in COPD irrespective of their vascular protective effects. Mancini and colleagues reported a similar reduction in mortality in both high-cardiovascular (CV) risk and low-CV risk groups after statin treatment. [205] Other studies also obtained a decrease in COPD-related mortality. [210-212] A retrospective study suggested that the treatment with statins prior to hospital admission was associated with decreasing 90-day mortality in patients with COPD exacerbation. [206]

References

[1] Greenwood J, Steinman L, Zamvil SS. Statin therapy and autoimmune disease: from protein prenylation to immunomodulation. Nature reviews. *Immunology* 2006; 6:358-70.

[2] Bu DX, Griffin G, Lichtman AH. Mechanisms for the anti-inflammatory effects of statins. *Current opinion in lipidology* 2011; 22:165-70.

[3] Stein DT, Devaraj S, Balis D, Adams-Huet B, Jialal I. Effect of statin therapy on remnant lipoprotein cholesterol levels in patients with combined hyperlipidemia. *Arteriosclerosis, thrombosis, and vascular biology* 2001; 21:2026-31.

[4] Prevention of cardiovascular events and death with pravastatin in patients with coronary heart disease and a broad range of initial cholesterol levels. The Long-Term Intervention with Pravastatin in Ischaemic Disease (LIPID) Study Group. *The New England journal of medicine* 1998; 339:1349-57.

[5] MRC/BHF Heart Protection Study of cholesterol lowering with simvastatin in 20,536 high-risk individuals: a randomised placebo-controlled trial. *Lancet* 2002; 360:7-22.

[6] Randomised trial of cholesterol lowering in 4444 patients with coronary heart disease: the Scandinavian Simvastatin Survival Study (4S). *Lancet* 1994; 344:1383-9.

[7] Downs JR, Clearfield M, Weis S, Whitney E, Shapiro DR, Beere PA, et al. Primary prevention of acute coronary events with lovastatin in men and women with average cholesterol levels: results of AFCAPS/TexCAPS. Air Force/Texas Coronary Atherosclerosis Prevention Study. *JAMA : the journal of the American Medical Association* 1998; 279:1615-22.

[8] Sacks FM, Pfeffer MA, Moye LA, Rouleau JL, Rutherford JD, Cole TG, et al. The effect of pravastatin on coronary events after myocardial infarction in patients with average cholesterol levels. Cholesterol and Recurrent Events Trial investigators. *The New England journal of medicine* 1996; 335:1001-9.

[9] Sever PS, Dahlof B, Poulter NR, Wedel H, Beevers G, Caulfield M, et al. Prevention of coronary and stroke events with atorvastatin in hypertensive patients who have average or lower-than-average cholesterol concentrations, in the Anglo-Scandinavian Cardiac

Outcomes Trial--Lipid Lowering Arm (ASCOT-LLA): a multicentre randomised controlled trial. Lancet 2003; 361:1149-58.

[10] Shepherd J, Cobbe SM, Ford I, Isles CG, Lorimer AR, MacFarlane PW, et al. Prevention of coronary heart disease with pravastatin in men with hypercholesterolemia. West of Scotland Coronary Prevention Study Group. *The New England journal of medicine* 1995; 333:1301-7.

[11] Ridker PM, Danielson E, Fonseca FA, Genest J, Gotto AM, Jr., Kastelein JJ, et al. Rosuvastatin to prevent vascular events in men and women with elevated C-reactive protein. *The New England journal of medicine* 2008; 359:2195-207.

[12] Liu PY, Liu YW, Lin LJ, Chen JH, Liao JK. Evidence for statin pleiotropy in humans: differential effects of statins and ezetimibe on rho-associated coiled-coil containing protein kinase activity, endothelial function, and inflammation. *Circulation* 2009; 119:131-8.

[13] Robinson JG, Smith B, Maheshwari N, Schrott H. Pleiotropic effects of statins: benefit beyond cholesterol reduction? A meta-regression analysis. *Journal of the American College of Cardiology* 2005; 46:1855-62.

[14] Landmesser U, Bahlmann F, Mueller M, Spiekermann S, Kirchhoff N, Schulz S, et al. Simvastatin versus ezetimibe: pleiotropic and lipid-lowering effects on endothelial function in humans. *Circulation* 2005; 111:2356-63.

[15] Laufs U, La Fata V, Plutzky J, Liao JK. Upregulation of endothelial nitric oxide synthase by HMG CoA reductase inhibitors. *Circulation* 1998; 97:1129-35.

[16] Laufs U, Liao JK. Post-transcriptional regulation of endothelial nitric oxide synthase mRNA stability by Rho GTPase. *The Journal of biological chemistry* 1998; 273:24266-71.

[17] Kureishi Y, Luo Z, Shiojima I, Bialik A, Fulton D, Lefer DJ, et al. The HMG-CoA reductase inhibitor simvastatin activates the protein kinase Akt and promotes angiogenesis in normocholesterolemic animals. *Nature medicine* 2000; 6:1004-10.

[18] Wolfrum S, Dendorfer A, Rikitake Y, Stalker TJ, Gong Y, Scalia R, et al. Inhibition of Rho-kinase leads to rapid activation of phosphatidylinositol 3-kinase/protein kinase Akt and cardiovascular protection. *Arteriosclerosis, thrombosis, and vascular biology* 2004; 24:1842-7.

[19] Feron O, Dessy C, Desager JP, Balligand JL. Hydroxy-methylglutaryl-coenzyme A reductase inhibition promotes endothelial nitric oxide synthase activation through a decrease in caveolin abundance. *Circulation* 2001; 103:113-8.

[20] Plenz GA, Hofnagel O, Robenek H. Differential modulation of caveolin-1 expression in cells of the vasculature by statins. *Circulation* 2004; 109:e7-8; author reply e7-8.

[21] Vasa M, Fichtlscherer S, Adler K, Aicher A, Martin H, Zeiher AM, et al. Increase in circulating endothelial progenitor cells by statin therapy in patients with stable coronary artery disease. *Circulation* 2001; 103:2885-90.

[22] Spiel AO, Mayr FB, Leitner JM, Firbas C, Sieghart W, Jilma B. Simvastatin and rosuvastatin mobilize Endothelial Progenitor Cells but do not prevent their acute decrease during systemic inflammation. *Thrombosis research* 2008; 123:108-13.

[23] Dimmeler S, Aicher A, Vasa M, Mildner-Rihm C, Adler K, Tiemann M, et al. HMG-CoA reductase inhibitors (statins) increase endothelial progenitor cells via the PI 3-kinase/Akt pathway. The *Journal of clinical investigation* 2001; 108:391-7.

[24] Llevadot J, Murasawa S, Kureishi Y, Uchida S, Masuda H, Kawamoto A, et al. HMG-CoA reductase inhibitor mobilizes bone marrow--derived endothelial progenitor cells. *The Journal of clinical investigation* 2001; 108:399-405.
[25] Weis M, Heeschen C, Glassford AJ, Cooke JP. Statins have biphasic effects on angiogenesis. *Circulation* 2002; 105:739-45.
[26] Chandrasekar B, Mummidi S, Mahimainathan L, Patel DN, Bailey SR, Imam SZ, et al. Interleukin-18-induced human coronary artery smooth muscle cell migration is dependent on NF-kappaB- and AP-1-mediated matrix metalloproteinase-9 expression and is inhibited by atorvastatin. *The Journal of biological chemistry* 2006; 281:15099-109.
[27] Shimizu K, Aikawa M, Takayama K, Libby P, Mitchell RN. Direct anti-inflammatory mechanisms contribute to attenuation of experimental allograft arteriosclerosis by statins. *Circulation* 2003; 108:2113-20.
[28] Jakobisiak M, Bruno S, Skierski JS, Darzynkiewicz Z. Cell cycle-specific effects of lovastatin. *Proceedings of the National Academy of Sciences of the United States of America* 1991; 88:3628-32.
[29] Yang Z, Kozai T, van der Loo B, Viswambharan H, Lachat M, Turina MI, et al. HMG-CoA reductase inhibition improves endothelial cell function and inhibits smooth muscle cell proliferation in human saphenous veins. *Journal of the American College of Cardiology* 2000; 36:1691-7.
[30] Laufs U, Marra D, Node K, Liao JK. 3-Hydroxy-3-methylglutaryl-CoA reductase inhibitors attenuate vascular smooth muscle proliferation by preventing rho GTPase-induced down-regulation of p27(Kip1). *The Journal of biological chemistry* 1999; 274:21926-31.
[31] Li M, Liu Y, Dutt P, Fanburg BL, Toksoz D. Inhibition of serotonin-induced mitogenesis, migration, and ERK MAPK nuclear translocation in vascular smooth muscle cells by atorvastatin. American journal of physiology. *Lung cellular and molecular physiology* 2007; 293:L463-71.
[32] Lefer AM, Campbell B, Shin YK, Scalia R, Hayward R, Lefer DJ. Simvastatin preserves the ischemic-reperfused myocardium in normocholesterolemic rat hearts. *Circulation* 1999; 100:178-84.
[33] Matsuki A, Igawa A, Nozawa T, Nakadate T, Igarashi N, Nonomura M, et al. Early administration of fluvastatin, but not at the onset of ischemia or reperfusion, attenuates myocardial ischemia-reperfusion injury through the nitric oxide pathway rather than its antioxidant property. *Circulation journal : official journal of the Japanese Circulation Society* 2006; 70:1643-9.
[34] Bulhak A, Roy J, Hedin U, Sjoquist PO, Pernow J. Cardioprotective effect of rosuvastatin in vivo is dependent on inhibition of geranylgeranyl pyrophosphate and altered RhoA membrane translocation. American journal of physiology. *Heart and circulatory physiology* 2007; 292:H3158-63.
[35] D'Annunzio V, Donato M, Erni L, Miksztowicz V, Buchholz B, Carrion CL, et al. Rosuvastatin given during reperfusion decreases infarct size and inhibits matrix metalloproteinase-2 activity in normocholesterolemic and hypercholesterolemic rabbits. *Journal of cardiovascular pharmacology* 2009; 53:137-44.

[36] Laufs U, Fata VL, Liao JK. Inhibition of 3-hydroxy-3-methylglutaryl (HMG)-CoA reductase blocks hypoxia-mediated down-regulation of endothelial nitric oxide synthase. *The Journal of biological chemistry* 1997; 272:31725-9.

[37] Di Napoli P, Taccardi AA, Grilli A, De Lutiis MA, Barsotti A, Felaco M, et al. Chronic treatment with rosuvastatin modulates nitric oxide synthase expression and reduces ischemia-reperfusion injury in rat hearts. *Cardiovascular research* 2005; 66:462-71.

[38] Girgis RE, Li D, Zhan X, Garcia JG, Tuder RM, Hassoun PM, et al. Attenuation of chronic hypoxic pulmonary hypertension by simvastatin. American journal of physiology. *Heart and circulatory physiology* 2003; 285:H938-45.

[39] Girgis RE, Mozammel S, Champion HC, Li D, Peng X, Shimoda L, et al. Regression of chronic hypoxic pulmonary hypertension by simvastatin. American journal of physiology. *Lung cellular and molecular physiology* 2007; 292:L1105-10.

[40] Taraseviciene-Stewart L, Scerbavicius R, Choe KH, Cool C, Wood K, Tuder RM, et al. Simvastatin causes endothelial cell apoptosis and attenuates severe pulmonary hypertension. American journal of physiology. *Lung cellular and molecular physiology* 2006; 291:L668-76.

[41] Hsu HH, Ruan T, Ko WJ, Hsu JY, Chen JS, Lee YC, et al. Effects of simvastatin on pulmonary C-fiber sensitivity in rats with monocrotaline-induced pulmonary hypertension. *The Journal of heart and lung transplantation : the official publication of the International Society for Heart Transplantation* 2011; 30:332-40.

[42] Liu B, Wang XQ, Yu L, Zhou TF, Wang XM, Liu HM. Simvastatin restores down-regulated GATA-6 expression in pulmonary hypertensive rats. *Experimental lung research* 2009; 35:411-26.

[43] Satoh K, Fukumoto Y, Nakano M, Sugimura K, Nawata J, Demachi J, et al. Statin ameliorates hypoxia-induced pulmonary hypertension associated with down-regulated stromal cell-derived factor-1. *Cardiovascular research* 2009; 81:226-34.

[44] Nishimura T, Faul JL, Berry GJ, Vaszar LT, Qiu D, Pearl RG, et al. Simvastatin attenuates smooth muscle neointimal proliferation and pulmonary hypertension in rats. *American journal of respiratory and critical care medicine* 2002; 166:1403-8.

[45] Carlin CM, Peacock AJ, Welsh DJ. Fluvastatin inhibits hypoxic proliferation and p38 MAPK activity in pulmonary artery fibroblasts. *American journal of respiratory cell and molecular biology* 2007; 37:447-56.

[46] Nishimura T, Vaszar LT, Faul JL, Zhao G, Berry GJ, Shi L, et al. Simvastatin rescues rats from fatal pulmonary hypertension by inducing apoptosis of neointimal smooth muscle cells. *Circulation* 2003; 108:1640-5.

[47] Lee JH, Lee DS, Kim EK, Choe KH, Oh YM, Shim TS, et al. Simvastatin inhibits cigarette smoking-induced emphysema and pulmonary hypertension in rat lungs. *American journal of respiratory and critical care medicine* 2005; 172:987-93.

[48] Sjogren B, Hamblin MW, Svenningsson P. Cholesterol depletion reduces serotonin binding and signaling via human 5-HT(7(a)) receptors. *European journal of pharmacology* 2006; 552:1-10.

[49] Crespo MJ, Quidgley JA. Statins decrease serotonin-induced contractions in coronary arteries of swine in vitro. *Pharmacology* 2006; 76:141-7.

[50] Alnaeb ME, Thompson CS, Seifalian AM, Hamilton G, Mikhailidis DP. Regional differences in the expression of nitric oxide synthase and specific receptors in the vascular tissues of control and diabetic rabbits: a pilot study. *In Vivo* 2007; 21:1069-74.

[51] Kao PN. Simvastatin treatment of pulmonary hypertension: an observational case series. *Chest* 2005; 127:1446-52.
[52] Wilkins MR, Ali O, Bradlow W, Wharton J, Taegtmeyer A, Rhodes CJ, et al. Simvastatin as a treatment for pulmonary hypertension trial. *American journal of respiratory and critical care medicine* 2010; 181:1106-13.
[53] Lee TM, Chen CC, Shen HN, Chang NC. Effects of pravastatin on functional capacity in patients with chronic obstructive pulmonary disease and pulmonary hypertension. *Clinical science* 2009; 116:497-505.
[54] Proud D, Leigh R. Epithelial cells and airway diseases. *Immunological reviews* 2011; 242:186-204.
[55] Holgate ST. The sentinel role of the airway epithelium in asthma pathogenesis. *Immunological reviews* 2011; 242:205-19.
[56] Peden DB. The role of oxidative stress and innate immunity in O(3) and endotoxin-induced human allergic airway disease. *Immunological reviews* 2011; 242:91-105.
[57] Holgate ST, Roberts G, Arshad HS, Howarth PH, Davies DE. The role of the airway epithelium and its interaction with environmental factors in asthma pathogenesis. *Proceedings of the American Thoracic Society* 2009; 6:655-9.
[58] Kraynack NC, Corey DA, Elmer HL, Kelley TJ. Mechanisms of NOS2 regulation by Rho GTPase signaling in airway epithelial cells. American journal of physiology. *Lung cellular and molecular physiology* 2002; 283:L604-11.
[59] Schaafsma D, Dueck G, Ghavami S, Kroeker A, Mutawe MM, Hauff K, et al. The mevalonate cascade as a target to suppress extracellular matrix synthesis by human airway smooth muscle. *American journal of respiratory cell and molecular biology* 2011; 44:394-403.
[60] Ghavami S, Mutawe MM, Sharma P, Yeganeh B, McNeill KD, Klonisch T, et al. Mevalonate cascade regulation of airway mesenchymal cell autophagy and apoptosis: a dual role for p53. *PLoS One* 2011; 6:e16523.
[61] Takeda N, Kondo M, Ito S, Ito Y, Shimokata K, Kume H. Role of RhoA inactivation in reduced cell proliferation of human airway smooth muscle by simvastatin. *American journal of respiratory cell and molecular biology* 2006; 35:722-9.
[62] Zeki AA, Franzi L, Last J, Kenyon NJ. Simvastatin inhibits airway hyperreactivity: implications for the mevalonate pathway and beyond. *Am J Respir Crit Care Med* 2009; 180:731-40.
[63] Zeki AA, Bratt JM, Rabowsky M, Last JA, Kenyon NJ. Simvastatin inhibits goblet cell hyperplasia and lung arginase in a mouse model of allergic asthma: a novel treatment for airway remodeling? *Translational research : the journal of laboratory and clinical medicine* 2010; 156:335-49.
[64] Ou XM, Wen FQ, Uhal BD, Feng YL, Huang XY, Wang T, et al. Simvastatin attenuates experimental small airway remodelling in rats. *Respirology* 2009; 14:734-45.
[65] Baarsma HA, Spanjer AI, Haitsma G, Engelbertink LH, Meurs H, Jonker MR, et al. Activation of WNT / beta-Catenin Signaling in Pulmonary Fibroblasts by TGF-beta(1) Is Increased in Chronic Obstructive Pulmonary Disease. *PLoS One* 2011; 6:e25450.
[66] Wright JL, Zhou S, Preobrazhenska O, Marshall C, Sin DD, Laher I, et al. Statin Reverses Smoke-induced Pulmonary Hypertension and Prevents Emphysema but Not Airway Remodeling. *American journal of respiratory and critical care medicine* 2011; 183:50-8.

[67] Opper C, Clement C, Schwarz H, Krappe J, Steinmetz A, Schneider J, et al. Increased number of high sensitive platelets in hypercholesterolemia, cardiovascular diseases, and after incubation with cholesterol. *Atherosclerosis* 1995; 113:211-7.

[68] Laufs U, Gertz K, Huang P, Nickenig G, Bohm M, Dirnagl U, et al. Atorvastatin upregulates type III nitric oxide synthase in thrombocytes, decreases platelet activation, and protects from cerebral ischemia in normocholesterolemic mice. *Stroke; a journal of cerebral circulation* 2000; 31:2442-9.

[69] Haramaki N, Ikeda H, Takenaka K, Katoh A, Sugano R, Yamagishi S, et al. Fluvastatin alters platelet aggregability in patients with hypercholesterolemia: possible improvement of intraplatelet redox imbalance via HMG-CoA reductase. *Arteriosclerosis, thrombosis, and vascular biology* 2007; 27:1471-7.

[70] Aikawa M, Rabkin E, Sugiyama S, Voglic SJ, Fukumoto Y, Furukawa Y, et al. An HMG-CoA reductase inhibitor, cerivastatin, suppresses growth of macrophages expressing matrix metalloproteinases and tissue factor in vivo and in vitro. *Circulation* 2001; 103:276-83.

[71] Maher BM, Dhonnchu TN, Burke JP, Soo A, Wood AE, Watson RW. Statins alter neutrophil migration by modulating cellular Rho activity--a potential mechanism for statins-mediated pleotropic effects? *Journal of leukocyte biology* 2009; 85:186-93.

[72] Pingitore A, Gemignani A, Menicucci D, Di Bella G, De Marchi D, Passera M, et al. Cardiovascular response to acute hypoxemia induced by prolonged breath holding in air. American journal of physiology. *Heart and circulatory physiology* 2008; 294:H449-55.

[73] Murphy DM, Forrest IA, Corris PA, Johnson GE, Small T, Jones D, et al. Simvastatin attenuates release of neutrophilic and remodeling factors from primary bronchial epithelial cells derived from stable lung transplant recipients. American journal of physiology. *Lung cellular and molecular physiology* 2008; 294:L592-9.

[74] Foldes G, von Haehling S, Okonko DO, Jankowska EA, Poole-Wilson PA, Anker SD. Fluvastatin reduces increased blood monocyte Toll-like receptor 4 expression in whole blood from patients with chronic heart failure. *International journal of cardiology* 2008; 124:80-5.

[75] Dinarello CA. Anti-inflammatory Agents: Present and Future. *Cell* 2010; 140:935-50.

[76] Chen JC, Wu ML, Huang KC, Lin WW. HMG-CoA reductase inhibitors activate the unfolded protein response and induce cytoprotective GRP78 expression. *Cardiovascular research* 2008; 80:138-50.

[77] Ke PY, Chen SS. Activation of the unfolded protein response and autophagy after hepatitis C virus infection suppresses innate antiviral immunity in vitro. *The Journal of clinical investigation* 2011; 121:37-56.

[78] Richardson CE, Kooistra T, Kim DH. An essential role for XBP-1 in host protection against immune activation in C. elegans. *Nature* 2010; 463:1092-5.

[79] Amuro H, Ito T, Miyamoto R, Sugimoto H, Torii Y, Son Y, et al. Statins, inhibitors of 3-hydroxy-3-methylglutaryl-coenzyme A reductase, function as inhibitors of cellular and molecular components involved in type I interferon production. *Arthritis and rheumatism* 2010; 62:2073-85.

[80] An G, Wang H, Tang R, Yago T, McDaniel JM, McGee S, et al. P-selectin glycoprotein ligand-1 is highly expressed on Ly-6Chi monocytes and a major determinant for Ly-

6Chi monocyte recruitment to sites of atherosclerosis in mice. *Circulation* 2008; 117:3227-37.

[81] Libby P, Ridker PM, Hansson GK. Inflammation in atherosclerosis: from pathophysiology to practice. *Journal of the American College of Cardiology* 2009; 54:2129-38.

[82] Kawakami A, Osaka M, Aikawa M, Uematsu S, Akira S, Libby P, et al. Toll-like receptor 2 mediates apolipoprotein CIII-induced monocyte activation. *Circulation research* 2008; 103:1402-9.

[83] Croce K, Libby P. Intertwining of thrombosis and inflammation in atherosclerosis. *Current opinion in hematology* 2007; 14:55-61.

[84] Healy AM, Pickard MD, Pradhan AD, Wang Y, Chen Z, Croce K, et al. Platelet expression profiling and clinical validation of myeloid-related protein-14 as a novel determinant of cardiovascular events. *Circulation* 2006; 113:2278-84.

[85] Morrow DA, Wang Y, Croce K, Sakuma M, Sabatine MS, Gao H, et al. Myeloid-related protein 8/14 and the risk of cardiovascular death or myocardial infarction after an acute coronary syndrome in the Pravastatin or Atorvastatin Evaluation and Infection Therapy: Thrombolysis in Myocardial Infarction (PROVE IT-TIMI 22) trial. *American heart journal* 2008; 155:49-55.

[86] Vogl T, Tenbrock K, Ludwig S, Leukert N, Ehrhardt C, van Zoelen MA, et al. Mrp8 and Mrp14 are endogenous activators of Toll-like receptor 4, promoting lethal, endotoxin-induced shock. *Nature medicine* 2007; 13:1042-9.

[87] Viemann D, Barczyk K, Vogl T, Fischer U, Sunderkotter C, Schulze-Osthoff K, et al. MRP8/MRP14 impairs endothelial integrity and induces a caspase-dependent and -independent cell death program. *Blood* 2007; 109:2453-60.

[88] McGown CC, Brown NJ, Hellewell PG, Reilly CS, Brookes ZL. Beneficial microvascular and anti-inflammatory effects of pravastatin during sepsis involve nitric oxide synthase III. *British journal of anaesthesia* 2010; 104:183-90.

[89] Planaguma A, Pfeffer MA, Rubin G, Croze R, Uddin M, Serhan CN, et al. Lovastatin decreases acute mucosal inflammation via 15-epi-lipoxin A4. *Mucosal immunology* 2010; 3:270-9.

[90] Birnbaum Y, Ye Y, Lin Y, Freeberg SY, Nishi SP, Martinez JD, et al. Augmentation of myocardial production of 15-epi-lipoxin-a4 by pioglitazone and atorvastatin in the rat. *Circulation* 2006; 114:929-35.

[91] Ye Y, Lin Y, Perez-Polo JR, Uretsky BF, Ye Z, Tieu BC, et al. Phosphorylation of 5-lipoxygenase at ser523 by protein kinase A determines whether pioglitazone and atorvastatin induce proinflammatory leukotriene B4 or anti-inflammatory 15-epi-lipoxin a4 production. *Journal of immunology* 2008; 181:3515-23.

[92] Spite M, Serhan CN. Novel lipid mediators promote resolution of acute inflammation: impact of aspirin and statins. *Circulation research* 2010; 107:1170-84.

[93] Claria J, Serhan CN. Aspirin triggers previously undescribed bioactive eicosanoids by human endothelial cell-leukocyte interactions. *Proceedings of the National Academy of Sciences of the United States of America* 1995; 92:9475-9.

[94] Claria J, Lee MH, Serhan CN. Aspirin-triggered lipoxins (15-epi-LX) are generated by the human lung adenocarcinoma cell line (A549)-neutrophil interactions and are potent inhibitors of cell proliferation. *Molecular medicine* 1996; 2:583-96.

[95] Takano T, Fiore S, Maddox JF, Brady HR, Petasis NA, Serhan CN. Aspirin-triggered 15-epi-lipoxin A4 (LXA4) and LXA4 stable analogues are potent inhibitors of acute inflammation: evidence for anti-inflammatory receptors. *The Journal of experimental medicine* 1997; 185:1693-704.

[96] Fukunaga K, Kohli P, Bonnans C, Fredenburgh LE, Levy BD. Cyclooxygenase 2 plays a pivotal role in the resolution of acute lung injury. *Journal of immunology* 2005; 174:5033-9.

[97] Bannenberg G, Moussignac RL, Gronert K, Devchand PR, Schmidt BA, Guilford WJ, et al. Lipoxins and novel 15-epi-lipoxin analogs display potent anti-inflammatory actions after oral administration. *British journal of pharmacology* 2004; 143:43-52.

[98] Levy BD, Lukacs NW, Berlin AA, Schmidt B, Guilford WJ, Serhan CN, et al. Lipoxin A4 stable analogs reduce allergic airway responses via mechanisms distinct from CysLT1 receptor antagonism. *The FASEB journal : official publication of the Federation of American Societies for Experimental Biology* 2007; 21:3877-84.

[99] Levy BD, De Sanctis GT, Devchand PR, Kim E, Ackerman K, Schmidt BA, et al. Multi-pronged inhibition of airway hyper-responsiveness and inflammation by lipoxin A(4). *Nat Med* 2002; 8:1018-23.

[100] Planaguma A, Kazani S, Marigowda G, Haworth O, Mariani TJ, Israel E, et al. Airway lipoxin A4 generation and lipoxin A4 receptor expression are decreased in severe asthma. *American journal of respiratory and critical care medicine* 2008; 178:574-82.

[101] Bhavsar PK, Levy BD, Hew MJ, Pfeffer MA, Kazani S, Israel E, et al. Corticosteroid suppression of lipoxin A4 and leukotriene B4 from alveolar macrophages in severe asthma. *Respiratory research* 2010; 11:71.

[102] Yamaguchi H, Higashi N, Mita H, Ono E, Komase Y, Nakagawa T, et al. Urinary concentrations of 15-epimer of lipoxin A(4) are lower in patients with aspirin-intolerant compared with aspirin-tolerant asthma. *Clinical and experimental allergy : journal of the British Society for Allergy and Clinical Immunology* 2011; 41:1711-8.

[103] Young RP, Hopkins R, Eaton TE. Pharmacological actions of statins: potential utility in COPD. *European respiratory review : an official journal of the European Respiratory Society* 2009; 18:222-32.

[104] Youssef S, Stuve O, Patarroyo JC, Ruiz PJ, Radosevich JL, Hur EM, et al. The HMG-CoA reductase inhibitor, atorvastatin, promotes a Th2 bias and reverses paralysis in central nervous system autoimmune disease. *Nature* 2002; 420:78-84.

[105] Aktas O, Waiczies S, Smorodchenko A, Dorr J, Seeger B, Prozorovski T, et al. Treatment of relapsing paralysis in experimental encephalomyelitis by targeting Th1 cells through atorvastatin. *The Journal of experimental medicine* 2003; 197:725-33.

[106] Greenwood J, Walters CE, Pryce G, Kanuga N, Beraud E, Baker D, et al. Lovastatin inhibits brain endothelial cell Rho-mediated lymphocyte migration and attenuates experimental autoimmune encephalomyelitis. *The FASEB journal : official publication of the Federation of American Societies for Experimental Biology* 2003; 17:905-7.

[107] Nath N, Giri S, Prasad R, Singh AK, Singh I. Potential targets of 3-hydroxy-3-methylglutaryl coenzyme A reductase inhibitor for multiple sclerosis therapy. *Journal of immunology* 2004; 172:1273-86.

[108] Liu W, Li WM, Gao C, Sun NL. Effects of atorvastatin on the Th1/Th2 polarization of ongoing experimental autoimmune myocarditis in Lewis rats. *Journal of autoimmunity* 2005; 25:258-63.

[109] Gegg ME, Harry R, Hankey D, Zambarakji H, Pryce G, Baker D, et al. Suppression of autoimmune retinal disease by lovastatin does not require Th2 cytokine induction. *Journal of immunology* 2005; 174:2327-35.

[110] Thomas PB, Albini T, Giri RK, See RF, Evans M, Rao NA. The effects of atorvastatin in experimental autoimmune uveitis. *The British journal of ophthalmology* 2005; 89:275-9.

[111] Leung BP, Sattar N, Crilly A, Prach M, McCarey DW, Payne H, et al. A novel anti-inflammatory role for simvastatin in inflammatory arthritis. *Journal of immunology* 2003; 170:1524-30.

[112] Neuhaus O, Strasser-Fuchs S, Fazekas F, Kieseier BC, Niederwieser G, Hartung HP, et al. Statins as immunomodulators: comparison with interferon-beta 1b in MS. *Neurology* 2002; 59:990-7.

[113] Vollmer T, Key L, Durkalski V, Tyor W, Corboy J, Markovic-Plese S, et al. Oral simvastatin treatment in relapsing-remitting multiple sclerosis. *Lancet* 2004; 363:1607-8.

[114] Dunn SE, Youssef S, Goldstein MJ, Prod'homme T, Weber MS, Zamvil SS, et al. Isoprenoids determine Th1/Th2 fate in pathogenic T cells, providing a mechanism of modulation of autoimmunity by atorvastatin. *The Journal of experimental medicine* 2006; 203:401-12.

[115] Imamura M, Okunishi K, Ohtsu H, Nakagome K, Harada H, Tanaka R, et al. Pravastatin attenuates allergic airway inflammation by suppressing antigen sensitisation, interleukin 17 production and antigen presentation in the lung. *Thorax* 2009; 64:44-9.

[116] McKay A, Leung BP, McInnes IB, Thomson NC, Liew FY. A novel anti-inflammatory role of simvastatin in a murine model of allergic asthma. *J Immunol* 2004; 172:2903-8.

[117] Kim DY, Ryu SY, Lim JE, Lee YS, Ro JY. Anti-inflammatory mechanism of simvastatin in mouse allergic asthma model. *Eur J Pharmacol* 2007; 557:76-86.

[118] Maneechotesuwan K, Xin Y, Ito K, Jazrawi E, Lee KY, Usmani OS, et al. Regulation of Th2 cytokine genes by p38 MAPK-mediated phosphorylation of GATA-3. *J Immunol* 2007; 178:2491-8.

[119] Zhang X, Tao Y, Troiani L, Markovic-Plese S. Simvastatin inhibits IFN regulatory factor 4 expression and Th17 cell differentiation in CD4+ T cells derived from patients with multiple sclerosis. *Journal of immunology* 2011; 187:3431-7.

[120] Bluestone JA, Abbas AK. Natural versus adaptive regulatory T cells. Nature reviews. *Immunology* 2003; 3:253-7.

[121] Sakaguchi S, Wing K, Miyara M. Regulatory T cells - a brief history and perspective. *European journal of immunology* 2007; 37 Suppl 1:S116-23.

[122] Hori S, Nomura T, Sakaguchi S. Control of regulatory T cell development by the transcription factor Foxp3. *Science* 2003; 299:1057-61.

[123] Fontenot JD, Gavin MA, Rudensky AY. Foxp3 programs the development and function of CD4+CD25+ regulatory T cells. *Nature immunology* 2003; 4:330-6.

[124] Khattri R, Cox T, Yasayko SA, Ramsdell F. An essential role for Scurfin in CD4+CD25+ T regulatory cells. *Nature immunology* 2003; 4:337-42.

[125] Wan YY, Flavell RA. Regulatory T-cell functions are subverted and converted owing to attenuated Foxp3 expression. *Nature* 2007; 445:766-70.

[126] Sakaguchi S, Powrie F. Emerging challenges in regulatory T cell function and biology. *Science* 2007; 317:627-9.

[127] Onishi Y, Fehervari Z, Yamaguchi T, Sakaguchi S. Foxp3+ natural regulatory T cells preferentially form aggregates on dendritic cells in vitro and actively inhibit their maturation. *Proceedings of the National Academy of Sciences of the United States of America* 2008; 105:10113-8.

[128] Maneechotesuwan K, Wamanuttajinda V, Kasetsinsombat K, Huabprasert S, Yaikwawong M, Barnes PJ, et al. Der p 1 suppresses indoleamine 2, 3-dioxygenase in dendritic cells from house dust mite-sensitive patients with asthma. *J Allergy Clin Immunol* 2009; 123:239-48.

[129] Verhasselt V, Milcent V, Cazareth J, Kanda A, Fleury S, Dombrowicz D, et al. Breast milk-mediated transfer of an antigen induces tolerance and protection from allergic asthma. *Nature medicine* 2008; 14:170-5.

[130] Polte T, Hansen G. Maternal tolerance achieved during pregnancy is transferred to the offspring via breast milk and persistently protects the offspring from allergic asthma. *Clinical and experimental allergy : journal of the British Society for Allergy and Clinical Immunology* 2008; 38:1950-8.

[131] Ray A, Khare A, Krishnamoorthy N, Qi Z, Ray P. Regulatory T cells in many flavors control asthma. *Mucosal immunology* 2010; 3:216-29.

[132] Tone Y, Furuuchi K, Kojima Y, Tykocinski ML, Greene MI, Tone M. Smad3 and NFAT cooperate to induce Foxp3 expression through its enhancer. *Nature immunology* 2008; 9:194-202.

[133] Kim HP, Leonard WJ. CREB/ATF-dependent T cell receptor-induced FoxP3 gene expression: a role for DNA methylation. *The Journal of experimental medicine* 2007; 204:1543-51.

[134] Kim YC, Kim KK, Shevach EM. Simvastatin induces Foxp3+ T regulatory cells by modulation of transforming growth factor-beta signal transduction. *Immunology* 2010; 130:484-93.

[135] Hartl D, Koller B, Mehlhorn AT, Reinhardt D, Nicolai T, Schendel DJ, et al. Quantitative and functional impairment of pulmonary CD4+CD25hi regulatory T cells in pediatric asthma. *The Journal of allergy and clinical immunology* 2007; 119:1258-66.

[136] Buckley AF, Kuo CT, Leiden JM. Transcription factor LKLF is sufficient to program T cell quiescence via a c-Myc--dependent pathway. *Nature immunology* 2001; 2:698-704.

[137] Wu J, Lingrel JB. KLF2 inhibits Jurkat T leukemia cell growth via upregulation of cyclin-dependent kinase inhibitor p21WAF1/CIP1. *Oncogene* 2004; 23:8088-96.

[138] Schober SL, Kuo CT, Schluns KS, Lefrancois L, Leiden JM, Jameson SC. Expression of the transcription factor lung Kruppel-like factor is regulated by cytokines and correlates with survival of memory T cells in vitro and in vivo. *Journal of immunology* 1999; 163:3662-7.

[139] Grayson JM, Murali-Krishna K, Altman JD, Ahmed R. Gene expression in antigen-specific CD8+ T cells during viral infection. *Journal of immunology* 2001; 166:795-9.

[140] Wu J, Lingrel JB. Kruppel-like factor 2, a novel immediate-early transcriptional factor, regulates IL-2 expression in T lymphocyte activation. *Journal of immunology* 2005; 175:3060-6.

[141] Li Z, Zhang Y, Liu Z, Wu X, Zheng Y, Tao Z, et al. ECM1 controls T(H)2 cell egress from lymph nodes through re-expression of S1P(1). *Nature immunology* 2011; 12:178-85.
[142] Bu DX, Tarrio M, Grabie N, Zhang Y, Yamazaki H, Stavrakis G, et al. Statin-induced Kruppel-like factor 2 expression in human and mouse T cells reduces inflammatory and pathogenic responses. *The Journal of clinical investigation* 2010; 120:1961-70.
[143] Sinclair LV, Finlay D, Feijoo C, Cornish GH, Gray A, Ager A, et al. Phosphatidylinositol-3-OH kinase and nutrient-sensing mTOR pathways control T lymphocyte trafficking. *Nature immunology* 2008; 9:513-21.
[144] Wagner RJ, Martin KA, Powell RJ, Rzucidlo EM. Lovastatin induces VSMC differentiation through inhibition of Rheb and mTOR. American journal of physiology. *Cell physiology* 2010; 299:C119-27.
[145] Korsgren M, Persson CG, Sundler F, Bjerke T, Hansson T, Chambers BJ, et al. Natural killer cells determine development of allergen-induced eosinophilic airway inflammation in mice. *The Journal of experimental medicine* 1999; 189:553-62.
[146] Hillyard DZ, Cameron AJ, McDonald KJ, Thomson J, MacIntyre A, Shiels PG, et al. Simvastatin inhibits lymphocyte function in normal subjects and patients with cardiovascular disease. *Atherosclerosis* 2004; 175:305-13.
[147] Katznelson S, Wang XM, Chia D, Ozawa M, Zhong HP, Hirata M, et al. The inhibitory effects of pravastatin on natural killer cell activity in vivo and on cytotoxic T lymphocyte activity in vitro. *The Journal of heart and lung transplantation : the official publication of the International Society for Heart Transplantation* 1998; 17:335-40.
[148] Katznelson S, Kobashigawa JA. Dual roles of HMG-CoA reductase inhibitors in solid organ transplantation: lipid lowering and immunosuppression. *Kidney international. Supplement* 1995; 52:S112-5.
[149] Blanco-Colio LM, Munoz-Garcia B, Martin-Ventura JL, Lorz C, Diaz C, Hernandez G, et al. 3-hydroxy-3-methylglutaryl coenzyme A reductase inhibitors decrease Fas ligand expression and cytotoxicity in activated human T lymphocytes. *Circulation* 2003; 108:1506-13.
[150] Kurakata S, Kada M, Shimada Y, Komai T, Nomoto K. Effects of different inhibitors of 3-hydroxy-3-methylglutaryl coenzyme A (HMG-CoA) reductase, pravastatin sodium and simvastatin, on sterol synthesis and immunological functions in human lymphocytes in vitro. *Immunopharmacology* 1996; 34:51-61.
[151] Coskey LA, Bitting J, Roth MD. Inhibition of natural killer cell activity by therapeutic levels of theophylline. *American journal of respiratory cell and molecular biology* 1993; 9:659-65.
[152] Timonen T, Stenius-Aarniala B. Natural killer cell activity in asthma. *Clinical and experimental immunology* 1985; 59:85-90.
[153] Jira M, Antosova E, Vondra V, Strejcek J, Mazakova H, Prazakova J. Natural killer and interleukin-2 induced cytotoxicity in asthmatics. I. Effect of acute antigen-specific challenge. *Allergy* 1988; 43:294-8.
[154] Krejsek J, Kral B, Vokurkova D, Derner V, Touskova M, Parakova Z, et al. Decreased peripheral blood gamma delta T cells in patients with bronchial asthma. *Allergy* 1998; 53:73-7.

[155] Urbanowicz RA, Lamb JR, Todd I, Corne JM, Fairclough LC. Enhanced effector function of cytotoxic cells in the induced sputum of COPD patients. *Respiratory research* 2010; 11:76.

[156] Fairclough L, Urbanowicz RA, Corne J, Lamb JR. Killer cells in chronic obstructive pulmonary disease. *Clinical science* 2008; 114:533-41.

[157] Nobes C, Marsh M. Dendritic cells: new roles for Cdc42 and Rac in antigen uptake? *Current biology :* CB 2000; 10:R739-41.

[158] Kuipers HF, Biesta PJ, Groothuis TA, Neefjes JJ, Mommaas AM, van den Elsen PJ. Statins affect cell-surface expression of major histocompatibility complex class II molecules by disrupting cholesterol-containing microdomains. *Human immunology* 2005; 66:653-65.

[159] Moreira AP, Hogaboam CM. Macrophages in allergic asthma: fine-tuning their pro- and anti-inflammatory actions for disease resolution. *Journal of interferon & cytokine research : the official journal of the International Society for Interferon and Cytokine Research* 2011; 31:485-91.

[160] Byers DE, Holtzman MJ. Alternatively activated macrophages and airway disease. *Chest* 2011; 140:768-74.

[161] Kim EY, Battaile JT, Patel AC, You Y, Agapov E, Grayson MH, et al. Persistent activation of an innate immune response translates respiratory viral infection into chronic lung disease. *Nat Med* 2008; 14:633-40.

[162] Chupp GL, Lee CG, Jarjour N, Shim YM, Holm CT, He S, et al. A chitinase-like protein in the lung and circulation of patients with severe asthma. *The New England journal of medicine* 2007; 357:2016-27.

[163] Reese TA, Liang HE, Tager AM, Luster AD, Van Rooijen N, Voehringer D, et al. Chitin induces accumulation in tissue of innate immune cells associated with allergy. *Nature* 2007; 447:92-6.

[164] Muzzarelli RA. Human enzymatic activities related to the therapeutic administration of chitin derivatives. *Cellular and molecular life sciences : CMLS* 1997; 53:131-40.

[165] Da Silva CA, Hartl D, Liu W, Lee CG, Elias JA. TLR-2 and IL-17A in chitin-induced macrophage activation and acute inflammation. *Journal of immunology* 2008; 181:4279-86.

[166] Shibata Y, Metzger WJ, Myrvik QN. Chitin particle-induced cell-mediated immunity is inhibited by soluble mannan: mannose receptor-mediated phagocytosis initiates IL-12 production. *Journal of immunology* 1997; 159:2462-7.

[167] Fujita E, Shimizu A, Masuda Y, Kuwahara N, Arai T, Nagasaka S, et al. Statin attenuates experimental anti-glomerular basement membrane glomerulonephritis together with the augmentation of alternatively activated macrophages. *The American journal of pathology* 2010; 177:1143-54.

[168] Maneechotesuwan K, Ekjiratrakul W, Kasetsinsombat K, Wongkajornsilp A, Barnes PJ. Statins enhance the anti-inflammatory effects of inhaled corticosteroids in asthmatic patients through increased induction of indoleamine 2, 3-dioxygenase. *J Allergy Clin Immunol* 2010; 126:754-62 e1.

[169] Munn DH, Shafizadeh E, Attwood JT, Bondarev I, Pashine A, Mellor AL. Inhibition of T cell proliferation by macrophage tryptophan catabolism. *J Exp Med* 1999; 189:1363-72.

[170] Frumento G, Rotondo R, Tonetti M, Damonte G, Benatti U, Ferrara GB. Tryptophan-derived catabolites are responsible for inhibition of T and natural killer cell proliferation induced by indoleamine 2,3-dioxygenase. *J Exp Med* 2002; 196:459-68.
[171] Terness P, Bauer TM, Rose L, Dufter C, Watzlik A, Simon H, et al. Inhibition of allogeneic T cell proliferation by indoleamine 2,3-dioxygenase-expressing dendritic cells: mediation of suppression by tryptophan metabolites. *J Exp Med* 2002; 196:447-57.
[172] Hayashi T, Beck L, Rossetto C, Gong X, Takikawa O, Takabayashi K, et al. Inhibition of experimental asthma by indoleamine 2,3-dioxygenase. *J Clin Invest* 2004; 114:270-9.
[173] Maneechotesuwan K, Supawita S, Kasetsinsombat K, Wongkajornsilp A, Barnes PJ. Sputum indoleamine-2, 3-dioxygenase activity is increased in asthmatic airways by using inhaled corticosteroids. *J Allergy Clin Immunol* 2008; 121:43-50.
[174] Hothersall E, McSharry C, Thomson NC. Potential therapeutic role for statins in respiratory disease. *Thorax* 2006; 61:729-34.
[175] Morimoto K, Janssen WJ, Fessler MB, McPhillips KA, Borges VM, Bowler RP, et al. Lovastatin enhances clearance of apoptotic cells (efferocytosis) with implications for chronic obstructive pulmonary disease. *Journal of immunology* 2006; 176:7657-65.
[176] Hodge S, Hodge G, Scicchitano R, Reynolds PN, Holmes M. Alveolar macrophages from subjects with chronic obstructive pulmonary disease are deficient in their ability to phagocytose apoptotic airway epithelial cells. *Immunology and cell biology* 2003; 81:289-96.
[177] Zhang X, Jin J, Peng X, Ramgolam VS, Markovic-Plese S. Simvastatin inhibits IL-17 secretion by targeting multiple IL-17-regulatory cytokines and by inhibiting the expression of IL-17 transcription factor RORC in CD4+ lymphocytes. *J Immunol* 2008; 180:6988-96.
[178] Barnes PJ. Immunology of asthma and chronic obstructive pulmonary disease. Nature reviews. *Immunology* 2008; 8:183-92.
[179] Zeiser R, Maas K, Youssef S, Durr C, Steinman L, Negrin RS. Regulation of different inflammatory diseases by impacting the mevalonate pathway. *Immunology* 2009; 127:18-25.
[180] Ray KK, Cannon CP, Ganz P. Beyond lipid lowering: What have we learned about the benefits of statins from the acute coronary syndromes trials? *The American journal of cardiology* 2006; 98:18P-25P.
[181] Quist-Paulsen P. Statins and inflammation: an update. *Current opinion in cardiology* 2010; 25:399-405.
[182] Ortego M, Bustos C, Hernandez-Presa MA, Tunon J, Diaz C, Hernandez G, et al. Atorvastatin reduces NF-kappaB activation and chemokine expression in vascular smooth muscle cells and mononuclear cells. *Atherosclerosis* 1999; 147:253-61.
[183] Edwards MR, Bartlett NW, Clarke D, Birrell M, Belvisi M, Johnston SL. Targeting the NF-kappaB pathway in asthma and chronic obstructive pulmonary disease. *Pharmacology & therapeutics* 2009; 121:1-13.
[184] Charokopos N, Apostolopoulos N, Kalapodi M, Leotsinidis M, Karamanos N, Mouzaki A. Bronchial asthma, chronic obstructive pulmonary disease and NF-kappaB. *Current medicinal chemistry* 2009; 16:867-83.

[185] Christman JW, Sadikot RT, Blackwell TS. The role of nuclear factor-kappa B in pulmonary diseases. *Chest* 2000; 117:1482-7.
[186] Hart LA, Krishnan VL, Adcock IM, Barnes PJ, Chung KF. Activation and localization of transcription factor, nuclear factor-kappaB, in asthma. *Am J Respir Crit Care Med* 1998; 158:1585-92.
[187] Liu SF, Haddad EB, Adcock I, Salmon M, Koto H, Gilbey T, et al. Inducible nitric oxide synthase after sensitization and allergen challenge of Brown Norway rat lung. *British journal of pharmacology* 1997; 121:1241-6.
[188] Papi A, Johnston SL. Rhinovirus infection induces expression of its own receptor intercellular adhesion molecule 1 (ICAM-1) via increased NF-kappaB-mediated transcription. *The Journal of biological chemistry* 1999; 274:9707-20.
[189] Biagioli MC, Kaul P, Singh I, Turner RB. The role of oxidative stress in rhinovirus induced elaboration of IL-8 by respiratory epithelial cells. *Free radical biology & medicine* 1999; 26:454-62.
[190] Mastronarde JG, He B, Monick MM, Mukaida N, Matsushima K, Hunninghake GW. Induction of interleukin (IL)-8 gene expression by respiratory syncytial virus involves activation of nuclear factor (NF)-kappa B and NF-IL-6. *The Journal of infectious diseases* 1996; 174:262-7.
[191] Garofalo R, Sabry M, Jamaluddin M, Yu RK, Casola A, Ogra PL, et al. Transcriptional activation of the interleukin-8 gene by respiratory syncytial virus infection in alveolar epithelial cells: nuclear translocation of the RelA transcription factor as a mechanism producing airway mucosal inflammation. *Journal of virology* 1996; 70:8773-81.
[192] Fiedler MA, Wernke-Dollries K, Stark JM. Mechanism of RSV-induced IL-8 gene expression in A549 cells before viral replication. *The American journal of physiology* 1996; 271:L963-71.
[193] Bitko V, Velazquez A, Yang L, Yang YC, Barik S. Transcriptional induction of multiple cytokines by human respiratory syncytial virus requires activation of NF-kappa B and is inhibited by sodium salicylate and aspirin. *Virology* 1997; 232:369-78.
[194] Barnes PJ. New therapies for chronic obstructive pulmonary disease. Medical principles and practice : international journal of the Kuwait University, *Health Science Centre* 2010; 19:330-8.
[195] Chung KF. p38 mitogen-activated protein kinase pathways in asthma and COPD. Chest 2011; 139:1470-9.
[196] Springer J, Scholz FR, Peiser C, Groneberg DA, Fischer A. SMAD-signaling in chronic obstructive pulmonary disease: transcriptional down-regulation of inhibitory SMAD 6 and 7 by cigarette smoke. *Biological chemistry* 2004; 385:649-53.
[197] Keddissi JI, Younis WG, Chbeir EA, Daher NN, Dernaika TA, Kinasewitz GT. The use of statins and lung function in current and former smokers. *Chest* 2007; 132:1764-71.
[198] Alexeeff SE, Litonjua AA, Sparrow D, Vokonas PS, Schwartz J. Statin use reduces decline in lung function: VA Normative Aging Study. *American journal of respiratory and critical care medicine* 2007; 176:742-7.
[199] Kim SE, Thanh Thuy TT, Lee JH, Ro JY, Bae YA, Kong Y, et al. Simvastatin inhibits induction of matrix metalloproteinase-9 in rat alveolar macrophages exposed to cigarette smoke extract. *Experimental & molecular medicine* 2009; 41:277-87.
[200] Takahashi S, Nakamura H, Seki M, Shiraishi Y, Yamamoto M, Furuuchi M, et al. Reversal of elastase-induced pulmonary emphysema and promotion of alveolar

epithelial cell proliferation by simvastatin in mice. American journal of physiology. *Lung cellular and molecular physiology* 2008; 294:L882-90.

[201] Ahmad T, Mabalirajan U, Sharma A, Aich J, Makhija L, Ghosh B, et al. Simvastatin improves epithelial dysfunction and airway hyperresponsiveness: from asymmetric dimethyl-arginine to asthma. *American journal of respiratory cell and molecular biology* 2011; 44:531-9.

[202] Agrawal A, Mabalirajan U, Ahmad T, Ghosh B. Emerging interface between metabolic syndrome and asthma. *American journal of respiratory cell and molecular biology* 2011; 44:270-5.

[203] Menzies D, Nair A, Meldrum KT, Fleming D, Barnes M, Lipworth BJ. Simvastatin does not exhibit therapeutic anti-inflammatory effects in asthma. *J Allergy Clin Immunol* 2007; 119:328-35.

[204] Hothersall EJ, Chaudhuri R, McSharry C, Donnelly I, Lafferty J, McMahon AD, et al. Effects of atorvastatin added to inhaled corticosteroids on lung function and sputum cell counts in atopic asthma. *Thorax* 2008; 63:1070-5.

[205] Mancini GB, Etminan M, Zhang B, Levesque LE, FitzGerald JM, Brophy JM. Reduction of morbidity and mortality by statins, angiotensin-converting enzyme inhibitors, and angiotensin receptor blockers in patients with chronic obstructive pulmonary disease. *Journal of the American College of Cardiology* 2006; 47:2554-60.

[206] Soyseth V, Brekke PH, Smith P, Omland T. Statin use is associated with reduced mortality in COPD. *The European respiratory journal : official journal of the European Society for Clinical Respiratory Physiology* 2007; 29:279-83.

[207] Blamoun AI, Batty GN, DeBari VA, Rashid AO, Sheikh M, Khan MA. Statins may reduce episodes of exacerbation and the requirement for intubation in patients with COPD: evidence from a retrospective cohort study. In*ternational journal of clinical practice* 2008; 62:1373-8.

[208] Barnes PJ, Celli BR. Systemic manifestations and comorbidities of COPD. *The European respiratory journal : official journal of the European Society for Clinical Respiratory Physiology* 2009; 33:1165-85.

[209] Janda S, Park K, FitzGerald JM, Etminan M, Swiston J. Statins in COPD: a systematic review. *Chest* 2009; 136:734-43.

[210] Lawes CM, Thornley S, Young R, Hopkins R, Marshall R, Chan WC, et al. Statin use in COPD patients is associated with a reduction in mortality: a national cohort study. *Primary care respiratory journal : journal of the General Practice Airways Group 2012.*

[211] Frost FJ, Petersen H, Tollestrup K, Skipper B. Influenza and COPD mortality protection as pleiotropic, dose-dependent effects of statins. *Chest* 2007; 131:1006-12.

[212] Ishida W, Kajiwara T, Ishii M, Fujiwara F, Taneichi H, Takebe N, et al. Decrease in mortality rate of chronic obstructive pulmonary disease (COPD) with statin use: a population-based analysis in Japan. *The Tohoku journal of experimental medicine* 2007; 212:265-73.

In: Statins ISBN: 978-1-62081-367-6
Editors: Benedetta La Grua and Alessandro Molinelli

Chapter IV

Statins as Anticancer Agents

Paul W. Sylvester, Abhita Malaviya, Suryatheja Ananthula, Parash Parajuli and Roshan V. Tiwari
College of Pharmacy, University of Louisiana at Monroe, Monroe, LA, US

Abstract

Statins are potent inhibitors of 3-hydroxy-3-methylglutaryl-coenzyme A (HMGCoA) reductase, the rate limiting enzyme in the mevalonate biosynthetic pathway for cholesterol synthesis. The mevalonate pathway is extremely important because it is also involved in the synthesis of sterol and non-sterol intermediates that are essential for tumor cell survival and growth.

Specifically, HMGCoA reductase catalyze the conversion of 3-hydroxy-3-methylglutaryl-coenzyme A to mevalonate, which subsequently produces isoprenoid intermediates such as farnesyl pyrophosphate and geranylgeranyl pyrophosphate that are required for posttranslational modification (isoprenylation) of various small GTP-binding proteins and heterotrimeric G-protein γ-subunit. Isoprenylation is needed for anchoring these signaling proteins to the cell membrane in close proximity to growth factor receptors so that these signaling proteins can be activated following receptor activation, and subsequently participate in turning on downstream mitogenic signaling pathways such as MAPK and Akt. HMGCoA reductase activity is characteristically elevated and/or unregulated in many forms of cancer and thereby, acts to promote cancer cell survival and proliferation by providing an abundance of non-sterol intermediates.

As a result, a great deal of attention has been focused on the development of agents that target and inhibit HMGCoA reductase activity for use in cancer chemotherapy. This review will focus on the growing body of research that demonstrates a role for statins as anticancer agents, starting with the origins of statin development as cholesterol lowering therapy and following the unique path they have taken towards anticancer agents. Finally, recent developments in the field will be discussed that indicate statins are poised to make the next step towards providing significant health benefits in the prevention and treatment of various forms of cancer.

Introduction

Statins constitute a class of drugs widely used in health care for the treatment of hypercholesterolemia. Statins such as simvastatin, lovastatin, mevastatin, pravastatin are naturally produced by certain fungi, whereas cerivastatin, atorvastatin, fluvastatin, rosuvastatin and pitvastatin are derived synthetically. Irrespective of their source, statins are known to decrease high blood cholesterol levels by suppressing the biosynthesis of cholesterol in the liver. Statins share a structural resemblance with 3-hydroxy-3-methylglutaryl-coenzyme A (HMGCoA) and competitively inhibit HMGCoA reductase, the rate limiting enzyme in the mevalonate pathway for cholesterol synthesis [1]. Interestingly, activity of the mevalonate pathway is constitutively active in various types of malignant cells due to elevated and unregulated HMGCoA reductase activity [2]. In addition to cholesterol, the mevalonate pathway produces abundant nonsterol products which are required for isoprenylation of key signaling proteins like Ras, Rap and Rab. Isoprenylation results in the anchoring of these proteins to the interior of the plasma membrane and allows for their activation and initiation of downstream mitogenic signaling. Furthermore, a higher portion of HMGCoA reductase activity is directed towards the synthesis of nonsterol intermediates in cancer cells as compared to normal cells. Statins act to block the mevalonate pathway by inhibiting HMGCoA reductase activity and subsequently preventing isoprenylation and activation of Ras proteins [3]. In addition, mutant forms of Ras proteins have also been found to be present in more than 30% of human tumors. These and other findings have lead to extensive research into the potential of statins as anticancer agents.

Historical Background

Following the elucidation of the biosynthetic pathway for cholesterol, many compounds were subsequently identified as competitive antagonists in the pathway. Tiparanol (MER/29) was one of the first such compounds that was found to inhibit the later stages of cholesterol synthesis. However, use of this compound induced many serious side effects including cataract and as such, this compound was withdrawn from the market [4, 5]. However, researchers screening microbial extracts at the Sankyo Research Laboratories discovered a HMGCoA reductase inhibitor and named this compound, citrinin [5]. Although citrinin strongly inhibited HMGCoA reductase and lowered serum cholesterol levels in rats, this compound was also found to induce severe kidney toxicity in a number of different species [5]. Subsequent screening studies lead to the identification of compactin/ML-236B or mevastatin [5]. Mevastatin was isolated from rice contaminated with the blue/green mold *Penicillium citrinum* (Pen-51). Mevastatin was found to strongly inhibited sterol synthesis from acetyl-CoA at relatively low treatment doses (IC_{50}=0.4 ng/ml) in a variety of cultured mammalian cells, including those obtained from patients with familial hypercholesterolemia. While mevastatin showed promising results in cell culture studies, this compound failed to produce similar results is rodents because multiple dosing of mevastatin induced an 8-10 fold elevation in HMGCoA reductase levels, nullifying the inhibitory effects of this compound [5].

Researchers at GlaxoSmithKline independently isolated the same compound from another blue/green fungus called *Penicillium brevicompacutum*, and these investigators also showed that mevastatin was ineffective in reducing cholesterol levels in rats [5]. However, additional studies in the chicken, dog and monkey did find that mevastatin was effective in significantly lowering circulating levels of LDL-cholesterol [4, 5], and these findings provided the necessary evidence needed to justify testing this compound in clinical trials. However, Phase II clinical trials with mevastatin were discontinued due to reports of increased incidence of lymphoma in dogs treated with doses 200-fold higher doses than those used in human patients [4, 5]. Nevertheless, these initial findings stimulated the search for other naturally occurring statins that had less adverse side effects. Later, collaborative research between Sankyo Research Laboratories in Japan and the Merck Research Laboratories in the United States lead to the isolation of a compound from two different fungi, *Aspergillus terreus* and *Monascus ruber,* that was structurally similar to mevastatin and later became known as lovastatin [4, 5]. Later studies showed that the cholesterol lowering effects of lovastatin were mediated by its action to significantly increase expression of hepatic LDL receptor levels in both dogs and Japanese patients with heterozygous familial hypercholesterolemia [4, 5].

Eventually, lovastatin received FDA approval in 1987, making it the first statin to be marketed in the United States [4, 5]. Following the success of lovastatin, other semisynthetic and synthetic statins with different pharmacokinetic and pharmacodynamic parameters were developed and are now available for clinical use.

Statin Classification Parameters

Structure: Statins can be classified based on a variety of parameters, including structure and their source of origin [6, 7]. Structurally, statins have a HMG-like moiety attached covalently to a hydrophobic group. Lovastatin, simvastatin and pravastatin are all characterized by having a polar head and a hydrophobic decalin ring. These statins are referred to as first generation or Type I statins. Lovastatin and simvastatin are lactone prodrugs that are hydrolyzed to 3, 5-dihydroheptanoic acid *in vivo*, whereas pravastatin is an open ring derivative of mevastatin that is obtained by microsomal hydroxylation [6, 7]. Fluvastatin, cerivastatin, atorvastatin, and rosuvastatin are pure synthetic compounds and are referred as Type II or second generation statins. Type II statins are devoid of an asymmetrical center and decalin ring, but they do have very large hydrophobic groups. These hydrophobic rings determine the physiological and chemical properties of these individual drugs [6, 7]. Figure 1 shows the chemical structure of various open and closed ringed statins.

Chemical Properties: Atorvastatin, fluvastatin, lovastatin, simvastatin and cerivastatin are lipophilic, while pravastatin and rosuvastatin are hydrophilic. In general, statins with high lipid solubility display the most rapid uptake into hepatic and other tissues [7, 8]. Although cerivastatin displays the highest octanol/water coefficient, an indication of high lipophilicity, this compound was taken off the market because it caused serious side effects including rhabdomyolysis.

In addition, highly lipophilic drugs tend to have a much greater dependency on cytochrome P-450 enzymes for oxidative metabolism and clearance from the body.

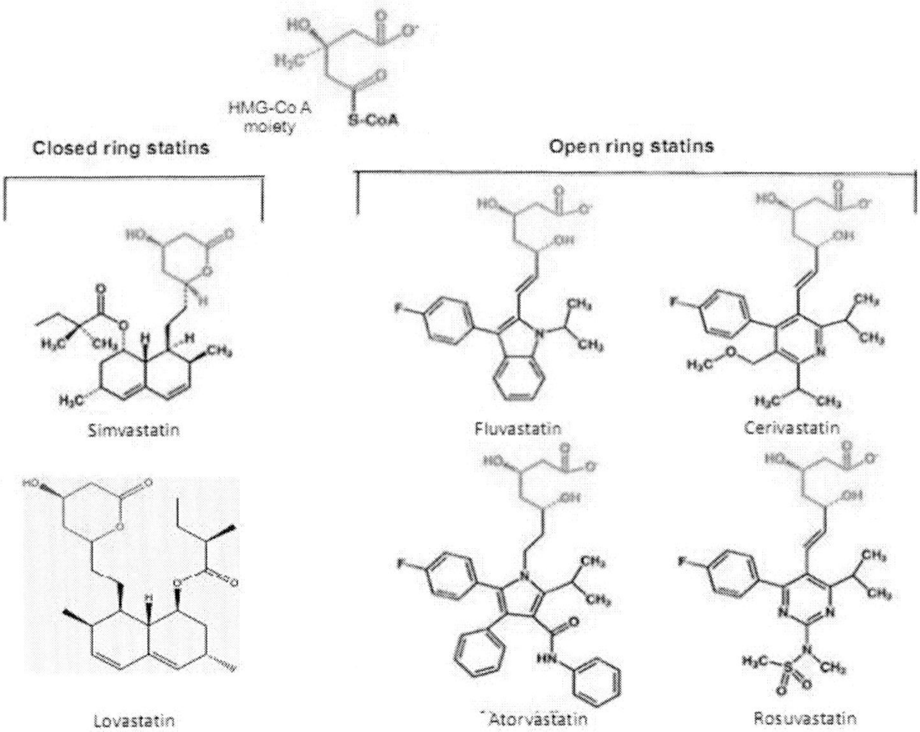

Figure 1. General chemical structure of statins based on the open and closed ring. The HMG like moiety (ring structure) is conserved in all statins and as illustrated at the top of the Figure.

Combined treatment of cerivastatin with gemfibrozil, a fibrate drug that is used to reduce elevated triglycerides and cholesterol levels and acts to inhibit P-450 activity, is associated with causing fatal rhabdomyolysis due to reduced hepatic metabolism and clearance of cerivastatin from the circulation [7, 8].

Anticancer Action of Statins

In addition to lowering circulating cholesterol levels, it is now evident that statins play a key role in modulating cellular processes such as cell activation, proliferation and apoptosis, all of which are critical in cancer development and progression. Although the exact mechanisms mediating the anticancer effects of statin are not completely understood, a large amount of data has accumulated related to the inhibitory effects of statins in tumorigenesis.

Growth Arrest: In vitro studies have shown that statins can alter the growth properties of tumor cells by interrupting growth-promoting signals [9]. Simvastatin was shown to inhibit the growth of human glioma cells, and this effect was completely reversed by co-administration with mevalonate [10]. Similarly, lovastatin was reported to inhibit ovarian cancer cell growth [11]. Subsequent, studies showed that simvastatin caused a dose-responsive decrease in cell proliferation in C6 glioma cells [12]. Pitavastatin and atorvastatin were also shown to significantly inhibit the growth of human extrahepatic cholangiocarcinoma (HuCCT1) and human intrahepatic cholangiocarcinoma (YSCCC) cells [13].

Various studies have shown that the antiproliferative effects of statins are mediated through the induction of cell cycle arrest [14]. Lovastatin was reported to induce blockade in G1 phase of the cell cycle by suppressing cyclin dependent kinase levels in breast cancer cells [15]. In U266 myeloma cells, mevastatin was shown to suppress the proliferation of cells by arresting their progression in G1 [16]. Similarly, short term, high-dose application of pravastatin induce growth inhibition in vascular smooth muscle cells [17]. Mevastatin also promoted growth arrest in pulmonary artery smooth muscle cells through inhibition of cyclin E kinase [18]. In the prostate cancer cell lines, PC3 and Du145, lovastatin and simvastatin were shown to induce arrest at G1 phase and increase the levels of p21 by suppressing activation of RhoA [19]. In whole animal models, lovastatin was reported to inhibit growth of EJ3-derived tumors in mice [20] and suppress the development of colorectal tumors in rats [21]. Statin treatment was also found to reduced the growth of fibrosarcoma and experimental lung metastases in rats [22], whereas pravastatin was shown to inhibit the incidence of nitrosourea and 1,2 dimethylhydrazine induced colon tumors in rats [23] and mice [24], respectively. Taken together, these finding in both *in vitro* and *in vivo* experimental tumor models clearly demonstrate the antiproliferative effects of statins.

Apoptosis: Statins treatment has also been shown initial apoptosis in a tumor cell specific manner. It has been proposed that statins can increase the pro-apoptotic potential of tumor cells by activating several apoptotic pathways. Studies have shown that statins can initiate apoptosis in a wide variety of tumor cell lines including B-16, MCF-7, Caco2, ovarian cancer cells and HL60, and this effect could be reversed by combined treatment with mevalonate [25, 26]. Lovastatin was shown to induce cell death in medullobalstoma cell lines [27], as well as effectively decreasing the viability of plasma cells from myeloma patients in a time- and dose-dependent manner [28]. Lovastatin was also shown to be cytotoxic to breast cancer cells that contained p53 mutations due to its ability to suppress DNA synthesis and induce p53-independent mitochondria-mediated apoptosis [29]. In addition, lovastatin was demonstrated to induce apoptosis in mesothelioma cells [30].

Statins have been reported to induce apoptosis in human myeloma cells [31] and prostate cancer cells [32, 33], pancreatic cancer cells [34], and glial cells [35]. Mevastatin was shown to induce apoptosis in JJ N-3 myeloma cells [31], while lovastatin was reported to induce apoptosis in pancreatic cancer [36], neuroblastoma [37], astocytoma [38], acute myelogenous leukemia [39] cells, and cells derived from juvenile monomyelocytic leukemia, pediatric solid malignancies (rhabdosarcoma and medullobalstoma), and squamous cell carcinoma of the cervix and head and neck [40]. Furthermore, cerivastatin was shown to have at least a 10-fold higher efficacy in triggering apoptosis in acute myeloid leukemia (AML) cells as compared to lovastatin and atorvastatin, while being equally effective in killing AML cells as lovastatin. In all these studies, cell death was shown to result from the initiation of apoptosis, and could be reversed by co-administration with mevalonate [41].

Some reports have suggested that the antiproliferative and apoptotic effects of statins may be mediated through different mechanisms. Specially, treatment with higher doses of mevastatin, fluvastatin or simvastatin was found to induce cell death by suppressing the Ras/ERK and Ras/Akt pathways, whereas lower doses of these agents were found to be cytostatic in C6 glioma cells [42]. Statin-induced apoptosis in tumor cells has been attributed to the downregulation of bcl-2 mRNA and protein [43]. In addition, simvastatin-induced apoptosis in human breast cancer cells [44] and C6 glioma cells [12] was reported to be mediated by c-jun N-terminal kinase pathway, while in human osteosarcoma cells, simvastatin promoted apoptosis by inhibiting RhoA activity and phospho-p42/p44 levels [45].

Angiogenesis: Angiogenesis is crucial for the growth of solid tumors. It involves endothelial cell proliferation, migration, extracellular matrix degradation and control of angiogenic factors. Vascular endothelial growth factor (VEGF) and basic fibroblast growth factor (bFGF) are growth factors that are involved in the progression of hematological malignancies. Therefore, targeting the formation of blood vessels is a promising strategy in cancer therapy [46, 47]. Interestingly, statins have been reported to exhibit both anti- and pro-angiogenic effects [48-50]. Simvastatin and cerivastatin were found to inhibit capillary growth in VEGF stimulated chick chorioallantoic membranes. In addition, both simvastatin and cerivastatin were shown to inhibit the growth of microvascular endothelial cells *in vitro* [51, 52]. Lovastatin potentiated the antitumor activity of TNF-α against tumor cells via inhibition of tumor-induced blood-vessel formation [53]. In the *in vivo* Lewis cancer lung model, cerivastatin was reported to decrease tumor growth and vascularization by 59% and 51% respectively [17]. Statins have been shown to inhibit angiogenesis by preventing binding of lipophilic anchors such as Ras, GTP-binding proteins [54] and geranylgeranyl pyrophosphate for RhoA for translocation to the cell membrane and ultimately alter mitogenic signaling [55].

A biphasic effect of statins on angiogenesis has also been demonstrated in various studies. Cerivastatin [17] and atorvastatin [56] were demonstrated to inhibit angiogenesis at high doses and increase angiogenesis at low doses. Simvastatin was reported to enhance phosphorylation of the endogenous Akt substrate endothelial nitric oxide synthase (eNOS) and accelerate vascular structure formation in an Akt-dependent manner and these effects were found to be similar to those induced by VEGF, suggesting that long-term statin treatment may enhance vascularization in developing tumors [57]. In addition, at high concentrations stains have been found to induce endothelial cell apoptosis under hypoxic conditions [58, 59].

The effects of statins on angiogenesis have been associated with increased activity in eNOS [57, 60]. Calveolin-1 is negatively regulated by eNOS and calveolin-1 expressions is downregulated by statin therapy. Furthermore, the relationship between eNOS and calveolin-1 differs depending on the type of endothelial cell that is examined. For example, it was shown that statin treatment results in nitric oxide mediated pro-angiogenic effects only in cells with low calveolin-1 expression [48] and these differences in calveolin-1 expression may be explained, at least in part, why the findings that the effects of statins vary in different types of endothelial cell lines [3].

Metastasis and Invasion: A serious and deadly characteristic in malignant cell progression is that cells will detach from the primary tumor, enter and exit the circulation, and start growing in a secondary site. This process requires protease activity, invasion of the basement membrane, cell migration, angiogenesis and attachment and detachment from the extracellular matrix. Statins have been shown to block metastasis at the level of cell attachment, migration and invasion in solid tumors [22, 61, 62]. Cerivastatin was shown to inhibit expression of urokinase-type plasminogen activator (uPA), uPA receptor (u-PAR), and matrix metalloproteinase-9 (MMP-9) in monocytes [63]. In addition, reduced monocytic MMP-9 secretion was also seen after simvastatin treatment [64]. In other studies, lovastatin inhibited *in vitro* growth and migration of the colonic adenocarcinoma cell lines SW480 and SW620 and suppressed the number of tumor colonies that were found in the liver [65].

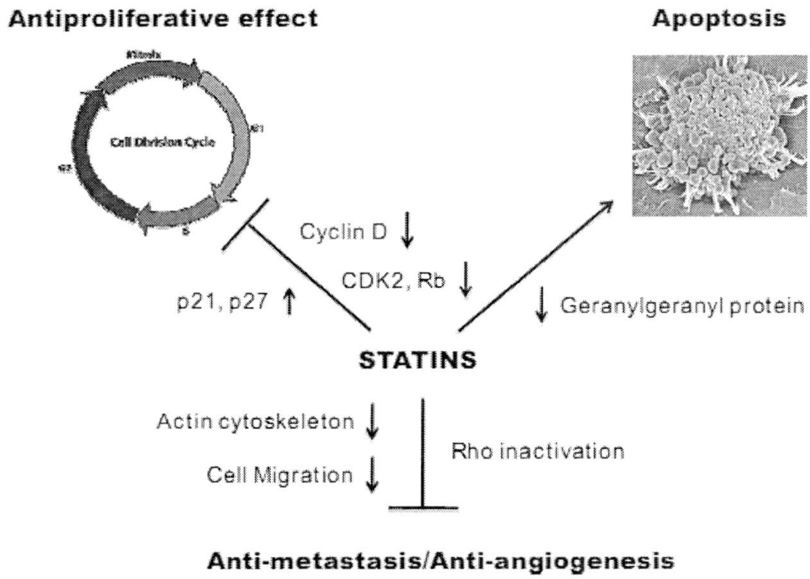

Figure 2. Summary of the anticancer actions of statins.

Lovastatin treatment also inhibited migration of lymphoma [68], F3II mammary carcinoma [66] and melanoma cells [67]. Similarly, simvastatin and cerivastatin reduced migration of human monocytic THP-1 [64] and endothelial [61] cells, respectively. Lovastatin was shown to reduce invasiveness of lymphoma cells [68], human glioma cells [69], melanoma cells [67] and NIH-3T3 [70] cells in matrigel. Cerivastatin reduced the invasiveness of a highly metastatic breast cancer cell line [71]. Fluvastatin was also shown to inhibit invasiveness of pancreatic cancer cells, colon and breast cancer cells [72].

The antimetastatic action of statins has also been confirmed *in vivo*. Lovastatin treatment was shown to reduce metastatic dissemination to the lungs in mice with established tumors of F311 mammary carcinoma cells [66]. Also, colon-derived MCA-26 cancer cells induced less liver metastasis in lovastatin treated mice, as compared to saline treatment in control mice. In addition, lovastatin significantly decreased the number of lymph nodes [67]. Fluvastatin treatment of mice injected with pancreatic tumor cells was reported to reduce the number and size of metastatic nodules in the liver [62]. In another study, when lovastatin and simvastatin were injected in B16F10 melanoma cells [67], and BN472 mammary adenocarcinoma cells [73], respectively, a decrease in lung metastasis was observed. A summary of the antitumor activity displayed by statins is summarized in Figure 2.

Mevalonate Pathway and Malignancy

Statins first attracted interest for cancer prevention as an unexpected finding of safety monitoring of clinical trials for statins and other lipid-lowering agents in preventing cardiovascular disease. The observation from randomized clinical trials indicated that the level of cholesterol in the blood was inversely correlated with cancer risk and cancer mortality and that long-term statin use showed a very favorable profile for cancer prevention [74]. As described previously, the mevalonate pathway is essential for the biosynthesis of cholesterol, ubiquinone and dolichol, which are required for the maintenance of cell membrane integrity, cell respiration and glycoprotein synthesis respectively. The other end products of mevalonate pathway include the downstream isoprenoids, farnesyl pyrophosphate (FPP) and geranylgeranyl pyrophosphate (GGPP). Isoprenoids are lipid moieties that are added to various proteins, such G-proteins and small GTPases subunits Ras, Rho and Rab during post-translational modification (prenylation) and anchor these proteins to the cell membrane [75, 76]. In the normal cells, HMGCoA reductase is subjected to complex feedback regulation at the transcriptional, translational and post-translational levels by both sterol and non-sterol products of the mevalonate pathway. In contrast, various types of tumor cells are resistant to sterol-dependent negative feedback [2, 26, 77]. Post-translational prenylation by FPP or GGPP is essential for small G-protein (Ras, Rho and Rab) function such as cell growth, proliferation, differentiation and migration. The inhibitory effects of statins are summarized in Figure 3.

Ras is activated by a very wide spectrum of extracellular stimuli (hormones, cytokines, growth factors, neurotransmitters, extracellular matrix components). Once activated, Ras communicates with the number of downstream targets involved in cell proliferation and function. Two of the major targets activated by Ras are the PI3K/PDK/Akt pathway and the Raf/MEK/ERK pathways, which are involved in cell cycle progression, survival, proliferation, migration and gene transcription. The C-terminus of Ras/Rho GTPases contains a region called CAAX in normal cells and CVLS in human H-Ras, CVVM in N-Ras and CIIM in K-Ras in malignant cells where FPP or GGPP are transferred to farnesylate or geranylgeranylate proteins by farnesyl transferase and geranylgeranyl transferase, respectively. CAAX prenylation is important for proper subcellular protein trafficking as it provides the lipid anchor for membrane association of proteins [3, 78, 79]. Disruption of normal CAAX prenylation will significantly alter the intracellular localization and biological functions of Ras and Rho.

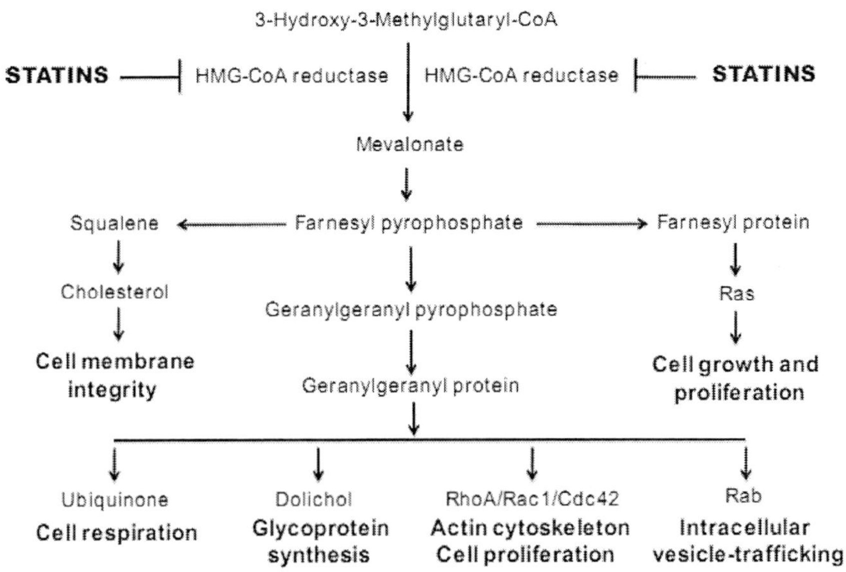

Figure 3. The inhibitory effects of statins on the mevalonate pathway and the synthesis of non-sterol intermediates.

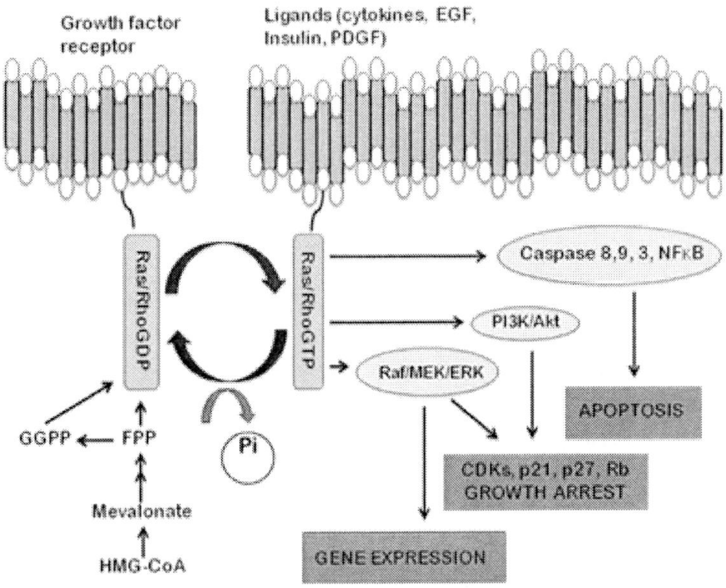

Figure 4. Summary of the inhibitory effects of statins on HMGCoA reductase and downstream mitogenic and survival pathways.

Ras mutations are commonly found in 90% of pancreas [80], 50% thyroid [81], 47% of colon, [82], 36% of melanoma [83], 30% of lung [84], and 44% of acute myeloid leukemia [85] cells. These findings strongly suggest that pharmacological interference with the mevalonate pathway may greatly impact Ras and Rho signaling and significantly inhibit tumor survival and metastasis. Statin inhibition of the Ras family member prenylation in malignant cells is believed to significantly attenuate proliferation, differentiation, angiogenesis and apoptosis, while reduced synthesis of other mevalonate pathway products such as cholesterol, dolichol and ubiquinone have also been implicated as potentially important compounds in mediating the anticancer effects of statins [86, 87]. Figure 4 summarizes the inhibitory effects of statins on HMGCoA reductase on intracellular mitogenic and survival pathways.

Epidemiological and Clinical Evidence

The earliest data that suggested a role for statins in cancer prevention was obtained from meta-analysis studies of patients receiving statin therapy to lowering blood cholesterol levels. Data obtained in Scandinavian Simvastatin Survival Study (4S) from patients with coronary heart disease and treated with simvastatin for a ten year period showed a strong correlation of statin use and a reduction in cancer incidence and mortality [88]. In contrast, results from the Cholesterol and Recurrent Events (CARE) study, which was a randomized double-blind trial showed an excess of breast cancer incidence among postmenopausal women treated with pravastatin as compared with placebo [89], while meta-analysis of other randomized trials demonstrated no association between the use of statins and the risk of fatal and nonfatal cancers [90, 91].

The first clinical study investigating the anticancer effect of statin was a phase I study in 88 patients with solid tumors (median age, 57 +/- 14 years) that were treated with 7-day courses of lovastatin at doses ranging from 2 to 45 mg/kg/day for a one month period [92]. The inhibitory effects of lovastatin on serum cholesterol and ubiquinone levels were monitored throughout the experimental period. Afterwards it was concluded that administration of 25 mg/kg lovastatin at a dose of daily for 7 consecutive days is well tolerated by cancer patients. However, a single patient did have recurrent high grade glioma [92]. The follow-up phase II study was conducted to determine the antitumor activity and to assess the toxicities and the pharmacokinetic features of lovastatin in patients with advanced measurable gastric adenocarcinoma. This phase II study was carried out in 16 patients using high-dose (35mg/kg/day) lovastatin treatment for a 7 day period. Results showed that anorexia was the most common adverse side effect [93]. However, two patients developed myalgia with elevated creatine kinase enzyme levels. These findings showed that when used in this dosage and schedule, lovastatin does not appear to be effective for patients with advanced gastric adenocarcinoma [93].

In another phase I/II trial examining the effects of lovastatin in patients with anaplastic astrocytoma and glioblastoma multiforme, patients were given high-dose lovastatin (30mg/kg/day) for 7 days with or without radiation [94]. Results showed that high doses lovastatin was well tolerated with concurrent radiation suggesting that central nervous system toxicity will not be a significant limiting factor as more selective farnesyl transferase inhibitors are tested as radiation sensitizers [94]. Other studies showed that treatment with low dose lovastatin in combination with standard therapeutic agents improved the survival of the patients [95-98], whereas long-term use of statins was associated with a reduced incidence in adenomatous colon polyps [99]. Taken together, these findings strongly suggested that further testing of the statins to fully evaluate the therapeutic effectiveness as potential anticancer drug at low doses when given alone or in combination with other chemotherapy is clearly needed.

Differential Effects of Individual Statins

The statin family is composed of nine unique compounds that are naturally derived or chemically synthesized. Mevastatin and lovastatin were the first active compounds isolated from fungi and modification of these natural statins led to the development of more potent semi-synthetic and synthetic statins, including simvastatin, pravastatin, fluvastatin, atorvastatin, cerivastatin, pitavastatin, and rosuvastatin [100]. There are currently seven individual statins on the market in the United States including: lovastatin (Mevacor, Merck Frosst); simvastatin (Zocor, Merck Frosst); atorvastatin (Lipitor, Pfizer); pravastatin (Pravachol, Bristol Meyer-Squibb); fluvastatin (Lescol, Novartis); rosuvastatin (Crestor, Astra Zeneca); and pitavastatin (Livalo, Kowa Company). Cerivastatin has been withdrawn from the market because it was found to cause severe side effects including fatal rhabdomyolysis [46].

The common structural feature of all statins is a side chain that exists either in a closed ring (inactive, lactone) or an open ring (active, acid) form. The closed ring structure undergoes activation *in vivo* by carboxyesterases in the plasma and liver. The open ring conformation of this drug blocks catalytically active HMG-CoA reductase by functioning as a molecular mimic of a reaction intermediate formed within the active site of the enzyme [6, 101]. Table 1 summarized the unique binding affinities, pharmacokinetics and bioavailability of the various members in the statin family of compounds [102-105]. Statins inhibit HMGCoA reductase by binding to the HMGCoA pocket with a common hydrophobic bulk, whereas the other substitute groups are positioned in a nonpolar groove [106]. Small differences in the chemical structure account for the different kinetic properties of the drug [6]. Furthermore, not all statins are equal, with individual statins displaying differential anticancer activity and potency.

Studies examining the antiproliferative activity of different statins on endothelial cells derived from human umbilical cord veins (HUVEC) showed that cerivastatin, simvastatin and fluvastatin caused a dose-dependent inhibition of endothelial cell growth, but the greatest growth inhibition was achieved with 0.1 μM cerivastatin, whereas higher treatment doses were required to obtain the same inhibition with simvastatin (2.5 μM) and fluvastatin (1 μM) [107]. Similar findings were observed in other studies using different cancer cell types [108, 109].

Additional studies show differential engulfing property of statins. Experiments examined the effects of 50 μM of hydrophobic, atorvastatin, lovastatin and simvastatin or 50 μM of hydrophilic, pravastatin on phagocytic index of peripheral white blood cells obtained from healthy normal individuals [110]. Results showed that only cells exposed to lovastatin, atorvastatin or simvastatin displayed a dose-responsive increase, whereas pravastatin treatment had no effect on white blood cell phagocytic index [110]. In other experiments, the antiproliferative effects of atorvastatin, lovastatin and simvastatin, and fluvastatin on human endothelial cells were compared and these four compounds displayed a wide range growth inhibiting potency [111].

In anti-inflammatory studies examining the differential effects of hydrophilic pravastatin and hydrophobic simvastatin on colon cancer cell-induced cytokine secretion by peripheral blood mononuclear cells, secretion of the pro-inflammatory cytokines IL-1β and IFNγ and that of the anti-inflammatory cytokines IL-1ra and IL-10 by colon cancer cells was decreased by simvastatin treatment, but not pravastatin [112].

Table 1. Chemical and HMGCoA reductase (HMGCoAR) binding characteristics of individual statins

Statin	Source	Lipophilic	Form	Bioavailability (%)	Ki HMGCoAR (nM)	IC_{50} (nM)
Lovastatin	Fungi	Yes	Lactone	<5	0.6 [36]	20 [40]
Simvastatin	Fungi	Yes	Lactone	<5	0.12 [36]	18.1 [46]
Pravastatin	Fungi (modified)	No	Acid	17	2.3 [36]	55.1 [46]
Fluvastatin	Synthetic	Yes	Acid	24	0.3 [36]	17.9 [46]
Atorvastatin	Synthetic	Yes	Acid	14	NA	15.2 [46]
Cerivastatin	Synthetic	Yes	Acid	60	1.3 [45]	13.1 [46]
Rosuvastatin	Synthetic	No	Acid	NA	0.1 [46]	11.8 [46]
Pitavastatin	Synthetic	Yes	Acid	NA	1.7 [47]	6.8 [47]

Treatment with simvastatin, but not pravastatin was also shown to inhibit colon cancer cell proliferation, and suggest that simvastatin appears to inhibit inflammation-induced colon cancer proliferation by altering the ratio between pro- and anti-inflammatory cytokines [112]. In another study by these same investigators, the effect of three hydrophobic statins - atorvastatin, lovastatin and simvastatin on the production of IL-1β, IL-1ra, IL-2, IL-6 and IFN-γ by peripheral blood mononuclear cells was examined. Results showed that lovastatin and simvastatin inhibited, whereas atorvastatin had no effect on IL-1β, demonstrating that different hydrophobic statins display differential anti-inflammatory potencies [113].

The effects of different statins were also tested on the viability of cultured rat pulmonary vein endothelial cells. Lovastatin, simvastatin, atorvastatin, fluvastatin and cerivastatin, which are hydrophobic statins, markedly reduced cell viability associated with DNA fragmentation, DNA laddering and activation of caspase-3, suggesting apoptotic cell death. Pravastatin, which is a hydrophilic statin, however, did not induce cell apoptosis. Apoptosis induced by hydrophobic statins was associated with activation of apoptosis-related intracellular signal transduction systems; attenuation of localization of RhoA to the membrane, induction of Rac1, and increase in phosphorylation of c-Jun N-terminal kinase and c-Jun. Endothelial cell apoptosis is underlying the improvement of the endothelial dysfunction with hydrophobic statins [114]. These studies suggest that the anticancer effects of individual statin are mediated by different intracellular signaling mechanisms.

Statin Use in Combination Therapy

It is now appreciated that anticancer chemotherapy is most effective when multiple drugs with complimentary mechanisms of action are given in combination. Combination chemotherapy optimizes the effectiveness of each drug to bring about a complimentary and synergistic therapeutic response, while at the same time reducing toxic adverse side effects associated with high dose monotherapy. Various investigations have shown that combined low dose treatment with complimentary chemotherapeutic agents displays significantly enhance anticancer effects, as compared to that observed from individual treatments alone [115].

Statin and Prenylation Inhibitor Combination Therapy: Statins act to block the mevalonate pathway by inhibiting HMGCoA reductase and subsequent isoprenylation of Ras family proteins, which is required for the anchoring of these proteins to the interior of the plasma membrane, and attenuate their activation and downstream mitogenic signaling [3]. Prenyl transferases are the enzymes responsible for attaching the prenyl groups to Ras proteins [116]. Specifically, members of the Ras family can be prenylated by either farnesyl transferases or geranylgeranyl transferases [117]. Farnesyl transferase inhibitors block the farnesylation of Ras and other members of the Ras family and treatment with these agents has been shown to inhibit the growth several types of tumor cells that are characterized by having Ras overexpression [118, 119]. Farnesyl transferase inhibitors have also been shown to suppress vascular endothelial growth factor (VEGF) expression in mice and reduced angiogenesis [120, 121]. However, the anticancer effects of farnesyl transferase inhibitors has been found to be somewhat limited because some mutated forms of Ras, such as N-Ras and K-Ras, undergo geranylgeranylation when the availability of farnesyl molecules is limited, and as such, tumor cells expressing high levels of N- and K-Ras mutation levels show response to treatment with farnesyl transferase inhibitors. In contrast, H-Ras does not undergo geranylgeranylation and tumor cells characterized by H-Ras mutation respond very well to farnesyl transferase inhibitors. RhoB is also a member of the Ras family and similar to Ras, RhoB also undergoes farnesylated and geranylgeranylated. Treatment with farnesyl transfer inhibitors has been shown to be effective in reducing farnesylated RhoB levels and tumor cell growth [122]. However, RhoB in leukemia cells exposed to farnesyl transfer inhibitors may undergo alternative geranylgeranylation and escape the anticancer effects of these drugs [3].

Studies have shown that combined treatment of statins with prenylation inhibitors results in a synergistic antiproliferative effect because of the complimentary actions of statins decreasing the pool of isoprenyl subunits in the cell, while prenylation inhibitors decrease transfer of any isoprenyl units to the proteins [3]. Combined treatment of statins with inhibitors of either farnesyl or geranylgeranyl transferase has been shown to synergistically inhibit tumor cell growth and survival [117, 123]. However, combination treatment with statins and geranylgeranyl transferase inhibitors is more effective in suppressing growth in tumor cells capable of escaping from the anticancer effects of farnesyl transferase inhibition alone, as is the case in tumor cells characterized by N-Ras, K-Ras and RhoB mutations [117, 123]. Statins have also been shown to decrease the geranylgeranylation of proteins like Rac1 and Rap1 [124, 125]. Combined treatment lovastatin and the geranylgeranyl transferase inhibitor, GGTI-2Z, has been shown to act synergistically to inhibit the growth of STS-26T malignant peripheral nerve sheath tumor cells [116]. Combined treatment with these agents was found to induce cell cycle arrest in G0/G1 [116]. Furthermore, other studies showed that autophagy also contributes for anticancer activity of this combination in MCF10.DCIS of human breast carcinoma and 1c1c7 murine hepatoma cells [116]. Cerivastatin and simvastatin have also been shown to induce autophagy in rhabdomyosarcoma cells [126].

Statins and γ-Tocotrienol Combination Therapy: γ-Tocotrienol is a member of the vitamin E family of compounds that displays potent anticancer activity [115, 127-131]. The anticancer effects of γ-tocotrienol is mediated in part through its action to induce the posttranscriptional down regulation of HMGCoA reductase [132]. Specifically, tocotrienols appear to reduce HMGCoA reductase activity by triggering both the retention of sterol regulatory element binding proteins (SREBP) on the endoplasmic reticulum and the degradation of HMGCoA reductase, thereby inducing the reduction of both mRNA and protein HMGCoA reductase levels [133]. In contrast, statins are competitive inhibitors of HMGCoA reductase and act to directly inhibit HMGCoA reductase activity. This effect of statins causes a reduction in cholesterol the negative feedback and subsequently induces SREBP cleavage and inhibits HMGCoA reductase degradation, resulting in an increase in both mRNA and protein HMGCoA reductase expression [133]. Since statins and γ-tocotrienol suppress HMGCoA reductase activity through independent mechanisms, there combined use was found to produce synergistic anticancer effects [134-136]. Results showed that treatment 2-8 μM simvastatin, lovastatin or mevastatin alone significantly inhibited, whereas treatment with high doses of pravastatin alone had no effect on EGF-dependent +SA mammary tumor cell growth [136]. Combined treatment with a subeffective doses (0.25 μM) of simvastatin, lovastatin or mevastatin with subeffective doses (0.25-2.0 μM) of γ-tocotrienol resulted in a synergistic inhibition of +SA cell growth [136]. These findings may have very important clinical implications in that combined low dose statin and γ-tocotrienol treatment may not only provide synergistic anticancer activity in the treatment of breast cancer, but also may be devoid of the adverse side effects and severe myotoxicity that is associated with high dose statin use.

Subsequent studies showed that this combination treatments caused a marked suppression in the activity of mitogenic signaling proteins including phosphorylated (activated) p44 MAPK, p54/46 JNK, p38 and Akt [136] and these effects were associated with cell cycle arrest in G1 phase [134]. Cell cycle analysis by flow cytometry showed that combined γ-tocotrienol and statin treatment induced cell cycle arrest without inducing apoptosis [134]. These findings are in agreement with previous studies that showed that similar treatments with statins and γ-tocotrienol were found to be cytostatic, but not cytotoxic to these cells [136].

Furthermore, these cytostatic effects were associated with a large decrease in the relative levels of cyclin D1, CDK2, and hyperphosphorylated Rb protein, and a corresponding increase in p27 levels [134]. Since similar effects were observed when γ-tocotrienol was combined with simvastatin, lovastatin, mevastatin, or pravastatin; these effects appear to be common to all statins and not a unique characteristic displayed by an individual statin family member. Combined statin and tocotrienol treatment was also found to induce a relatively large reduction in cyclin D1 expression in malignant +SA mammary epithelial cells [134]. Active cyclin D1-CDK4/6 and cyclin E-CDK2 complexes sequentially phosphorylate and inactivate the Rb protein to initiate E2F dependent transcription, a requirement for progression into S-phase, and combined γ-tocotrienol and statin treatment resulted in a marked reduction in CDK2 levels, and a reduction in Rb phosphorylation in +SA mammary tumor cells [134].

Experimental results also showed that the growth inhibitory affects of combined low dose statin and γ-tocotrienol treatment on +SA mammary tumor cells are directly related to suppression in HMGCoA reductase activity [135]. Specially, combined treatment with these agents resulted in a significant inhibition in +SA cell growth, and corresponding decrease in total HMGCoA reductase, Rap1A and Rab6 prenylation, and MAPK signaling, and supplementation with mevalonate reversed these effects [135].

However, these studies also showed that the growth inhibitory effects resulting from treatment with a moderated dose (4 μM) of γ-tocotrienol is not dependent on a reduction in HMGCoA reductase activity because this treatment had little or no effect on protein prenylation and mevalonate supplementation did not reverse these antiproliferative effects [135]. These findings clearly demonstrate that the synergistic antiproliferative effects of combined low dose statin and γ-tocotrienol treatment result directly from an inhibition in HMGCoA reductase activity and subsequent suppression in mevalonate synthesis. Similarly, combined treatment of γ-tocotrienol with atorvastatin has also been shown to synergistically inhibit growth of colon cancer cells [137]. This combination decreased RhoA protein concentration in the cell membrane by inhibiting the geranylgeranylation of RhoA and caused cell cycle arrest.

Statins with NSAIDS Combination Therapy: Several studies have shown that the nonsteroidal anti-inflammatory drugs (NSAIDS) can be used not only as anti-inflammatory agents but also as anticancer drugs, particularly in colorectal cancer [138-140]. NSAIDS are the cyclooxygenase (COX) inhibitors and treatment with COX inhibitors has been shown to inhibit tumor cell growth, survival, angiogenesis and metastasis [141, 142]. NSAIDS also work through COX-independent mechanisms [143]. In a population based case control study, aspirin used in combination with atorvastatin and simvastatin reduced the risk of colorectal cancer by 62% if used for 5 or more years [144]. Furthermore, combined use of NSAIDS with statins was also found to lowers the risk of prostate cancer if used for 5 years [145]. Combined low dose treatment of celecoxib with atorvastatin increased tumor latency, and decreased tumor sized of PC-3 prostate cancer cells growth in nude male mice [146]. In the azoxymethane-induced colon carcinogenesis rat model, low dose combination of atorvastatin and celecoxib decreased the incidence of adenocarcinomas by 71% [147]. At present, the exact mechanism mediating the synergistic anticancer effects of combined low dose statin and NSAIDS is unknown.

Statins and Doxorubicin Combination Therapy: The P-glycoprotein inhibitory properties of statins is useful for its it use in combination treatment with other chemotherapeutic agents to treat drug resistance cancers [25]. P-glycoprotein is an efflux pump located on the surface of cell membranes, and cancer cells that overexpress P-glycoprotein characteristically display multidrug resistance [148].

Doxorubicin is an antibiotic and used in the chemotherapy of variety of cancers. Combined treatment of lovastatin and doxorubicin in resistant ovarian cancer cells was found to sensitize the cells to doxorubicin and potentiated its anticancer activity [148]. Combined treatment of lovastatin with doxorubicin significantly inhibited the growth of multidrug resistant SKOV3 cells. Simvastatin, atorvastatin and lovastatin were also found to inhibit P-glycoprotein activity in other types of cancer cells [149-151].

Statins and FOLFIRI Combination Therapy: In a recent Phase-II clinical study, combined treatment of simvastatin with conventional FLOFIRI chemotherapy significantly reduced the progression of the colorectal cancer [152]. FOLFIRI chemotherapy includes the administration of irinotecan, 5-fluorouracil and leucovorin and is used as a first line treatment against colorectal cancer. Since high dose statins therapy is associated with severe adverse side effects, researchers in this study used very low concentration of simvastatin in combination with FOLFIRI. Combination resulted in a positive patient outcome, with no increased toxicity related to addition of simvastatin [152].

Statins and Tumor Biomarkers

Prostate specific antigen (PSA) is present in the serum of healthy men, but levels of this protein are usually significantly increased in prostate cancer patients. As such, PSA screening has become a useful tool for the early diagnosis of prostate cancer. Long term statin use has been shown to reduce the risk of advanced prostate cancer in men [153, 154]. One study reported that long term use of statins decreased the PSA levels by 42% [155]. However, the role of statin-induced reductions in PSA levels in reducing the risk of advanced prostate cancer is unclear [156]. Furthermore, reduced PSA levels resulting from statin use might also indicate a false negative result during prostate cancer screening. Further studies are needed to understand the direct relationship between statin use and PSA levels in men.

Conclusion

Although statins were initially developed as a treatment to lower high circulating cholesterol levels, it is now clearly evident that these agents have significant potential as anticancer agents. The inhibitory effect of statins on the mevalonate pathway is now understood to have a significant impact in attenuating many of the processes involved in tumor cell development, growth, and progression. The research findings highlighted in this present review not only demonstrate the effectiveness and potency of statins as anticancer agents, but also illustrate the tumor-selective nature of these agents. Since combination therapy of statins with other chemotherapeutic agents results not only in an enhanced therapeutic response, but also requires significantly lower treatment doses to suppress cancer cell growth and survival, an additional benefit that can be realized as in corresponding reduction in adverse side effects and toxicity characteristically associated with high-dose chemotherapy.

References

[1] Goldstein JL, Brown MS: Regulation of the mevalonate pathway. *Nature* 343, 425-430, 1990.

[2] Mo H, Elson CE: Studies of the isoprenoid-mediated inhibition of mevalonate synthesis applied to cancer chemotherapy and chemoprevention. *Exp. Biol. Med. (Maywood)* 229, 567-585, 2004.

[3] Graaf MR, Richel DJ, van Noorden CJ, Guchelaar HJ: Effects of statins and farnesyltransferase inhibitors on the development and progression of cancer. *Cancer Treat. Rev.* 30, 609-641, 2004.

[4] Stossel TP: The discovery of statins. *Cell* 134, 903-905, 2008.

[5] Endo A: A historical perspective on the discovery of statins. *Proc. Jpn. Acad. Ser. B. Phys. Biol. Sci.* 86, 484-493, 2010.

[6] Istvan ES, Deisenhofer J: Structural mechanism for statin inhibition of HMG-CoA reductase. *Science* 292, 1160-1164, 2001.

[7] Schachter M: Chemical, pharmacokinetic and pharmacodynamic properties of statins: an update. *Fundam. Clin. Pharmacol.* 19, 117-125, 2005.

[8] Stancu C, Sima A: Statins: mechanism of action and effects. *J. Cell Mol. Med.* 5, 378-387, 2001.

[9] Castellano F, Bruscalupi G, Columba S, Di Croce L, Trentalance A, Augusti-Tocco G: Characterization of the response of growth and differentiation to lipoproteins and agents affecting cholesterol metabolism in murine neuroblastoma cells. *Int. J. Dev. Neurosci.* 12, 77-84, 1994.

[10] Soma MR, Pagliarini P, Butti G, Paoletti R, Paoletti P, Fumagalli R: Simvastatin, an inhibitor of cholesterol biosynthesis, shows a synergistic effect with N,N'-bis(2-chloroethyl)-N-nitrosourea and beta-interferon on human glioma cells. *Cancer Res.* 52, 4348-4355, 1992.

[11] Melichar B, Ferrandina G, Verschraegen CF, Loercher A, Abbruzzese JL, Freedman RS: Growth inhibitory effects of aromatic fatty acids on ovarian tumor cell lines. *Clin. Cancer Res.* 4, 3069-3076, 1998.

[12] Koyuturk M, Ersoz M, Altiok N: Simvastatin induces proliferation inhibition and apoptosis in C6 glioma cells via c-jun N-terminal kinase. *Neurosci. Lett.* 370, 212-217, 2004.

[13] Kamigaki M, Sasaki T, Serikawa M, Inoue M, Kobayashi K, Itsuki H, Minami T, Yukutake M, Okazaki A, Ishigaki T, Ishii Y, Kosaka K, Chayama K: Statins induce apoptosis and inhibit proliferation in cholangiocarcinoma cells. *Int. J. Oncol.* 39, 561-568, 2011.

[14] Keyomarsi K, Sandoval L, Band V, Pardee AB: Synchronization of tumor and normal cells from G1 to multiple cell cycles by lovastatin. *Cancer Res.* 51, 3602-3609, 1991.

[15] Rao S, Lowe M, Herliczek TW, Keyomarsi K: Lovastatin mediated G1 arrest in normal and tumor breast cells is through inhibition of CDK2 activity and redistribution of p21 and p27, independent of p53. *Oncogene* 17, 2393-2402, 1998.

[16] Janosi J, Sebestyen A, Bocsi J, Barna G, Nagy K, Valyi-Nagy I, Kopper L: Mevastatin-induced apoptosis and growth suppression in U266 myeloma cells. *Anticancer Res.* 24, 1817-1822, 2004.

[17] Weis M, Heeschen C, Glassford AJ, Cooke JP: Statins have biphasic effects on angiogenesis. *Circulation* 105, 739-745, 2002.

[18] Fouty BW, Rodman DM: Mevastatin can cause G1 arrest and induce apoptosis in pulmonary artery smooth muscle cells through a p27Kip1-independent pathway. *Circ Res.* 92, 501-509, 2003.

[19] Hoque A, Chen H, Xu XC: Statin induces apoptosis and cell growth arrest in prostate cancer cells. *Cancer Epidemiol. Biomarkers Prev.* 17, 88-94, 2008.

[20] Sebti SM, Tkalcevic GT, Jani JP: Lovastatin, a cholesterol biosynthesis inhibitor, inhibits the growth of human H-ras oncogene transformed cells in nude mice. *Cancer Commun.* 3, 141-147, 1991.

[21] Iishi H, Tatsuta M, Baba M, Yano H, Sakai N, Uehara H, Nakaizumi A: ras p21 Isoprenylation inhibition induces flat colon tumors in Wistar rats. *Dis. Colon. Rectum.* 43, 70-75, 2000.

[22] Matar P, Rozados VR, Roggero EA, Scharovsky OG: Lovastatin inhibits tumor growth and metastasis development of a rat fibrosarcoma. *Cancer Biother. Radiopharm.* 13, 387-393, 1998.

[23] Narisawa T, Morotomi M, Fukaura Y, Hasebe M, Ito M, Aizawa R: Chemoprevention by pravastatin, a 3-hydroxy-3-methylglutaryl-coenzyme A reductase inhibitor, of N-methyl-N-nitrosourea-induced colon carcinogenesis in F344 rats. *Jpn. J. Cancer Res.* 87, 798-804, 1996.

[24] Narisawa T, Fukaura Y, Tanida N, Hasebe M, Ito M, Aizawa R: Chemopreventive efficacy of low dose of pravastatin, an HMG-CoA reductase inhibitor, on 1,2-dimethylhydrazine-induced colon carcinogenesis in ICR mice. *Tohoku J. Exp. Med.* 180, 131-138, 1996.

[25] Martirosyan A, Clendening JW, Goard CA, Penn LZ: Lovastatin induces apoptosis of ovarian cancer cells and synergizes with doxorubicin: potential therapeutic relevance. *BMC Cancer* 10, 1-13, 2010.

[26] Wong WW, Dimitroulakos J, Minden MD, Penn LZ: HMG-CoA reductase inhibitors and the malignant cell: the statin family of drugs as triggers of tumor-specific apoptosis. *Leukemia* 16, 508-519, 2002.

[27] Macaulay RJ, Wang W, Dimitroulakos J, Becker LE, Yeger H: Lovastatin-induced apoptosis of human medulloblastoma cell lines in vitro. *J. Neurooncol.* 42, 1-11, 1999.

[28] Van de Donk NW, Kamphuis MM, Lokhorst HM, Bloem AC: The cholesterol lowering drug lovastatin induces cell death in myeloma plasma cells. *Leukemia* 16, 1362-1371, 2002.

[29] Shibata MA, Ito Y, Morimoto J, Otsuki Y: Lovastatin inhibits tumor growth and lung metastasis in mouse mammary carcinoma model: a p53-independent mitochondrial-mediated apoptotic mechanism. *Carcinogenesis* 25, 1887-1898, 2004.

[30] Rubins JB, Greatens T, Kratzke RA, Tan AT, Polunovsky VA, Bitterman P: Lovastatin induces apoptosis in malignant mesothelioma cells. *Am. J. Respir. Crit. Care Med.* 157, 1616-1622, 1998.

[31] Shipman CM, Croucher PI, Russell RG, Helfrich MH, Rogers MJ: The bisphosphonate incadronate (YM175) causes apoptosis of human myeloma cells in vitro by inhibiting the mevalonate pathway. *Cancer Res.* 58, 5294-5297, 1998.

[32] Marcelli M, Cunningham GR, Haidacher SJ, Padayatty SJ, Sturgis L, Kagan C, Denner L: Caspase-7 is activated during lovastatin-induced apoptosis of the prostate cancer cell line LNCaP. *Cancer Res.* 58, 76-83, 1998.

[33] Marcelli M, Cunningham GR, Walkup M, He Z, Sturgis L, Kagan C, Mannucci R, Nicoletti I, Teng B, Denner L: Signaling pathway activated during apoptosis of the prostate cancer cell line LNCaP: overexpression of caspase-7 as a new gene therapy strategy for prostate cancer. *Cancer Res.* 59, 382-390, 1999.

[34] Muller C, Bockhorn AG, Klusmeier S, Kiehl M, Roeder C, Kalthoff H, Koch OM: Lovastatin inhibits proliferation of pancreatic cancer cell lines with mutant as well as with wild-type K-ras oncogene but has different effects on protein phosphorylation and induction of apoptosis. *Int. J. Oncol.* 12, 717-723, 1998.

[35] Choi JW, Jung SE: Lovastatin-induced proliferation inhibition and apoptosis in C6 glial cells. *J. Pharmacol. Exp. Ther.* 289, 572-579, 1999.

[36] Sumi S, Beauchamp RD, Townsend CM, Jr., Uchida T, Murakami M, Rajaraman S, Ishizuka J, Thompson JC: Inhibition of pancreatic adenocarcinoma cell growth by lovastatin. *Gastroenterology* 103, 982-989, 1992.

[37] Dimitroulakos J, Yeger H: HMG-CoA reductase mediates the biological effects of retinoic acid on human neuroblastoma cells: lovastatin specifically targets P-glycoprotein-expressing cells. *Nat. Med.* 2, 326-333, 1996.

[38] Bouterfa HL, Sattelmeyer V, Czub S, Vordermark D, Roosen K, Tonn JC: Inhibition of Ras farnesylation by lovastatin leads to downregulation of proliferation and migration in primary cultured human glioblastoma cells. *Anticancer Res.* 20, 2761-2771, 2000.

[39] Clutterbuck RD, Millar BC, Powles RL, Newman A, Catovsky D, Jarman M, Millar JL: Inhibitory effect of simvastatin on the proliferation of human myeloid leukaemia cells in severe combined immunodeficient (SCID) mice. *Br. J. Haematol.* 102, 522-527, 1998.

[40] Dimitroulakos J, Ye LY, Benzaquen M, Moore MJ, Kamel-Reid S, Freedman MH, Yeger H, Penn LZ: Differential sensitivity of various pediatric cancers and squamous

cell carcinomas to lovastatin-induced apoptosis: therapeutic implications. *Clin. Cancer Res.* 7, 158-167, 2001.

[41] Wong WW, Tan MM, Xia Z, Dimitroulakos J, Minden MD, Penn LZ: Cerivastatin triggers tumor-specific apoptosis with higher efficacy than lovastatin. *Clin. Cancer Res.* 7, 2067-2075, 2001.

[42] Yanae M, Tsubaki M, Satou T, Itoh T, Imano M, Yamazoe Y, Nishida S: Statin-induced apoptosis via the suppression of ERK1/2 and Akt activation by inhibition of the geranylgeranyl-pyrophosphate biosynthesis in glioblastoma. *J. Exp. Clin. Cancer Res.* 30, 74, 2011.

[43] Dimitroulakos J, Thai S, Wasfy GH, Hedley DW, Minden MD, Penn LZ: Lovastatin induces a pronounced differentiation response in acute myeloid leukemias. *Leuk. Lymphoma* 40, 167-178, 2000.

[44] Koyuturk M, Ersoz M, Altiok N: Simvastatin induces apoptosis in human breast cancer cells: p53 and estrogen receptor independent pathway requiring signalling through JNK. *Cancer Lett.* 250, 220-228, 2007.

[45] Fromigue O, Hay E, Modrowski D, Bouvet S, Jacquel A, Auberger P, Marie PJ: RhoA GTPase inactivation by statins induces osteosarcoma cell apoptosis by inhibiting p42/p44-MAPKs-Bcl-2 signaling independently of BMP-2 and cell differentiation. *Cell Death Differ.* 13, 1845-1856, 2006.

[46] Dulak J, Jozkowicz A: Anti-angiogenic and anti-inflammatory effects of statins: relevance to anti-cancer therapy. *Curr. Cancer Drug Targets* 5, 579-594, 2005.

[47] Holash J, Maisonpierre PC, Compton D, Boland P, Alexander CR, Zagzag D, Yancopoulos GD, Wiegand SJ: Vessel cooption, regression, and growth in tumors mediated by angiopoietins and VEGF. *Science* 284, 1994-1998, 1999.

[48] Brouet A, Sonveaux P, Dessy C, Moniotte S, Balligand JL, Feron O: Hsp90 and caveolin are key targets for the proangiogenic nitric oxide-mediated effects of statins. *Circ. Res.* 89, 866-873, 2001.

[49] Miura S, Matsuo Y, Saku K: Simvastatin suppresses coronary artery endothelial tube formation by disrupting Ras/Raf/ERK signaling. *Atherosclerosis* 175, 235-243, 2004.

[50] Tang D, Park HJ, Georgescu SP, Sebti SM, Hamilton AD, Galper JB: Simvastatin potentiates tumor necrosis factor alpha-mediated apoptosis of human vascular endothelial cells via the inhibition of the geranylgeranylation of RhoA. *Life Sci.* 79, 1484-1492, 2006.

[51] Park HJ, Kong D, Iruela-Arispe L, Begley U, Tang D, Galper JB: 3-hydroxy-3-methylglutaryl coenzyme A reductase inhibitors interfere with angiogenesis by inhibiting the geranylgeranylation of RhoA. *Circ. Res.* 91, 143-150, 2002.

[52] Vincent L, Soria C, Mirshahi F, Opolon P, Mishal Z, Vannier JP, Soria J, Hong L: Cerivastatin, an inhibitor of 3-hydroxy-3-methylglutaryl coenzyme a reductase, inhibits endothelial cell proliferation induced by angiogenic factors in vitro and angiogenesis in in vivo models. *Arterioscler. Thromb. Vasc. Biol.* 22, 623-629, 2002.

[53] Feleszko W, Balkowiec EZ, Sieberth E, Marczak M, Dabrowska A, Giermasz A, Czajka A, Jakobisiak M: Lovastatin and tumor necrosis factor-alpha exhibit potentiated antitumor effects against Ha-ras-transformed murine tumor via inhibition of tumor-induced angiogenesis. *Int. J. Cancer* 81, 560-567, 1999.

[54] Elson CE, Peffley DM, Hentosh P, Mo H: Isoprenoid-mediated inhibition of mevalonate synthesis: potential application to cancer. *Proc. Soc. Exp. Biol. Med.* 221, 294-311, 1999.

[55] Yoshida Y, Kawata M, Katayama M, Horiuchi H, Kita Y, Takai Y: A geranylgeranyltransferase for rhoA p21 distinct from the farnesyltransferase for ras p21S. *Biochem. Biophys. Res. Commun.* 175, 720-728, 1991.

[56] Urbich C, Dernbach E, Zeiher AM, Dimmeler S: Double-edged role of statins in angiogenesis signaling. *Circ. Res.* 90, 737-744, 2002.

[57] Kureishi Y, Luo Z, Shiojima I, Bialik A, Fulton D, Lefer DJ, Sessa WC, Walsh K: The HMG-CoA reductase inhibitor simvastatin activates the protein kinase Akt and promotes angiogenesis in normocholesterolemic animals. *Nat. Med.* 6, 1004-1010, 2000.

[58] Rowinsky EK, Windle JJ, Von Hoff DD: Ras protein farnesyltransferase: A strategic target for anticancer therapeutic development. *J. Clin. Oncol.* 17, 3631-3652, 1999.

[59] Dimmeler S, Zeiher AM: Endothelial cell apoptosis in angiogenesis and vessel regression. *Circ. Res.* 87, 434-439, 2000.

[60] Laufs U, Fata VL, Liao JK: Inhibition of 3-hydroxy-3-methylglutaryl (HMG)-CoA reductase blocks hypoxia-mediated down-regulation of endothelial nitric oxide synthase. *J. Biol. Chem.* 272, 31725-31729, 1997.

[61] Vincent L, Chen W, Hong L, Mirshahi F, Mishal Z, Mirshahi-Khorassani T, Vannier JP, Soria J, Soria C: Inhibition of endothelial cell migration by cerivastatin, an HMG-CoA reductase inhibitor: contribution to its anti-angiogenic effect. *FEBS Lett.* 495, 159-166, 2001.

[62] Kusama T, Mukai M, Iwasaki T, Tatsuta M, Matsumoto Y, Akedo H, Inoue M, Nakamura H: 3-hydroxy-3-methylglutaryl-coenzyme a reductase inhibitors reduce human pancreatic cancer cell invasion and metastasis. *Gastroenterology* 122, 308-317, 2002.

[63] Ganne F, Vasse M, Beaudeux JL, Peynet J, Francois A, Mishal Z, Chartier A, Tobelem G, Vannier JP, Soria J, Soria C: Cerivastatin, an inhibitor of HMG-CoA reductase, inhibits urokinase/urokinase-receptor expression and MMP-9 secretion by peripheral blood monocytes--a possible protective mechanism against atherothrombosis. *Thromb. Haemost.* 84, 680-688, 2000.

[64] Wong B, Lumma WC, Smith AM, Sisko JT, Wright SD, Cai TQ: Statins suppress THP-1 cell migration and secretion of matrix metalloproteinase 9 by inhibiting geranylgeranylation. *J. Leukoc. Biol.* 69, 959-962, 2001.

[65] Mehta N, Hordines J, Sykes D, Doerr RJ, Cohen SA: Low density lipoproteins and Lovastatin modulate the organ-specific transendothelial migration of primary and metastatic human colon adenocarcinoma cell lines in vitro. *Clin. Exp. Metastasis* 16, 587-594, 1998.

[66] Alonso DF, Farina HG, Skilton G, Gabri MR, De Lorenzo MS, Gomez DE: Reduction of mouse mammary tumor formation and metastasis by lovastatin, an inhibitor of the mevalonate pathway of cholesterol synthesis. *Breast Cancer Res. Treat.* 50, 83-93, 1998.

[67] Jani JP, Specht S, Stemmler N, Blanock K, Singh SV, Gupta V, Katoh A: Metastasis of B16F10 mouse melanoma inhibited by lovastatin, an inhibitor of cholesterol biosynthesis. *Invasion Metastasis* 13, 314-324, 1993.

[68] Matar P, Rozados VR, Binda MM, Roggero EA, Bonfil RD, Scharovsky OG: Inhibitory effect of Lovastatin on spontaneous metastases derived from a rat lymphoma. *Clin. Exp. Metastasis* 17, 19-25, 1999.
[69] Prasanna P, Thibault A, Liu L, Samid D: Lipid metabolism as a target for brain cancer therapy: synergistic activity of lovastatin and sodium phenylacetate against human glioma cells. *J. Neurochem.* 66, 710-716, 1996.
[70] Wang IK, Lin-Shiau SY, Lin JK: Suppression of invasion and MMP-9 expression in NIH 3T3 and v-H-Ras 3T3 fibroblasts by lovastatin through inhibition of ras isoprenylation. *Oncology* 59, 245-254, 2000.
[71] Denoyelle C, Vasse M, Korner M, Mishal Z, Ganne F, Vannier JP, Soria J, Soria C: Cerivastatin, an inhibitor of HMG-CoA reductase, inhibits the signaling pathways involved in the invasiveness and metastatic properties of highly invasive breast cancer cell lines: an in vitro study. *Carcinogenesis* 22, 1139-1148, 2001.
[72] Kusama T, Mukai M, Iwasaki T, Tatsuta M, Matsumoto Y, Akedo H, Nakamura H: Inhibition of epidermal growth factor-induced RhoA translocation and invasion of human pancreatic cancer cells by 3-hydroxy-3-methylglutaryl-coenzyme a reductase inhibitors. *Cancer Res.* 61, 4885-4891, 2001.
[73] Kort WJ, Hulsmann WC, Stehman TE: Modulation of metastatic ability by inhibition of cholesterol synthesis. *Clin. Exp. Metastasis* 7, 517-523, 1989.
[74] Oliver MF: Might treatment of hypercholesterolaemia increase non-cardiac mortality? *Lancet* 337, 1529-1531, 1991.
[75] Zhang FL, Casey PJ: Protein prenylation: molecular mechanisms and functional consequences. *Annu. Rev. Biochem.* 65, 241-269, 1996.
[76] Fritz G: Targeting the mevalonate pathway for improved anticancer therapy. *Curr. Cancer Drug Targets* 9, 626-638, 2009.
[77] Houten SM, Frenkel J, Waterham HR: Isoprenoid biosynthesis in hereditary periodic fever syndromes and inflammation. *Cell Mol. Life Sci.* 60, 1118-1134, 2003.
[78] Siperstein MD: Cholesterol, cholesterogenesis and cancer. *Adv. Exp. Med. Biol.* 369, 155-166, 1995.
[79] Campbell PM, Der CJ: Oncogenic Ras and its role in tumor cell invasion and metastasis. *Semin. Cancer Biol.* 14, 105-114, 2004.
[80] Almoguera C, Shibata D, Forrester K, Martin J, Arnheim N, Perucho M: Most human carcinomas of the exocrine pancreas contain mutant c-K-ras genes. *Cell* 53, 549-554, 1988.
[81] Lemoine NR, Mayall ES, Wyllie FS, Williams ED, Goyns M, Stringer B, Wynford-Thomas D: High frequency of ras oncogene activation in all stages of human thyroid tumorigenesis. *Oncogene* 4, 159-164, 1989.
[82] Vogelstein B, Fearon ER, Hamilton SR, Kern SE, Preisinger AC, Leppert M, Nakamura Y, White R, Smits AM, Bos JL: Genetic alterations during colorectal-tumor development. *N. Engl. J. Med.* 319, 525-532, 1988.
[83] Ball NJ, Yohn JJ, Morelli JG, Norris DA, Golitz LE, Hoeffler JP: Ras mutations in human melanoma: a marker of malignant progression. *J. Invest. Dermatol.* 102, 285-290, 1994.
[84] Rodenhuis S, Slebos RJ, Boot AJ, Evers SG, Mooi WJ, Wagenaar SS, van Bodegom PC, Bos JL: Incidence and possible clinical significance of K-ras oncogene activation in adenocarcinoma of the human lung. *Cancer Res.* 48, 5738-5741, 1988.

[85] Janssen JW, Steenvoorden AC, Lyons J, Anger B, Bohlke JU, Bos JL, Seliger H, Bartram CR: RAS gene mutations in acute and chronic myelocytic leukemias, chronic myeloproliferative disorders, and myelodysplastic syndromes. *Proc. Natl. Acad. Sci. U S A* 84, 9228-9232, 1987.

[86] McCarty MF: Suppression of dolichol synthesis with isoprenoids and statins may potentiate the cancer-retardant efficacy of IGF-I down-regulation. *Med. Hypotheses* 56, 12-16, 2001.

[87] Wachtershauser A, Akoglu B, Stein J: HMG-CoA reductase inhibitor mevastatin enhances the growth inhibitory effect of butyrate in the colorectal carcinoma cell line Caco-2. *Carcinogenesis* 22, 1061-1067, 2001.

[88] Strandberg TE, Pyorala K, Cook TJ, Wilhelmsen L, Faergeman O, Thorgeirsson G, Pedersen TR, Kjekshus J: Mortality and incidence of cancer during 10-year follow-up of the Scandinavian Simvastatin Survival Study (4S). *Lancet* 364, 771-777, 2004.

[89] Sacks FM, Pfeffer MA, Moye LA, Rouleau JL, Rutherford JD, Cole TG, Brown L, Warnica JW, Arnold JM, Wun CC, Davis BR, Braunwald E: The effect of pravastatin on coronary events after myocardial infarction in patients with average cholesterol levels. Cholesterol and Recurrent Events Trial investigators. *N. Engl. J. Med.* 335, 1001-1009, 1996.

[90] Bjerre LM, LeLorier J: Do statins cause cancer? A meta-analysis of large randomized clinical trials. *Am. J. Med.* 110, 716-723, 2001.

[91] Downs JR, Clearfield M, Tyroler HA, Whitney EJ, Kruyer W, Langendorfer A, Zagrebelsky V, Weis S, Shapiro DR, Beere PA, Gotto AM: Air Force/Texas Coronary Atherosclerosis Prevention Study (AFCAPS/TEXCAPS): additional perspectives on tolerability of long-term treatment with lovastatin. *Am. J. Cardiol.* 87, 1074-1079, 2001.

[92] Thibault A, Samid D, Tompkins AC, Figg WD, Cooper MR, Hohl RJ, Trepel J, Liang B, Patronas N, Venzon DJ, Reed E, Myers CE: Phase I study of lovastatin, an inhibitor of the mevalonate pathway, in patients with cancer. *Clin. Cancer Res.* 2, 483-491, 1996.

[93] Kim WS, Kim MM, Choi HJ, Yoon SS, Lee MH, Park K, Park CH, Kang WK: Phase II study of high-dose lovastatin in patients with advanced gastric adenocarcinoma. *Invest. New Drugs* 19, 81-83, 2001.

[94] Larner J, Jane J, Laws E, Packer R, Myers C, Shaffrey M: A phase I-II trial of lovastatin for anaplastic astrocytoma and glioblastoma multiforme. *Am. J. Clin. Oncol.* 21, 579-583, 1998.

[95] Schmidt F, Groscurth P, Kermer M, Dichgans J, Weller M: Lovastatin and phenylacetate induce apoptosis, but not differentiation, in human malignant glioma cells. *Acta Neuropathol.* 101, 217-224, 2001.

[96] Kawata S, Yamasaki E, Nagase T, Inui Y, Ito N, Matsuda Y, Inada M, Tamura S, Noda S, Imai Y, Matsuzawa Y: Effect of pravastatin on survival in patients with advanced hepatocellular carcinoma. A randomized controlled trial. *Br. J. Cancer* 84, 886-891, 2001.

[97] Miller AC, Kariko K, Myers CE, Clark EP, Samid D: Increased radioresistance of EJras-transformed human osteosarcoma cells and its modulation by lovastatin, an inhibitor of p21ras isoprenylation. *Int. J. Cancer* 53, 302-307, 1993.

[98] Agarwal B, Rao CV, Bhendwal S, Ramey WR, Shirin H, Reddy BS, Holt PR: Lovastatin augments sulindac-induced apoptosis in colon cancer cells and potentiates chemopreventive effects of sulindac. *Gastroenterology* 117, 838-847, 1999.

[99] Siddiqui AA, Nazario H, Mahgoub A, Pandove S, Cipher D, Spechler SJ: The long-term use of statins is associated with a decreased incidence of adenomatous colon polyps. *Digestion* 79, 17-22, 2009.

[100] Corsini A, Maggi FM, Catapano AL: Pharmacology of competitive inhibitors of HMG-CoA reductase. *Pharmacol. Res.* 31, 9-27, 1995.

[101] Istvan ES,Palnitkar M, Buchanan SK, Deisenhofer J: Crystal structure of the catalytic portion of human HMGCoA reductase; insights into regulation of activity and catalysis. *EMBO J* 19, 819-830, 2000.

[102] Bischoff H, Angerbauer R, Bender J, Bischoff E, Faggiotto A, Petzinna D, Pfitzner J, Porter MC, Schmidt D, Thomas G: Cerivastatin: pharmacology of a novel synthetic and highly active HMG-CoA reductase inhibitor. *Atherosclerosis* 135, 119-130, 1997.

[103] McTaggart F, Buckett L, Davidson R, Holdgate G, McCormick A, Schneck D, Smith G, Warwick M: Preclinical and clinical pharmacology of Rosuvastatin, a new 3-hydroxy-3-methylglutaryl coenzyme A reductase inhibitor. *Am. J. Cardiol.* 87, 28B-32B, 2001.

[104] Kajinami K, Mabuchi H, Saito Y: NK-104: a novel synthetic HMG-CoA reductase inhibitor. *Expert. Opin. Investig Drugs* 9, 2653-2661, 2000.

[105] Olson RE, Rudney H: Biosynthesis of ubiquinone. *Vitam. Horm.* 40, 1-43, 1983.

[106] Liao JK, Laufs, U: Pleiotropic effects of statins: *Annu Rev Pharmacol Toxicol* 45, 89-118, 2005.

[107] Schaefer CA, Kuhlmann CR, Gast C, Weiterer S, Li F, Most AK, Neumann T, Backenkohler U, Tillmanns H, Waldecker B, Wiecha J, Erdogan A: Statins prevent oxidized low-density lipoprotein- and lysophosphatidylcholine-induced proliferation of human endothelial cells. *Vascul. Pharmacol.* 41, 67-73, 2004.

[108] Sato I, Ma L, Ikeda M, Morita I, Murota S: Simvastatin, a potent HMG-CoA reductase inhibitor, inhibits the proliferation of human and bovine endothelial cells in vitro. *J. Atheroscler. Thromb.* 4, 102-106, 1998.

[109] Negre-Aminou P, van Vliet AK, van Erck M, van Thiel GC, van Leeuwen RE, Cohen LH: Inhibition of proliferation of human smooth muscle cells by various HMG-CoA reductase inhibitors; comparison with other human cell types. *Biochim. Biophys. Acta* 1345, 259-268, 1997.

[110] Salman H, Bergman M, Djaldetti M, Bessler H: Hydrophobic but not hydrophilic statins enhance phagocytosis and decrease apoptosis of human peripheral blood cells in vitro. *Biomed. Pharmacother.* 62, 41-45, 2008.

[111] Muck AO, Seeger H, Wallwiener D: Class-specific pro-apoptotic effect of statins on human vascular endothelial cells. *Z. Kardiol.* 93, 398-402, 2004.

[112] Bergman M, Salman H, Djaldetti M, Bessler H: Statins as modulators of colon cancer cells induced cytokine secretion by human PBMC. *Vascul. Pharmacol.* 54, 88-92, 2011.

[113] Bessler H, Salman H, Bergman M, Straussberg R, Djaldetti M: In vitro effect of statins on cytokine production and mitogen response of human peripheral blood mononuclear cells. *Clin. Immunol.* 117, 73-77, 2005.

[114] Kaneta S, Satoh K, Kano S, Kanda M, Ichihara K: All hydrophobic HMG-CoA reductase inhibitors induce apoptotic death in rat pulmonary vein endothelial cells. *Atherosclerosis* 170, 237-243, 2003.

[115] Sylvester PW: Synergistic anticancer effects of combined gamma-tocotrienol with statin or receptor tyrosine kinase inhibitor treatment. *Genes Nutr.* 7, 63-74, 2012.

[116] Sane KM, Mynderse M, Lalonde DT, Dean IS, Wojtkowiak JW, Fouad F, Borch RF, Reiners JJ, Jr., Gibbs RA, Mattingly RR: A novel geranylgeranyl transferase inhibitor in combination with lovastatin inhibits proliferation and induces autophagy in STS-26T MPNST cells. *J. Pharmacol. Exp. Ther.* 333, 23-33, 2010.

[117] Konstantinopoulos PA, Karamouzis MV, Papavassiliou AG: Post-translational modifications and regulation of the RAS superfamily of GTPases as anticancer targets. *Nat. Rev. Drug Discov.* 6, 541-555, 2007.

[118] Sun J, Qian Y, Hamilton AD, Sebti SM: Ras CAAX peptidomimetic FTI 276 selectively blocks tumor growth in nude mice of a human lung carcinoma with K-Ras mutation and p53 deletion. *Cancer Res.* 55, 4243-4247, 1995.

[119] Rose WC, Lee FY, Fairchild CR, Lynch M, Monticello T, Kramer RA, Manne V: Preclinical antitumor activity of BMS-214662, a highly apoptotic and novel farnesyltransferase inhibitor. *Cancer Res.* 61, 7507-7517, 2001.

[120] Cox AD, Garcia AM, Westwick JK, Kowalczyk JJ, Lewis MD, Brenner DA, Der CJ: The CAAX peptidomimetic compound B581 specifically blocks farnesylated, but not geranylgeranylated or myristylated, oncogenic ras signaling and transformation. *J. Biol. Chem.* 269, 19203-19206, 1994.

[121] Rak J, Mitsuhashi Y, Bayko L, Filmus J, Shirasawa S, Sasazuki T, Kerbel RS: Mutant ras oncogenes upregulate VEGF/VPF expression: implications for induction and inhibition of tumor angiogenesis. *Cancer Res.* 55, 4575-4580, 1995.

[122] Lebowitz PF, Casey PJ, Prendergast GC, Thissen JA: Farnesyltransferase inhibitors alter the prenylation and growth-stimulating function of RhoB. *J. Biol. Chem.* 272, 15591-15594, 1997.

[123] Lerner EC, Zhang TT, Knowles DB, Qian Y, Hamilton AD, Sebti SM: Inhibition of the prenylation of K-Ras, but not H- or N-Ras, is highly resistant to CAAX peptidomimetics and requires both a farnesyltransferase and a geranylgeranyltransferase I inhibitor in human tumor cell lines. *Oncogene* 15, 1283-1288, 1997.

[124] Hamadmad SN, Hohl RJ: Lovastatin suppresses erythropoietin receptor surface expression through dual inhibition of glycosylation and geranylgeranylation. *Biochem. Pharmacol.* 74, 590-600, 2007.

[125] Kou R, Sartoretto J, Michel T: Regulation of Rac1 by simvastatin in endothelial cells: differential roles of AMP-activated protein kinase and calmodulin-dependent kinase kinase-beta. *J. Biol. Chem.* 284, 14734-14743, 2009.

[126] Araki M, Motojima K: Hydrophobic statins induce autophagy in cultured human rhabdomyosarcoma cells. *Biochem. Biophys. Res. Commun.* 367, 462-467, 2008.

[127] Sylvester PW, Theriault A: Role of tocotrienols in the prevention of cardiovascular disease and breast cancer. *Curr. Top Nutraceutical. Res.* 1, 121-136, 2003.

[128] Sylvester PW, Shah SJ: Mechanisms mediating the antiproliferative and apoptotic effects of vitamin E in mammary cancer cells. *Front. Biosci.* 10, 699-709, 2005.

[129] Sylvester PW, Kaddoumi A, Nazzal S, El Sayed KA: The value of tocotrienols in the prevention and treatment of cancer. *J. Am. Coll. Nutr.* 29, 324S-333S, 2010.

[130] Sylvester PW, Wali VB, Bachawal SV, Shirode AB, Ayoub NM, Akl MR: Tocotrienol combination therapy results in synergistic anticancer response. *Front. Biosci.* 17, 3183-3195, 2011.

[131] Sylvester PW: Synergistic anticancer effects of combined gamma-tocotrienol with statin or receptor tyrosine kinase inhibitor treatment. *Genes Nutr.* 2011.

[132] Parker RA, Pearce BC, Clark RW, Gordon DA, Wright JJ: Tocotrienols regulate cholesterol production in mammalian cells by post- transcriptional suppression of 3-hydroxy-3-methylglutaryl-coenzyme A reductase. *J. Biol. Chem.* 268, 11230-11238, 1993.

[133] Goldstein JL, DeBose-Boyd RA, Brown MS: Protein sensors for membrane sterols. *Cell* 124, 35-46, 2006.

[134] Wali VB, Bachawal SV, Sylvester PW: Combined treatment of gamma-tocotrienol with statins induce mammary tumor cell cycle arrest in G1. *Exp. Biol. Med. (Maywood)* 234, 639-650, 2009.

[135] Wali VB, Bachawal SV, Sylvester PW: Suppression in Mevalonate Synthesis Mediates Antitumor Effects of Combined Statin and gamma-Tocotrienol Treatment. *Lipids* 44, 925-934, 2009.

[136] Wali VB, Sylvester PW: Synergistic antiproliferative effects of gamma-tocotrienol and statin treatment on mammary tumor cells. *Lipids* 42, 1113-1123, 2007.

[137] Yang Z, Xiao H, Jin H, Koo PT, Tsang DJ, Yang CS: Synergistic actions of atorvastatin with gamma-tocotrienol and celecoxib against human colon cancer HT29 and HCT116 cells. *Int. J. Cancer* 126, 852-863, 2010.

[138] Rosenberg L, Palmer JR, Zauber AG, Warshauer ME, Stolley PD, Shapiro S: A hypothesis: nonsteroidal anti-inflammatory drugs reduce the incidence of large-bowel cancer. *J. Natl. Cancer Inst.* 83, 355-358, 1991.

[139] Thun MJ, Namboodiri MM, Calle EE, Flanders WD, Heath CW, Jr.: Aspirin use and risk of fatal cancer. *Cancer Res.* 53, 1322-1327, 1993.

[140] Muscat JE, Stellman SD, Wynder EL: Nonsteroidal antiinflammatory drugs and colorectal cancer. *Cancer* 74, 1847-1854, 1994.

[141] Tsujii M, Kawano S, DuBois RN: Cyclooxygenase-2 expression in human colon cancer cells increases metastatic potential. *Proc. Natl. Acad. Sci. U S A* 94, 3336-3340, 1997.

[142] Sheng H, Shao J, Morrow JD, Beauchamp RD, DuBois RN: Modulation of apoptosis and Bcl-2 expression by prostaglandin E2 in human colon cancer cells. *Cancer Res.* 58, 362-366, 1998.

[143] Grosch S, Maier TJ, Schiffmann S, Geisslinger G: Cyclooxygenase-2 (COX-2)-independent anticarcinogenic effects of selective COX-2 inhibitors. *J. Natl. Cancer Inst.* 98, 736-747, 2006.

[144] Hoffmeister M, Chang-Claude J, Brenner H: Individual and joint use of statins and low-dose aspirin and risk of colorectal cancer: a population-based case-control study. *Int. J. Cancer* 121, 1325-1330, 2007.

[145] Flick ED, Habel LA, Chan KA, Van Den Eeden SK, Quinn VP, Haque R, Orav EJ, Seeger JD, Sadler MC, Quesenberry CP, Jr., Sternfeld B, Jacobsen SJ, Whitmer RA, Caan BJ: Statin use and risk of prostate cancer in the California Men's Health Study cohort. *Cancer Epidemiol. Biomarkers Prev.* 16, 2218-2225, 2007.

[146] Zheng X, Cui XX, Avila GE, Huang MT, Liu Y, Patel J, Kong AN, Paulino R, Shih WJ, Lin Y, Rabson AB, Reddy BS, Conney AH: Atorvastatin and celecoxib inhibit prostate PC-3 tumors in immunodeficient mice. *Clin. Cancer Res.* 13, 5480-5487, 2007.

[147] Reddy BS, Wang CX, Kong AN, Khor TO, Zheng X, Steele VE, Kopelovich L, Rao CV: Prevention of azoxymethane-induced colon cancer by combination of low doses of atorvastatin, aspirin, and celecoxib in F 344 rats. *Cancer Res.* 66, 4542-4546, 2006.

[148] Stein WD: Kinetics of the multidrug transporter (P-glycoprotein) and its reversal. *Physiol. Rev.* 77, 545-590, 1997.

[149] Bogman K, Peyer AK, Torok M, Kusters E, Drewe J: HMG-CoA reductase inhibitors and P-glycoprotein modulation. *Br. J. Pharmacol.* 132, 1183-1192, 2001.

[150] Wang E, Casciano CN, Clement RP, Johnson WW: HMG-CoA reductase inhibitors (statins) characterized as direct inhibitors of P-glycoprotein. *Pharm. Res.* 18, 800-806, 2001.

[151] Sieczkowski E, Lehner C, Ambros PF, Hohenegger M: Double impact on p-glycoprotein by statins enhances doxorubicin cytotoxicity in human neuroblastoma cells. *Int. J. Cancer* 126, 2025-2035.

[152] Lee J, Jung KH, Park YS, Ahn JB, Shin SJ, Im SA, Oh do Y, Shin DB, Kim TW, Lee N, Byun JH, Hong YS, Park JO, Park SH, Lim HY, Kang WK: Simvastatin plus irinotecan, 5-fluorouracil, and leucovorin (FOLFIRI) as first-line chemotherapy in metastatic colorectal patients: a multicenter phase II study. *Cancer Chemother. Pharmacol.* 64, 657-663, 2009.

[153] Platz EA, Leitzmann MF, Visvanathan K, Rimm EB, Stampfer MJ, Willett WC, Giovannucci E: Statin drugs and risk of advanced prostate cancer. *J. Natl. Cancer Inst.* 98, 1819-1825, 2006.

[154] Murtola TJ, Tammela TL, Lahtela J, Auvinen A: Cholesterol-lowering drugs and prostate cancer risk: a population-based case-control study. *Cancer Epidemiol. Biomarkers Prev.* 16, 2226-2232, 2007.

[155] Cyrus-David MS, Weinberg A, Thompson T, Kadmon D: The effect of statins on serum prostate specific antigen levels in a cohort of airline pilots: a preliminary report. *J. Urol.* 173, 1923-1925, 2005.

[156] Hamilton RJ, Goldberg KC, Platz EA, Freedland SJ: The influence of statin medications on prostate-specific antigen levels. *J. Natl. Cancer Inst.* 100, 1511-1518, 2008.

In: Statins
Editors: Benedetta La Grua and Alessandro Molinelli
ISBN: 978-1-62081-367-6

Chapter V

Relevant Aspects of the Pleiotropic Properties and Review of Adverse Effects

***Jaime Gulín Dávila*[1,*], *Paloma Sempere Serrano*[1] *and Antonio García Sabina*[1]**
[1]Pharmacy Service, Lucus Augusti Hospital,
Lugo, Spain

Abstract

Statins are the most potent lipid-lowering agents available today in the pharmaceutical market. They are currently the drugs of choice for the treatment of hypercholesterolemia, several clinical trials have shown that statins substantially reduce cardiovascular morbidity and mortality in patients with and without existing coronary heart disease. Statins work by reducing cholesterol synthesis by inhibiting the enzyme HMG-CoA reductase.

The decrease in cholesterol levels is associated with increased expression of receptors of hepatocytes, with a greater extraction of plasma LDL-C and a lower diffusion of it into the tissues. In addition to its activity on LDL-C, statins increase levels of HDL-C and lead to a decrease in triglycerides.

These lipid-lowering activities must add a number of pleiotropic properties that together with the above make this group of drugs an important weapon for influencing the cardiovascular risk patient. We are in a family of substances with a good safety profile, but its potential toxicity is a fact that should not be ignored. The HMG-CoA reductase inhibitors may be associated with hepatotoxicity and myopathy, which normally do not occur, but in certain circumstances such as interactions, liver failure or differences in gene expression may manifest.

[*] Contact details: Jaime Gulín Dávila. C / San Cibrao s/n. 27004. Lugo (Spain). jaime.gulin.davila@sergas.es.

Introduction

Cardiovascular disease is undoubtedly the great epidemic of the 21st Century. Increasing life expectancy, especially in Western societies, and certain socio-cultural changes such as stress or the tendency to less healthy eating based on fast food has made coronary disease an important health issue.

High blood cholesterol levels markedly increase cardiovascular risk. Although the maintenance of adequate lipid profile should be based on a suitable diet, dietary measures are often insufficient and the patient has to resort to drugs. The use of lipid lowering drugs is even recommended in situations where cholesterol levels are normal in patients with a history of ischemic heart disease. It is important, therefore, that safe and effective drugs are available. Statins are both safe and effective.

Statins are a family of drugs that have revolutionized lipid-lowering therapy [1]. This new structural group was born in 1973, through the work of Endo [2], and was released in 1987 when Lovastatin was launched. Talking about statins means talking about molecules that greatly reduce plasma cholesterol levels; they are therefore drugs with a leading role in the treatment of cardiovascular disease.

Pharmacology

Brief Summary of the Pharmacological Properties

Mevastatin and lovastatin are two natural products derived from *Penicillium citrinum* and *Aspergillus terreus* respectively [2-4]. Their structure is similar to that of 3-hydroxy-3-methylglutaryl-coenzyme A (HMG-CoA), a precursor of mevalonic acid, which is essential for the synthesis of cholesterol [2]. Derivatives such as simvastatin and pravastatin were obtained from lovastatin, which demonstrated its ability to inhibit cholesterol synthesis. Subsequently fluvastatin, atorvastatin, rosuvastatin, and more recently pitavastatin were all synthesized [5].

Action Mechanism and Blood Cholesterol Lowering Activity

Statins have structural analogy with the HMGCoA metabolite (Figure 1), in this way they inhibit the HMGCoA reductase enzyme competitively and reversibly, blocking a limiting step in cholesterol synthesis. They behave as substances with high affinity for the enzyme, even higher than the natural substrate (approximately 10,000 times higher). Because of this activity, intracellular hepatic biosynthesis of cholesterol is reduced and intracellular deposit is decreased [5-7].

The intracellular concentration of LDL cholesterol (LDL-C) correlates inversely with the synthetic activity of plasma membrane receptors for LDL-C; the increase in number of these receptors increases extraction from the plasma not only of LDL-C, but also V-LDL; in this way, LDL-C cholesterol and that generated from the V-LDL cholesterol is reduced in the plasma [5-7].

It could be said that the lipid-lowering activity of statins is high; however, some differ from others. There is a wide range of possibilities in terms of cholesterol-lowering power: rosuvastatin and atorvastatin can reduce LDL-C in percentages above 50%, while lovastatin, fluvastatin and pravastatin, do not reach 35%.

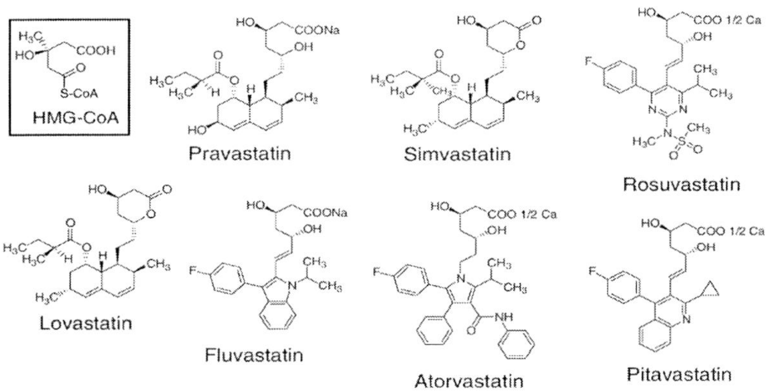

Figure 1. Structure of HMG-CoA and statins.

Table 1. Decrease of C-LDL levels with each statin

	Decrease =19%	Decrease 20-23%	Decrease 24-28%	Decrease 29-35%	Decrease 36-41%	Decrease 42-46%	Decrease 47-50%	Decrease 51-54%	Decrese 55-57%	Decrease 58-62%
Atorvastatin				5 mg	10 mg	20 mg	40 mg	80 mg		
Fluvastatin			20 mg	40 mg						
Lovastatin		10 mg	20 mg	40 mg						
Pitavastatin				1 mg	2 mg	4 mg				
Pravastatin	5 mg	10 mg	20 mg	40 mg						
Rosuvastatin					5 mg	10 mg	20 mg	10-20 mg	40 mg	80 mg
Simvastatin		5 mg	10 mg	20 mg	40 mg	80 mg				

Thus, we could talk about high potency statins and statins with limited power. Simvastatin, fluvastatin and the recent pitavastatin are intermediate. LDL-C reduction capacity is the main factor to consider when choosing the drug, because it determines beforehand the tool's contribution to achieving the therapeutic goal [8-14]. Table 1 shows each statin's capacity for reducing LDL-C.

Pleiotropic Properties

Apart from their lipid-lowering effects, statins are attributed antithrombotic, antiinflammatory and antioxidant properties. These features are known as the *pleiotropic effects* of statins [5]. The main mechanism that explains these effects (independent or not of lipid reduction, according to authors), is related to inhibition of the step from HMG-CoA to mevalonic acid. The reduction of mevalonate will decrease the formation of isoprenoids, which stimulate multiple proinflammatory pathways by activating migration, differentiation and cell proliferation mechanisms. Note that only some of these effects have been observed *in vitro* and that not all statins show the same effects [15]. Thus, the pleiotropic effects attributed to statins include:

- Modulation of endothelial function, by an increase in nitric acid production and a reduction in the synthesis and action of endothelin and angiotensin II.
- Antiinflammatory effects, due to the inhibition of various inflammatory cytokines. Because of their anti-inflammatory action, statins increase the stability of atheromatous plaque, reducing the accumulation of macrophages and by inhibiting the production of proteins related to thrombus formation.
- Antioxidant effects, reducing the expression of free radicals and preserving antioxidant capacity.
- Antithrombotic effects, reducing platelet aggregation and fibrinogen concentration acting through the nitric oxide pathway.

Table 2. Pleiotropic aplications of statins

System	Disorder
Cardiology	Heart failure Atrial fibrillation ventricular arrhythmias Acute coronary syndrome and percutaneous coronary intervention Aortic stenosis
Pulmonology	Asthma Chronic obstructive lung disease
Hematology/oncology	Prostate cancer Colon cancer Lung cancer Pancreatic cancer Renal cancer
Neurology	Stroke Intracranial hemorrhage Multiple sclerosis Alzheimer's disease Parkinson's disease
Nephrology	Glomerulonephritis Renal failure Renal transplantation Contrast-induced nephropathy
Rheumatology	Rheumatoid arthritis Osteoarthritis Osteoporosis Systemic sclerosis
Miscellaneous	Venous thromboembolism Polycystic ovary syndrome Macular degeneration Influenza Infection and sepsis

Several clinical trials have recently been published that open the door to a future with new applications for these drugs in therapy.

The GRACE [16] and MADIT-II [17] studies showed a lower incidence of arrhythmias in patients treated with statins. The results of STATIN STEMI [18] and ARMYDA [19] studies, showed a lower rate of complications in percutaneous angioplasty if individuals were receiving statin therapy during the previous days. *Blamoun et al* [20] obtained a lower incidence of exacerbations and need for intubation in a cohort of 185 patients diagnosed with chronic obstructive pulmonary disease and treated with statins. In oncology beneficial effects of statins were also observed; *Poytner et al* [21] in a case-control study found a 50% lower incidence of colorectal cancer and less metastatic disease in patients who had received statins for at least 5 years; in cancer lung and breast cancer, *Khurana et al* [22] obtained reductions of 55% and 67% in treatments of over 6 months with statins. Table 2 shows some of the applications of statins that arise from their pleiotropic properties.

All these properties and test results suggest a future for statins beyond coronary disease, and involve many medical disciplines including cardiology, neurology, pulmonology, nephrology and rheumatology. Thus, as has happened with other drugs such as aspirin, allopurinol or chloroquine [14], pharmacology research shows once again its dynamism.

Clinical Implications

Statins have a privileged position in lipid-lowering therapy because they are powerful and well tolerated. Their efficacy in reducing LDL-C is a highly valued quality because it fulfils therapeutic goals difficult to achieve with other drug groups [5, 14].

Clinical use of HMG-CoA reductase inhibitors is centred on two uses: in combination with a suitable diet, or when the diet is insufficient, to reduce cholesterol levels in patients with hypercholesterolemia, and as a cardiovascular preventive measure in patients with cardiovascular disease or those with risk factors such as diabetes mellitus, smoking or obesity [5, 14].

Brief Summary of Pharmacokinetic Properties

Table 3. Pharmacokinetics of statins

	Simvastatin	Lovastatin	Atorvastatin	Fluvastatin	Pravastatin	Rosuvastatin	Pitavastatin
Biodisponibility	5	5	12	20-30	18	20	51
Hepatic extraction	≥ 80	≥ 70	≥ 70	≥ 70	≤ 20	≤ 20	≤ 20
CYP3A4 metabolism	+++	+++	+++	-	+	-	-
CYP2C9 metabolism	-	-	-	+++	-	+	-

Statins are drugs that are absorbed when administered orally. Lovastatin and simvastatin are prodrugs administered as lactones.

The active hydroxy acids are formed in the cells of the intestinal mucosa and liver, whereas the other statins are active agents. They are taken orally, presenting a variable bioavailability ranging from <5% of simvastatin and lovastatin up to 75% in the case of rosuvastatin. Protein binding is high in all of them except for pravastatin and they have a very intense hepatic metabolism and high biliary excretion. All statins are metabolised by cytochrome P450, except for pitavastatin, which is metabolised through cytoplasmic enzymes. Lovastatin, simvastatin and atorvastatin are metabolised by CYP3A4, and fluvastatin by CYP2C9 *(complete with table).* It must be taken into account that many medications are metabolised through CYP3A4, and this may cause significant interactions. The plasma half-life is short, except in rosuvastatin and atorvastatin. Because of the circadian variation of HMG-CoA reductase, this short half-life makes them more effective when administered at night [5, 23]. In Table 3 are the most relevant pharmacokinetic properties of each of the statins.

Adverse Effects and Interactions

From the point of view of safety, well-documented evidence has shown that statins are generally well tolerated. Most reported side effects are mild, transient and common to many other drugs, such as skin rash, headache, and gastrointestinal upset ... Less common but more clinically relevant are the adverse effects on the muscles, liver, kidneys and nervous system. The adverse effects of statins are directly related to dosage, so that a recent meta-analysis relating the incremental risk of adverse effects with different intensities of statin dose, concluded that high doses of drugs such as atorvastatin or simvastatin 80mg were associated with a significantly increased risk of adverse effects (odds ratio(OR)=1.44; 95% IC, 1.33-1.55; $p < 0.001$) and these adverse effects led to discontinuation of treatment (OR=1.28; 95% CI, 1.18-1.39; $p<0.001$).

These doses were also associated with an increased risk of impaired liver function and significant CK elevations, with the final recommendation that intensive doses be reserved for high-risk cases, and that for most cardiovascular risk-reduction cases moderate doses are sufficient [24]. Also in patients in whom adverse effects such as myopathy cause the use of statins to be dropped, the use of low doses appears to be an option for continuing treatment [25]. Because of its greater relevance, muscle toxicity is discussed more extensively in the followings section.

- *Muscle toxicity* Approximately between 5% and 10% of patients have muscle pain without a rise in CK [26], making it the most important and documented adverse effects of statins and also the greatest reason for abandoning the treatment. Myopathy with increased CK appears in between 0.1% -0.2% of patients treated and this is multiplied by four when combining statins with fibrates [27]. The mechanism by which statins induce myotoxicity is unclear and there is no consensus of opinion. Several hypotheses suggest two mechanisms of muscle toxicity; a mechanism of toxic type (related mitochondrial reactions at intracellular level, depletion of metabolites and destabilization of cell membranes [27-29]) and other immunologically mediated causes [28-29]. It is a dose-dependent adverse effect [5] and has shown a higher incidence of myopathy in patients treated with high doses of simvastatin (160 mg) or atorvastatin (80 mg) versus low doses and/or placebo [30-32]. The muscular toxicity of statins moves in a range from mild muscle aches to severe and fatal cases of rhabdomyolysis (0.15 deaths/1000000 prescriptions) [33], with elevation of CK> 10 times the normal upper limit, tissue degradation, renal failure and death. This means that it becomes increasingly important to study the factors that may predispose a person to increased severity of muscle toxicity, relating demographic and genetic factors, existence or not of co-morbidities, concomitant medications and type and dose of statin, so that the occurrence of myopathy with a statin can be solved by more than half the patients by changing to a different one.

- *Demographic factors:* The frequency of myopathy is higher in older patients and women. Advanced age (> 80 years) is a major risk factor for myopathy in turn favoured by the inherent characteristics of elderly patients, such as polypharmacy and worsening renal function [34, 35]. Regarding myopathic risk differences between races, different studies show an increased risk in Asians, but there is only evidence of higher plasma concentrations of rosuvastatin in Asians compared to Caucasians, when both receive the same dose [36].
- *Genetic factors:* As for the influence of genetics in the occurrence of myotoxicity, we found the gene SLCO1B1 (OATP1B1 encoder) to be an important determinant of plasma statin levels [37]. It has been observed that in carriers of the SNP 521T> C, specifically the homozygous CC, peak plasma concentrations occur in the order of 274%, 221%, 144% and 65% compared to the wild genotype for pravastatin, simvastatin, atorvastatin and rosuvastatin, respectively [38-40]. The SLCO1B1 * 17 haplotype has been correlated with high concentrations of pravastatin [41, 42]. In a study in which a genome-wide scan was conducted in patients with different degrees of myopathy and who received high doses of simvastatin, it was found that 60% of cases of myopathy were attributed to a specific variant of gene SLCOB1, specifically the rs4149056C variant. Heterozygotes for this variant had four times greater incidence of myopathy, and in homozygotes, incidence was multiplied by seventeen [43]. Fluvastatin pharmacokinetics may be altered in patients with CYP2C9 * 3 and CYP2C9 * 2 in which a decrease occurs in the clearance of the drug. Also, coenzyme-Q10 is found in the interindividual variation in susceptibility to muscle toxicity of statins. Significant associations between levels of coenzyme-Q10, the gene COQ2 and patients intolerant to statin therapy have been found, but further studies [44] are needed.
- *Co-morbidities:* In the presence of renal failure, hypothyroidism, acute bacterial or viral infections [45, 46], and reduced body mass and post-critical states, risk of myotoxicity is increased [47]. Also in diabetic patients treated with statins, the incidence of myopathy is increased, particularly in elderly patients taking several kinds of drugs and with reduced kidney function [34]. For patients with pre-existing myopathy, either inherited (deficiency of carnitine-palmityl transferase II, McArdel's syndrome) or acquired (post-polio syndrome), statins can aggravate

myopathy and even increase the risk of rhabdomyolysis [48, 49]. The symptoms of myasthenia gravis may also be enhanced by the myotoxic effect of statins [50]. Liver dysfunction is considered one of the risk factors of increased plasma levels of statins due to decreased metabolism and excretion of statins. So is excessive alcohol consumption, which is itself a potential factor of muscle toxicity.

- *Type of statin:* Incidence of rhabdomyolysis has been reported more frequently to different drug control agencies in Europe and in America, in patients treated with lovastatin, simvastatin and atorvastatin, compared with the lowest incidence with fluvastatin and pravastatin [51, 52].
- *Concomitant medication:* Potent inhibitors of P-glycoprotein and the CYP3A4 cytochrome increase the risk of myopathy when combined with statins, due to increased plasma concentrations of atorvastatin, lovastatin and simvastatin mainly. One option for continuing treatment when myopathy occurs due to this interaction mechanism is the shift to fluvastatin or low doses of rosuvastatin [53]. Moderate inhibitors should be used cautiously, using the minimum possible dose and monitoring the treatment. Rosuvastatin has little affinity with cytochrome P450, so that interactions are not expected at this level, however, the product information for Rosuvastatin contraindicates combination with cyclosporine or protease inhibitors, as they can significantly increase AUC values due to inhibition of OATPB1 and / or P-glycoprotein [5, 54] Fluvastatin is metabolized by CYP2C9, but its affinity is low and the significance of the interactions is often lower. The affinity of pravastatin by cytochrome P450 is low and it is excreted virtually unmetabolised, so it is not to be associated with interactions at this level. OATP1B1 inhibitors, like gemfibrozil, cyclosporine or eltrombopag can increase plasma concentrations of statins and the risk of myotoxicity and this is more prevalent with simvastatin, lovastatin, pravastatin and rosuvastatin, due to their being hydrophilic in nature [55]. Another interaction mechanism has been described with the emergence of several cases of rhabdomyolysis in patients treated with atorvastatin and systemic fusidic acid in which the antibiotic inhibits the glucuronidation of statins, increasing plasma levels [33]. Given the seriousness of the potential interactions, it is advisable to take special precautions when using drugs with little experience of use, as is the case of sitagliptin and the recent case report of rhabdomyolysis in combination with lovastatin [56]. Regarding pharmacodynamic interactions, avoid simultaneous prescription of statins and other drugs that are directly related to the occurrence of myopathy, such as daptomycin or trabectedin [57, 58]. A myopathy case was described as caused by the interaction between atorvastatin and ezetimibe, whose mechanism is not clearly established [59]. Here too we find cases of rhabdomyolysis in patients taking large amounts of liquorice or red rice [60]. Perhaps the interaction of statins associated with muscle toxicity is that which occurs with other lipid-lowering drugs such as gemfibrozil. From the pharmacokinetic point of view, inhibition of OATPB1 by gemfibrozil will produce an increase in plasma statin levels except for fluvastatin; it can be doubled in the case of rosuvastatin [60]. However, the pharmacodynamic aspect of interaction is the best known, and shows an increased risk of adverse effects on the muscles, particularly rhabdomyolysis, by an additive mechanism at even moderate doses; this effect

was observed even after several months of combined treatment [61, 62]. The interaction of gemfibrozil with cerivastatin was what led to the suspension of sales of the latter in 2001 due to the occurrence of rhabdomyolysis whose seriousness caused the benefit / risk relationship of treatment with cerivastatin to become unfavorable.

Due to the potential seriousness that may entail the statin-induced myopathy, prevention is recommended, with particular attention given to conditions that produce elevations of CK (Table 4) and combinations with drugs that increase its plasma levels and risk of rhabdomyolysis (Table 5). If the combination with fibrates is unavoidable, fenofibrate should be preferred to gemfibrozil [63-65].

Table 4. Situations with CK elevation

Trauma
Intramuscular injections
Burn
Exercise
Rigidity
Spasm
Prolongued bed rest
Hyper and Hypothermia
Cardioversión
Stroke
Meningitis
Heart attack
Hypothyroidism
Asthma
Sepsis
Shock
Acute psycosis
Hypervitaminosis E and A
Idiopatic hyperCKemia (high CK with no demonstrable cause)

Table 5. High statin levels substances related

Ciclosporin
Macrolide Antibiotics (eritromycin, clathromycin, telithromycin)
Azole Antifungals (fluconazole, itraconazole, ketoconazole, posaconazole, voriconazole)
Calcium antagonist (verapamil, diltiazem)
Nefazodone
Protease Inhibitor (ritonavir, nelfinavir, indinavir, saquinavir)
Warfarin
Cimetidine,ranitidine
Omeprazole
Amiodarone
Fibrate (gemfibrozil)
Grapefruit juice

Fluvastatin may be the most suitable for combining with gemfibrozil [66], preferably taking the fibrate in the morning and the statin in the evening [67]. Among statin regimens least associated with myopathy are fluvastatin [68], low doses of rosuvastatin [69], atorvastatin every other day [70], or atorvastatin or rosuvastatin one or two times a week [71-76]. Depending on the intensity of clinical symptoms and the elevation of CK levels, the possible discontinuation of statin therapy should be evaluated. It is advisable to inform patients of the risk and signs of myopathy so they may recognise the symptoms and detect muscle toxicity at an early stage.

- *Neurological and neuropsychiatric symptoms and sleep disturbances:* Major neurological adverse effects described in relation to statins are the appearance of peripheral neuropathy and impaired cognitive function.

    - *Peripheral neuropathy,* the frequency of peripheral neuropathy with statins in patients is around 1/10,000 according to spontaneous reports to the Spanish Pharmacovigilance System. Peripheral neuropathy secondary to the use of statins appears after their introduction and is reversed after withdrawal. It can occur at any time with an increase in incidence from the fourth month [77]. In a cohort population-based survey and two case-control studies nested in population cohorts it was found that long-term exposure to statins may increase the risk of polyneuropathy. However, in another case-control study, no significant association between statin use and the occurrence of polyneuropathy [78] was found. Recently, an experimental study that found neurophysiological alterations in peripheral nerves of patients on long-term statin treatment was published [79]. Statin polyneuropathy is a rare problem, but it should be considered given the widespread use of this type of drug. In most cases, sensory or motor abnormalities are reduced after withdrawal of treatment.
    - *Cognitive impairment and other neuropsychiatric effects:* The effects of statins on cognitive decline are controversial. While some studies suggested beneficial effects on dementia, the number of cases associating statins with cognitive impairment [80] behavioural disorders and mood, aggression, depression [81, 82] or suicide [83] has increased. Some clinical trial data show that sleep disorders, such as nightmares or insomnia and memory loss are more common in some groups treated with statins than with placebo [84, 85], lovastatin being the one showing higher prevalence. This seems related to the higher lipophilicity of lovastatin and the ease with which it crosses the blood-brain barrier, but evidence is not conclusive and data should be interpreted with caution [84].

- *Liver toxicity:* Hepatotoxicity associated with statins contributes to their underuse and may constitute a cause of abandoning the therapy [86] at an early stage. It is manifested by elevated liver enzymes in the absence of pathophysiological changes. This hepatotoxicity is often of the hepatocellular type and very rarely cholestatic. The results of clinical trials show that elevated serum transaminases occurs in 1.2% of patients treated with high doses of statins [87]. Hepatotoxicity is considered a reversible, dose-dependent adverse effect, not related to any statin in particular but considered a class effect. Many cases of transaminase elevations resolve spontaneously without treatment withdrawal and the results of clinical trials show no significant differences in transaminase elevation with statin treatment compared with a placebo [80, 81]. Cases of liver failure directly related to the use of statins are extremely rare and its incidence is similar to what might be found in the general population [88, 89]. In patients with previous liver disorders such as non-alcoholic fatty liver disease, the incidence of elevated liver enzymes caused by treatment with statins does not appear significantly higher than in patients without lipid-lowering therapy, and these drugs can be considered safe in these patients [86, 93]. They are also seen to be safe drugs in patients with hepatitis B or C, although they can produce a marked elevation of liver enzymes in these patients [91, 92]. In patients with primary biliary cirrhosis treatment with statins, no adverse effects of relevance have been found in the liver [91, 93]. In the presence of previous liver disease, it is always necessary to consider the current degree of liver function, and its possible impact on the metabolism and excretion of statins; this means high doses of statins are not recommended in patients with moderate to severe hepatic impairment.

- *Renal toxicity:* All statins are associated with the appearance of a very low incidence of hematuria and proteinuria [94]. The occurrence of proteinuria in patients treated with statins appears to be due to the interference that the inhibition of the HMGCoA reductase produces in the process of protein re-uptake by the renal tubules [95] and many authors consider the effect of statins to be renoprotective [96], although there is no consistent evidence to this effect. Statins are not associated with acute renal failure, except in those cases where the primary cause is the occurrence of rhabdomyolysis. Their use is considered safe in patients with renal failure and in dialysis.
- *Diabetes:* HMG-CoA reductase inhibitors may increase the risk of diabetes mellitus (DM) in patients at risk of developing the disease. The benefit-risk balance of statins clearly remains favourable, although it is considered necessary to monitor these patients [97]. In December 2011, after conducting a risk assessment of onset of DM, European national drug agencies included in the statins technical specifications DM as a common adverse reaction.
- *Other side effects:* Statins are also associated with sexual dysfunction and interstitial lung disease.

References

[1] Steinberg D. The Statins in Preventive Cardiology. *N. Engl. J. Med.* 2009; 29: 541-2.

[2] Endo A. A historical perspective on the discovery of statins. *Proc. Jpn. Acad. Ser. B Phys. Biol. Sci.* 2010; 86:484-93.

[3] Brown, A.G., Smale, T.C., King, T.J., Hasenkamp, R. and Thompson, R.H. Crystal and molecular structure of compactin, a new antifungal metabolite from Penicillium brevicompactum. *J. Chem. Soc., Perkin Trans*. 1960; 1: 1165–1170.

[4] Alberts, A.W., Chen, J., Kuron, G., Hunt, V., Huff, J., Hoffman, C. et al. Mevinolin: a highly potent competitive inhibitor of hydroxymethylglutaryl-coenzyme A reductase and a cholesterol-lowering agent. *Proc. Natl. Acad. Sci. USA.* 1980; 77: 3957–3961.

[5] García-Sabina A, Gulín-Dávila J, Sempere-Serrano P, González-Juanatey C, Martínez-Pacheco R. Specific considerations on the prescription and therapeutic interchange of statins. *Farm. Hosp.* 2011 Aug 4. [Epub ahead of print].

[6] Schachter M. Chemical, pharmacokinetic and pharmacodynamic properties of statins: an update. *Fundam. Clin. Pharmacol.* 2005; 19:117-25.

[7] Liao JK. Beyond lipid lowering: the role of statins in vascular protection. *Int. J. Cardiol.* 2002; 86: 5-18.

[8] Cui Y, Watson DJ, Girman CJ, Shapiro DR, Gotto AM et al. Effects of increasing high-density lipoprotein cholesterol and decreasing low-density lipoprotein cholesterol on the incidence of first acute coronary events (from the Air Force/Texas Coronary Atherosclerosis Prevention Study). *Am. J. Cardiol.* 2009; 104: 829-34.

[9] Law MR, Wald NJ, Rudnicka AR. Quantifying effect of statins on low density lipoprotein cholesterol, ischaemic heart disease, and stroke: systematic review and meta-analysis. *BMJ.* 2003; 326: 1423-7.

[10] Juridique HJ, Hutten BA, Gagné C, Langslet G, McCrindle BW, Wiegman A, Hsia J, Kastelein JJ, Stein EA. Efficacy and safety of rosuvastatin therapy for children with familial hypercholesterolemia. *J. Am. Coll. Cardiol.* 2010; 55:1121-6.

[11] Jones PH, Davidson MH, Stein EA, Bays HE, McKenney JM, Miller E et al. Comparison of the efficacy and safety of rosuvastatin versus atorvastatin, simvastatin, and pravastatin across doses (STELLAR* Trial). *Am. J. Cardiol.* 2003; 92: 152-60.

[12] Brown WV, Bays HE, Hassman DR, McKenney J, Chitra R, Hutchinson H et al Efficacy and safety of rosuvastatin compared with pravastatin and simvastatin in patients with hypercholesterolemia: a randomized, double-blind, 52-week trial. *Am. Heart J.* 2002; 144: 1036-43.

[13] Edwards JE, Moore RA. Statins in hypercholesterolaemia: a dose-specific meta-analysis of lipid changes in randomised, double blind trials. *BMC Fam. Pract.* 2003; 4-18.

[14] García Sabina A. e-mecum. Ayuda en la toma de decisiones farmacoterapéuticas. *Editorial Médica* A.W.W.E. 2009.

[15] Mihos CG, Santana O. Pleiotropic effects of the HMG-CoA reductase inhibitors. *Int. J. Gen. Med.* 2011; 4:261-71.

[16] Vedre A, Gurm H, Froehlich J, et al. Impact of prior statin therapy on arrhythmic events in patients with acute coronary syndromes (from the Global Registry of Acute Coronary Events [GRACE]). *Am. J. Cardiol.* 2009;104:1613–1617.

[17] Vyas AK, Guo H, Moss AJ, et al. Reduction in ventricular tachyarrhythmias with statins in the Multicenter Automatic Defibrillator Implantation Trial (MADIT) II. *J. Am. Coll. Cardiol.* 2006;47:769–773.

[18] Kim JS, Kim J, Choi D, et al. Efficacy of high-dose atorvastatin loading before primary percutaneous coronary intervention in ST-segment relevation myocardial infarction: The STATIN STEMI trial. *JACC Cardiovasc. Interv.* 2010;3:332–339.

[19] Pasceri V, Patti G, Nusca A, Pristipino C, Richichi G, Di Sciascio G. Randomized trial of atorvastatin for reduction of myocardial damage during coronary intervention: Results from the ARMYDA (Atorvastatin for Reduction of MYocardial Damage during Angioplasty) trial. *Circulation.* 2004;110:674–678.

[20] Blamoun AI, Batty GN, DeBari VA, Rashid AO, Sheikh M, Khan MA. Statins may reduce episodes of exacerbation and the requirement for intubation in patients with

COPD: Evidence from a retrospective cohort study. *Int. J. Clin. Pract.* 2008; 62: 1373–1378.

[21] Poynter JN, Gruber SB, Higgins PD, et al. Statins and the risk of colorectal cancer. *N. Engl. J. Med.* 2005;352:2184–2192.

[22] Khurana V, Sheth A, Caldito G, Barkin JS. Statins reduce the risk of pancreatic cancer in humans: A case-control study of half a million veterans. *Pancreas.* 2007;34: 260–265.

[23] Schachter M. Chemical, pharmacokinetic and pharmacodynamic properties of statins: an update. *Fundam. Clin. Pharmacol.* 2005; 19:117-25.

[24] Silva M, Matheus ML, Jarvis C, Nolan NM, Belliveau P. Meta-analysis of drug-induced adverse events asociated with intensive-dose statin therapy. *Clin. Ther.* 2007; 29(2):253-60.

[25] Abd TT, Jacobson TA. Statin-induced myopathy: a review and update. *Expert Opin. Saf.* 2011; 10(3):373-87.

[26] Harris LJ, Thapa R, Brown M, Pabbathi S, Childress RD, Heimberg M, Braden R, Elam MB. Clinical and laboratory phenotype of patients experiencing statin intolerance attributable to myalgia. *J. Clin. Lipidol.* 2011; 5(4): 299-307.

[27] Kashani A, Phillips CO. Risks associated with statin therapy: a systematic overview of randomized clinical trials. *Circulation.* 2006. 114 (25): 2788-97.

[28] Needham M, Fabian V, Knezevic W, et al. Progressive myopathy with up-regulation of MHC-I associated with statin therapy. *Neuromuscular. Disord.* 2007; 17:194-200.

[29] Christopher-Stine L, Casciola-Rosen LA, Hong G, et al. A novel auto-antibody recognizing 200-Kd and 100-Kd proteins is associated with an immune-mediated necrotizing myopathy. *Arthritis Rheum.* 2010; 62: 2757-66.

[30] Davidson MH, Stein EA, Dujoune CA, et al. The efficacy and six-week tolerability of simvastatin 80 and 160mg/day. *Am. J. Cardiol.* 1997; 257(79): 38-42.

[31] De Lemo JA, Blazing MA, Wiviott SD, et al. Early intensive vs a delayed conservative simvastatin strategy in patientes with acute coronary síndromes: phase z of the A to Z trial. *JAMA.* 2005; 294: 2437-45.

[32] Pedersen TR, Faergeman O, Kastelein JP, et al. Hight-dose atorvastatin vs usual-dose simvastatin for secondary prevention after myocardial infaration.The IDEAL study: a randomized controlled trial. *JAMA.* 2005; 294: 2437-45.

[33] Magee CN, Medani SA, Leavey SF, Conlon PJ, Clarkson MR. Severe rhabdomyolysis as a onsequence of the interaction of fusidic acid and atorvastatin. *Am. J. Kidney Dis.* 2010; 56(5) e11-5.

[34] Pasternak RC, Smith SC Jr, Bairey-Merz CN, et al. and Writing Committee Members. ACC/AHA/NHLBI clinical advisory on the use and safety of statins. *Circulation.* 2002; 106: 1024-8.

[35] Armitage J. The safety of statins in clinical practice. *Lancet.* 2007; 370: 1781-90.

[36] Lee E, Ryan S, Birmingham B, et al. Rosuvastatin pharmacokinetics and pharmacogenetics in white and Asian subjects residing in the same environment. *Clin. Pharmacol. Ther.* 2005; 78(4): 330-41.

[37] Tirona RG, Leake BF, Merino G, et al. Polymorphisms in OATP-C; identification of multiple allelic variants associated with altered transport activity among European and Africa-Americans. *J. Biol. Chem.* 2001; 276: 35669-75.

[38] Niemi M, Pasanen MK, Neuvonen PJ. SLCO1B1 polymorphism and sex affect the pharmacokinetics of pravastatin but non fluvastatin. *Clin. Pharmacol. Ther.* 2006: 80(4): 356-366.

[39] Pasanen MK, Fredrikson H, Neuvonen PJ, Niemi M. Different effects of SLCO1B1 polymorphism on the pharmacokinetics of atorvastatin and rosuvastatin. *Clin. Pharmacol. Ther.* 2007: 82(6): 726-733.

[40] Pasanen MK, Neuvonen M, Neuvonen PJ, Niemi M. SLCO1B1 polymorphism markedly affects the pharmacokinetics of simvastatin acid. *Pharmacogenet Genomics.* 2006; 16(12): 873-879.

[41] Niemi M, Schaeffeler E, Lang T, Fromm MF, Neuvonen M, Kyrklund C, Backman JT, Kerb R, Scwab M, Neuvonen PJ, Eichelbaum M, Kivisto KT. High plasma pravastatin concentrations are associated with single nucleotide polymorphism and haplotypes of organic anion transporting polypeptide-C (OATP-C, SLCO1B1). *Pharmacogenetics.* 2004; 14(7): 429-440.

[42] Niemi M, Neuvonen PJ, Hofmann U, Backman JT, Schwab M, Lutjohann D, von Bergmann K, Eichelbaum M, Kivisto KT. Acute effects of pravastatin on cholesterol synthesis are associated with SLCO1B1 (encoding OATP1B1) haplotype *17. *Pharmacogenet Genomics.* 2005: 15(5): 303-309.

[43] The SEARCH Collaborative Group. SLCO1B1 variants and statin-induced myopathy; a genomewide study. *N. Engl. J. Med.* 2008; 359(8):789-99.

[44] Oh J, Ban MR, Miskie BA, et al. Genetic determinants of statin intolerance. *Lipids Health Dis.* 2007; 6:7.

[45] Wong WM, Wai-Hung Shek T, Chan KH. Rhabdomyolisis triggered by cytomegalovirus infection in a heart transplant patient on concomitant cyclosporine and atorvastatin theraphy. *Gastroenterol. Hepatol.* 2004; 19(8):952-3.

[46] Finsterer J, Zuntner G. Rhabdomyolysis from simvastatin triggered by infection and muscle exertion. *South Med. J.* 2005; 98(8):827-9.

[47] Wilhemi M, Winterhalter M, Fisher S, et al. Massive post operative rhabdomyolysis following combined CABG/addominal aortic replacement: a possible association with HMG-coA reductase inhibitors. Cardiovasc. *Drugs Ther.* 2002; 16(5): 471-5.

[48] Leung NM, Ooi TC, McQueen MJ. Use of statins and fibrates in hyperlipidemic patients with neuromuscular disorders. *Arch. Interm. Med.* 2000; 132: 418-9.

[49] Franc S, Bruckert E, Giral P, et al. Rhabdomyolysis in patients with preexisting myopathy, treated with antilipemic agents. *Presse Med.* 1997; 26: 1855-8.

[50] Oh SJ, Dhall R, Young A, et al. Statins may aggravate myasthenia gravis. *Muscle Nerve.* 2008; 38: 1101-7.

[51] Chang JT, Staffa JA, Parks M, Green L. Rhabdomyolysis with HMG coA reductase inhibitors and gemfibrozil combination therapy. *Pharmacoepidemiol Drug Saf.* 2004; 13: 417-426.

[52] Heart Protection Study Collaborative Group. MRC/BHF Heart Protection Study of cholesterol lowering with simvastatina in 20,536 high-risk individualist: a randomized placebo-controlled trila. *Lancet.* 2002; 360: 7-22.

[53] Joy TR, Hegele RA. Narrative review; statin related myopathy. *Am. Internd. Med.* 2009; 160(12): 885-6.

[54] Crestor®(Rosuvastatina). Ficha técnica. Disponible en: https://sinaem4.agemed.es/consaem.

[55] Neuvonen PJ, Backman JT, Niemi M. Pharmacokinetic comparison of the potential over-the-counter statins simvastatin, lovastatin, fluvastatin and pravastatin. *Clin. Pharmacokinetic*. 2008; 47(7): 463-74.
[56] Robert V, Digregorio, Pharm D. Rhabdomyolysis caused by a potential sitagliptin-lovastatin interaction. *Pharmacotherapy*. 2009; 29 (3): 352-6.
[57] Cubicin® (Daptomicina) Ficha técnica. Disponible en: http://www.ema.europa.eu/docs/es_ES/document_library/EPAR_-_Product_Information/human/000637/WC500036049.pdf.
[58] Yondelis® (Trabectedina) Ficha ténica. Disponible en: http://www.ema.europa.eu/docs/es_ES/document_library/EPAR_-_Product_Information/human/000773/WC500045832.pdf.
[59] Wefflad LA, Flach LA. Myopathy associated with atorvastain-ezetimiba combination therapy. *Pharmacotherapy*. 2007; 27(2): 309-11.
[60] Scneck DW, Birmingham BZ, Zalikowski JA, Mitchell PD, Wang Y, et al. The effect of gemfibrozil on the pharmacokinetics of rosuvastatin. *Clin. Pharmacol. Ther*. 2004; 75: 455-63.
[61] Unal A, Torun E, Sipahioglo MH, Torgoz B, Kaya MG, et al. Fenofibrato induced acute renal failure due to massive rhabdomyolysis after coadminitration of statin in two patiens. *Inetrn. Med.* 2008; 47 (11): 1017-9.
[62] Cummins D, Mackey M, Baker E. Recovery time in a case of gemfibrozil and simvastatin associated rhabdomyolysis. *Southern Medical Journal*. 2009;102: 858-60.
[63] Bottorff MB. Statin safety and drug interactions: clinical implications. *Am. J. Cardiol.* 2006; 97 Suppl: 27-31C.
[64] Franssen R, Vergeer M, Stroes ES, et al. Combination statin-fibrate therapy; safety aspects. *Diabetes Obes. Metab*. 2009; 11(2): 89-94.
[65] Davidson MH, Armani A, Mc Kenney JM, et al. Safety considerations with fibrate therapy. *Am. J. Cardiol*. 2007; 99 Suppl: 3-18C.
[66] Spence JD, Munoz CE, Hendricks L, et al. Pharmacokinetics of the combination of fluvastatin and gemfibrozil. *Am. J. Cardio*l. 1995; 76 Suppl: 80-3A.
[67] San Vicente Blanco R, Pérez Irazusta I, Ibarra Amarica J, Berraindo Zabalegui I, Uibe Oyarbida F, el al. Guía de práctica clínica sobre el manejo de los lípidos como factor de riesgo cardiovasculñar (internet). Vitoria-Gasteiz:osakidetza; 2008. Disponible en: www.guíasalud.es.
[68] Stein EA, Ballantyne CM, Windler E, et al. Efficacy and tolerability of fluvastatin XL 80mg alone, ezetimibe alona, and the combination of fluvastatin XL 80mg with ezetimibe in patients with a history of muscle-related side effects with other statins. *Am. J. Cardiol.* 2008; 101: 490-6.
[69] Glueck CJ, Aregawi D, Agloria M, et al. Rosuvastatin 5 and 10mg/d: a pilot study of the effects in hypercholesterolemic adults unable to tolerate other statins and reach LDLcholesterol goals with non statin lipid-lowering therapies. *Clin. Ther.* 2006; 28:733-42.
[70] Matalka MS, Raunan MC, Deedwania PC. Is alternate daily dose of atorvastatin effective in treating patients with hyperlypidemia? The alternate day versus daily dosing of atorvastatin study (ADDAS). *Am. Heart J.* 2002; 144: 674-7.
[71] Juszcyk MA, Seip RL, Thompson PD. Decreasing LDL cholesterol and medication cost with every-other-day statin therapy. *Prev. Cardiol.* 2005; 8:197-9.

[72] Athyros VG, Tzomalos K, Kkafika Al, Koumaras H, Karagiannia A, Mikhailidis DP. Effectiveness of ezetimibe alone or in combination with twice a week Atorvastatin (10mg) for statin intolerant high-risk patients. *Am. J. Cardiol.* 2008; 101(4): 483-5.

[73] Backes JM, Venero CV, Gibson CA, et al. Effectiveness and tolerability of every-other day rosuvastatin dosing in patients with prior statin intolerance. *Ann. Pharmacother.* 2008; 42: 341-16.

[74] Backes JM, Moriarty PM, Ruisinger JF, et al. Effects of one weekly rosuvastatin among patients with a prior statin intolerance. *Am. J. Cardiol.* 2007; 100: 554-5.

[75] Mackie BD, Satija S, Nell C, et al. Monday, Wednesday, and Friday dosing of rosuvastatin in patients previously intolerant to statin therapy (letter). *Am. J. Cardiol.* 2007; 99: 291.

[76] Gardale M, Kearns A, Thompson PD. Efficacy of rosuvastatin (5mg and 10mg) twice a week in patients intolerant to daily statins. *Am. Cardiol.* 2008; 10(12): 1747-8.

[77] Gaist D, García Rodriguez LA, Huerta C, Halls J, Sindrup SH. Are users lipid-lowering drugs at increased risk pf peripheral neuropathy? *Eur. J. Clin. Pharmacol.* 2001; 56:931-3.

[78] Law M, Rudnicka AR. Statin safety: a systematic review. *Am. J. Cardiol.* 2006; 97: 52-60.

[79] Otruba P, Kanovsky P, Hlustik P. Treatmente with statins and peripheral neuropathy: results of 36-months a prospective clinical and neurophysiological follow-up. *Neuro Endocrinol. Lett.* 2011; 32(5): 688-690.

[80] Evans MA, Golomb BA. Statin-associated adverse cognitive effects: survey results from 171 patients. *Pharmacotherapy*. 2009; 29 (7): 800-11.

[81] Davery Smith G, Song F, Sheldon TA. Cholestero llowering and mortality: the importance of considering initial level of risk. *BMJ.* 1993; 306:1367-73.

[82] Morgan R, Palinkas L, Barrett-Connor E, et al. Plasma cholesterol and depressive symptoms in older man. *Lancet.* 1993; 341: 75-9.

[83] Muldoon MF, Manuck SB, Matthews KA. Lowering cholesterol concentrations and mortality. *BMJ.* 1990; 301: 309-14.

[84] Tuccori M, Lapi F, Testi A, et al. Statin-associated psychiatric adverse events. *Drug Saft.* 2008; 31: 1115-23.

[85] Black DM, Lamkin G, Olivera EH, et al. Sleep disturbance and HMG co A reductase inhibitors. *JAMA*. 1990; 264:1105.

[86] Rzoug FS, Volk ML, Hatoum HH, et al. Hepatotoxicity fears contribute to underutilization of statin nedications by primary care physicians. *Am. J. Med. Sci.* 2010; 340: 89-93.

[87] LaRosa JC, Grundy SM, Waters DD, et al. Intensive lipid lowering with atorvastatin in patients with stable coronary disease. *N. Engl. J. Med.* 2005; 352: 1425-35.

[88] Calderon RM, Cubeddu LX, Golberg RB, et al. Statins in the treatment of dyslipidemia in the presence of elevated liver aminotranferase levels: a therapeutic dilemma. *Mayo Clin. Proc.* 2010; 85: 349-56.

[89] Bhardwaj SS. Lipid lowering agents that cause drug-induced hepatotoxicity. *Clin. Liver Dis.* 2007; 11: 597-613.

[90] Wiesinger HA, Shah J, White A, et al. Liver biochemistry abnormalities in a quaternary care lipid clinic database. *Ann. Hepatol.* 2008; 7: 63-6.

[91] Tandra S, Vuppalenchi R. Use of statins in patients with liver disease. *Curr. Treat. Options Cardiovasc. Med.* 2009; 11: 272-8.

[92] 3-hydroxyl-3methylglutaril coenzyme A reductasa inhibitor use in chronic liver disease:a therapeutic controversy. *J. Clin. Lipidol.* 2011; 5(6): 450-9.

[93] Aburajab MA, Kaplan MM.Statin use patients with primary biliary cirrhosis (PBC): are they safe? *Clin. Gastroenterol. Hepatol.* 2006; 4: 838-9.

[94] Bays H. Statin safety: an overview assessment of the data 2005. *Am. J. Cardiol.* 2006; 97: 6C-26C.

[95] Agarwal R. Statin induced proteinuria: renal injury or renoprotection? *J. Am. Soc. Nephrol.* 2004; 15: 2502-3.

[96] Brown WV. Safety of statins. *Cur. Opin. Lipidol.* 2008; 19: 558-62.

[97] http://www.aemps.gob.es/informa/informeMensual/211/diciembre/docs/informe-mensual_diciembre-2011.pdf.

In: Statins
Editors: Benedetta La Grua and Alessandro Molinelli
ISBN: 978-1-62081-367-6

Chapter VI

Statins: Pharmacology, Clinical Implications and Adverse Effects

Novo Salvatore and Mignano Antonino
Chair of Cardiovascular Diseases, Centre for the Early Diagnosis of Preclinical and Multifocal Atherosclerosis and for Secondary Prevention, Division of Cardiology, University Hospital "Paolo Giaccone", University of Palermo, Italy

Abstract

Statins, the most used lipid-lowering drugs, act classically like inhibitors of HMG-CoA reductase enzyme, blocking one of the most important cholesterol pathways. Reducing production of endogen cholesterol, statins determine an increased expression of LDL receptors that consent removal of "bad cholesterol" from blood by the liver; a reduction of VLDL hepatic production that induce an hipotrygliceridemic effect too; and at the same time an increased HDL production according to statin's different kind. Indeed, statins effectiveness is different and it is demonstrated that atorvastatin and rosuvastatina are more effective than simvastatin, pravastatin, lovastatin and fluvastatin. About their use in clinical practice, physicians exploit their classic effect and their pleiotropic effect too. Statins improve endothelial function, plaque stability and reduce inflammation and platelet aggregation. So today, statins are a very important weapon in the hand of physician. Specifically, importance of statins in secondary prevention of coronary heart disease (CHD) is established from a long time but their use in CHD primary prevention is still discussed because, if the protective effect is proven, on the other hand NNT and costs are so high. Statins find another important employment in prevention of periprocedural outcomes in patients that undergo PCI. For their capacity of plaque stabilization and inflammation lowering, and for an emerging direct effect on Central Nervous System (CNS), statins use is broadened to prevent ischemic stroke and, for the same reason, it is demonstrated their preventing role in CHF progression in particular in patients with metabolic syndrome. At least statins are helpful for management of patients with peripheral artery disease where symptoms reduction and progression are proved. Moreover it was tried to use them in subjects with aortic valve stenosis too, but it is unclear if there is an effective benefit in terms of progression of disease. On the other side, statins are burdened with important side effects that need accurate follow up, considering onset of symptoms, increased hepatic enzyme and attendant use of drugs that interact with P450 cytochrome or that increase myopathy possibility, like fibric acid derivates. Indeed, classical side effects of statins are hepatotoxicity and myopathy up to rhabdomyolysis. These side effects haven't an important incidence but they are more common in case of combination of statins and fibrates. It is also important underline like today research involves itself in study of correlation between statins and cancer and like this dispute is still open. The twelve years follow-up of the 4S studies showed not an increase but a decrease of new cases of cancer using simvastatin.

Introduction

Statins are one of the most used drugs in the world. In this chapter we want to stress statins pharmacology, their clinical use and side effects that they can determinate. So, writing about their history, their mechanism of action, their interactions, their typical and emerging use, we want to clarify how today statins represent an important weapon in the hands of physician, and in particular of cardiologist specialist, for the care of important genetic and acquired diseases like familial hypercholesterolemia, coronary artery disease, stroke, peripheral arterial disease and so on.

History

Akira Endo, researcher of Sankyo Company, is the discover of the first inhibitor of 3 hydroxyl—methyl glutaryl coenzyme A reductase that he named mevastatin. In 1976 he isolated this substance from a Penicillium Citrinum extract, studying its effect in rat liver and demonstrating its mechanism of action. However, at first time, these discovers haven't a clinical relevance because of side effects, presumed toxicity on cell wall and because cholesterol role in cardiovascular diseases weren't verified. We need to wait for Brown and Goldstein in the early 1970s that, studying patients with familial hypercholesterolemia, determined a decreased cholesterol production after statins use; in these patients usually cholesterol is high for lack of LDL receptors. After that Merck Sharp & Dohme develops lovastatin but, like Sankyo, stopped its researches for important toxic effects on gastrointestinal system and on cataract development. Only after extensive testing on animals, FDA approved statins in 1987 and only after 1994, 4S study, using Simvastatin, threw a light on role of study in secondary prevention of coronary disease for the first time. Today after withdrawn from the market of cerivastatin in 2001, statins on the market are fluvastatin, lovastatin, mevastatin, pitavastatin, pravastatin, rosuvastatin, simvastatin and atorvastatin that in 2003 became the most sell drug in history [1].

Pharmacology

Statins, inhibitors of HMGCoA reductase, act like reversible competitive inhibitor thanks to a lateral group that is similar to mevalonic acid.

Reducing conversion of HMGCoA to mevalonic acid, statins inhibit precociously this important pathway of cholesterol production at hepatic level and determine an increased expression of LDL receptors after SREBP split and relocation to nucleus. Once in the nucleus, SREBP can bind to specific DNA sequences (the sterol regulatory elements or SREs) that are found in the control regions of the genes that encode enzymes needed to lipids regulation. Specifically in the LDL receptor the recognition site is 5′-ATCACCCCAC-3′, which is designated sterol regulatory element 1 (SRE-1) [2]. Kim et al. showed that the ability of SREBPs to recognize a direct, rather than inverted, repeat depends on a tyrosine that replaces an arginine found in all other bHLH-Zip proteins [3, 4].

Increased LDL receptors reduce principally "bad cholesterol" and at the same time reduce VLDL hepatic production recognising ApoE that is an important component of VLDL. This effect can explain effective of statins in homozygous familial hypercholesterolemia where there is lack of LDL receptors [4, 5].

The same mechanism can explain reduced level of triglycerides that is more evident in patients with tryclicerides levels higher than 250 mg/dl [6].

Another important effect of statins is increment of HDL levels that can change depending on statin efficacy that is higher for simvastatin than atorvastatin but lower than rosuvastatin considering comparable dose [7, 8].

Considering LDL reduction, it emerge from literature like simvastatin is three times more effective than pravastatin and lovastatin, 2 times than fluvastatin but 2 times less than atorvastatin and 4 times than rosuvastatin [9].

As a result of the common biosynthetic pathway Coenzyme Q (ubiquinone) and dolichol levels are also affected, to a certain degree, by the treatment with these HMG-CoA reductase inhibitors. Plasma levels of CoQ_{10} are lowered in the course of statin treatment. This could be related to the fact that statins lower plasma LDL levels, and CoQ_{10} is mainly transported by LDL, but a decrease is also found in platelets and in lymphocytes of statin treated patients, therefore it could truly depend on inhibition of CoQ_{10} synthesis. There are also some indications that statin treatment affects muscle ubiquinone levels, although it is not yet clear to which extent this depends on some effect on mitochondrial biogenesis. Some papers indicate that CoQ_{10} depletion during statin therapy might be associated with subclinical cardiomyopathy and this situation is reversed upon CoQ_{10} treatment [10].

However, classic effects doesn't explain all of benefits that derive from their use and for this reason pharmacologists speak about pleiotropic effect of statins defining it like non depending on cholesterol lowering effect.

In particular these effects consist in a reduction of esterified cholesterol accumulation into macrophages; in an increased endothelial NO synthesis; in an increased stability of atherosclerotic plaque due to matrix metalloproteinase inhibition and to reduced smooth muscular cells proliferation; in an improved endothelial function and in a decreased inflammation, like demonstrated in different studies that correlate statins use with lower PCR; in a reduced oxidized LDL that are more cytotoxic and atherogenic like oxidative stress mediators; and in an inhibited platelet aggregation and so inhibited thrombogenic response [11-14].

In addiction to these effects on cardiovascular system, it is emerging how statins act on immune system, CNS and bone level by inhibition isoprenoids and so inhibition of small GTP binding proteins [15]. A case-control study, that was published on JAMA, demonstrated that use of statins the prior 180 days (adjusted OR, 0.50; 95% confidence interval, 0.33-0.76) or prior 3 years (adjusted OR, 0.57; 95% confidence interval, 0.40-0.82) was associated with a significant reduction in the risk of hip fracture, even after controlling for variables such as race, insurance status, psychoactive medications, estrogen and thiazide use, ischemic heart disease, cancer, and diabetes mellitus. No significant relationship was observed between use of nonstatin lipid-lowering agents and hip fracture risk [16].

It is important to consider that all of these described pleiotropic effects occur manly after use of an high dose as demonstrated from different studies like the ATHEROMA study where were studied effects of low-dose (10 mg) and high-dose (80 mg) of atorvastatin on carotid plaque inflammation as determined by ultrasmall super paramagnetic iron oxide (USPIO)-enhanced carotid magnetic resonance imaging (MRI), showing a reduction of macrophage activity [17].

About pharmacokinetics after oral administration, absorption changes from 30% to 85%. The majority of the statins have a low circulation concentration: 12% for atorvastatin, 17% for pravastatin, 20-30 % for fluvastatin, 5% for simvastatin and lovastatin. Important first passage effect by liver exists and excretion is hepatic after bio-transformation by different CYP Cytochrome depending on statin different kind. In particular for their liver metabolism, lovastatin, simvastatin, atorvastatin and cerivastatin follow the cytochrome P450 (CYP 3A4) pathway. Fluvastatin follows the CYP 2C9 pathway, and pravastatin is metabolized differently. Atorvastatin, cerivastatin, fluvastatin and pravastatin are administered as active compounds (acid form). Lovastatin and simvastatin are administered as inactive forms (lactone), which have to be enzymatically hydrolyzed to generate active forms [18].

It is important to consider that interindividual differences can exist about statins efficacy depending on genetic profile of patients that can change in relation to all of genes involved in pharmacokinetics of statins and so in genes that code for proteins that are involved in drug transport, drug target pathway and drug metabolism.

In a recent study DNA of 1536 individuals treated with pravastatin, 40 mg/d, was analyzed for 148 single-nucleotide polymorphisms (SNPs) within 10 candidate genes related to lipid metabolism. Variation within these genes was then examined for associations with changes in lipid levels observed with pravastatin therapy during a 24-week period. Two common and tightly linked SNPs (linkage disequilibrium $r^2 = 0.90$; heterozygote prevalence = 6.7% for both) were significantly associated with reduced efficacy of pravastatin therapy. Both of these SNPs were in the gene coding for 3-hydroxy-3-methylglutaryl-coenzyme A (HMG-CoA) reductase, the target enzyme that is inhibited by pravastatin. For example, compared with individuals homozygous for the major allele of one of the SNPs, individuals with a single copy of the minor allele had a 22% smaller reduction in total cholesterol (−32.8 vs −42.0 mg/dL [−0.85 vs −1.09 mmol/L]; $P = .001$; absolute difference, 9.2 mg/dL [95% confidence interval, 3.8-14.6 mg/dL] and a 19% smaller reduction in low-density lipoprotein (LDL) cholesterol (−27.7 vs −34.1 mg/dL [−0.72 vs −0.88 mmol/L]); $P = .005$; absolute difference, 6.4 mg/dL [95% CI, 2.2-10.6 mg/dL]. The association for total cholesterol reduction persisted even after adjusting for multiple tests on all 33 SNPs evaluated in the HMG-CoA reductase gene as well as for all 148 SNPs evaluated was similar in magnitude and direction among men and women and was present in the ethnically diverse total cohort as well as in the majority subgroup of white participants. No association for either SNPs was observed for the change in high-density lipoprotein (HDL) cholesterol ($P > .80$) and neither was associated with baseline lipid levels among those actively treated or among those who did not receive the drug. Among the remaining genes, less robust associations were found for squalene synthase and change in total cholesterol, apolipoprotein E and change in LDL cholesterol, and cholesteryl ester transfer protein and change in HDL cholesterol, although none of these met conservative criteria for purely pharmacogenetic effects [19].

And another study showed that after adjustment for covariates, carriers of the ABCB1 1236T variant allele had a greater reduction in total cholesterol and low-density lipoprotein cholesterol with simvastatin treatment, as compared with homozygotes with the wild-type allele (-29.0% [95% CI, -25.9 to -32.5]) versus -24.2% [95% CI, -19.0 to -29.3] [P = .042] and -39.6% [95% CI, -35.8 to -44.0] versus -33.8% [95% CI, -27.4 to -40.2] [P = .042], respectively). Similar results were observed for the 2677G >A/T polymorphism and haplotype data. The 1236T, 2677non-G, and 3435T alleles were less frequent in ADR cases than in the non-ADR group (P < .05 for all single-nucleotide polymorphisms). Haplotype analyses also demonstrated a reduction of the T-non-G-T haplotype frequency (20%) in patients in whom myalgia developed during simvastatin treatment, as compared with the non-ADR group (41.4%) (P = .03). No significant associations were observed between the CYP3A4 -392A>G and CYP3A5*3 allele variants and the efficacy or tolerability of simvastatin [20].

Clinical Use

Use of statins increased with increased indication in a lot of disease conditions.

Naturally statins born like drugs to use in every kind of hypercholesterolemia, in particular for the familiar one, but it is important consider that we can use statins for heterozygous form because in the homozygous form their effect is reduced for lack of LDL receptors expression.

Certainly after more then 30 years from their discovery, statins role is sure for secondary prevention of coronary disease.

Like demonstrated in a lot of trials like 4S study that is the first one, or the ASCOT-LLA study, statins reduce significantly possibility of a secondary event in patients that had a first coronary event. In particular 4S study demonstrated like use of simvastatin in patients with angina pectoris or previous CHD guarantee a 37% reduction in the risk of undergoing revascularization procedures and improves survival. Exactly the relative risk of death in the simvastatin group was 0.70 (95% CI 0.58-0.85, p = 0.0003) and 0.58 (95% CI 0.46-0.73) for coronary death. About incidence of major coronary events. The relative risk was 0.66 (95% CI 0.59-0.75, p < 0.00001), and the respective probabilities of escaping such events were 70.5% and 79.6% [21].

ASCOTT-LLA study, in the same way, underlines a reduction of total cardiovascular events and in particular in a population of 19342 hypertensive patients, 100 primary events had occurred in the atorvastatin group compared with 154 events in the placebo group with an hazard ratio of 0,64 (95% CI 0.50–0.83, p=0.0005) and this benefit emerged in the first year of follow-up [22].

All of these considerations are the base of current guidelines of American College of Cardiology/ American Heart Association that provide a class 1, level of evidence A for initiating statins in pre-discharge stage and for LDL target of <100 and the same is for ESC guidelines for STEMI. For NSTEMI European Society of Cardiology recommends a target of

<70 mg/dL with a class 1, level of evidence B. All of these guidelines underline that statin therapy should be initiated as soon as possible [23-24].

Role of statins is more discussed for primary prevention because is unclear real benefit that statins can have in patients with high cardiovascular risk [25-27].

A Cochrane review demonstrated reduction of the most relevant outcomes, considering 14 randomised controlled trials dating from 1994 to 2006. In this review 34,272 participants were included. Eleven trials recruited patients with specific conditions (raised lipids, diabetes, hypertension, and microalbuminuria). All-cause mortality was reduced by statins (RR 0.84, 95% CI 0.73 to 0.96) as was combined fatal and non-fatal CVD endpoints (RR 0.70, 95% CI 0.61 to 0.79). Benefits were also seen in the reduction of revascularisation rates (RR 0.66, 95% CI 0.53 to 0.83). Total cholesterol and LDL cholesterol were reduced in all trials but there was evidence of heterogeneity of effects. There was no clear evidence of any significant harm caused by statin prescription or of effects on patient quality of life [28].

Another prospective meta-analysis of data from 90056 participants in 14 randomised trials of statins shows a 12% proportional reduction in all-cause mortality per mmol/L reduction in LDL cholesterol (rate ratio [RR] 0.88, 95% CI 0.84–0.91; $p < 0.0001$). This reflected a 19% reduction in coronary mortality (0.81, 0.76–0.85; $p<0.0001$), and non-significant reductions in non-coronary vascular mortality (0.93, 0.83–1.03; $p=0.2$) and non-vascular mortality (0.95, 0.90–1.01; $p=0.1$). These benefits were significant within the first year, but were greater in subsequent years [29].

Similar results are confirmed in an important recent trial, the JUPITER that demonstrated reduction of incidence of major cardiovascular events and death, in 17802 healthy patients with high PCR, marker of systemic inflammation, and with LDL cholesterol <130 mg/dl and so in patients without classical indications to rosuvastatin treatment.

Specifically rosuvastatin reduced LDL cholesterol levels by 50% and high-sensitivity C-reactive protein levels by 37%. The rates of the primary end point were 0.77 and 1.36 per 100 person-years of follow-up in the rosuvastatin and placebo groups, respectively (hazard ratio for rosuvastatin, 0.56; 95% confidence interval, 0.46 to 0.69; $p<0.00001$), with corresponding rates of 0.17 and 0.37 for myocardial infarction (hazard ratio, 0.46; 95% CI, 0.30 to 0.70; $p=0.0002$), 0.18 and 0.34 for stroke (hazard ratio, 0.52; 95% CI, 0.34 to 0.79; $p=0.002$), 0.41 and 0.77 for revascularization or unstable angina (hazard ratio, 0.53; 95% CI, 0.40 to 0.70; $p<0.00001$), 0.45 and 0.85 for the combined end point of myocardial infarction, stroke, or death from cardiovascular causes (hazard ratio, 0.53; 95% CI, 0.40 to 0.69; $p<0.00001$), and 1.00 and 1.25 for death from any cause (hazard ratio, 0.80; 95% CI, 0.67 to 0.97; $p=0.02$) [30-31].

And these aren't the only one works in literature that underline this new emerging employment possibility of statins.

To complete this overview on role of statins in management of patients with CHD, it is important to consider that statins have important beneficial effects in patients that undergoes to percutaneous coronary interventions.

Thanks to capacity of plaque stabilization and to effect on platelet aggregability, statins periprocedural use permits improvement of all of outcomes, a reduction of myocardial damage during angioplasty.

These data are clear in the ARMYDA-Recaptured study that demonstrated how statins use have important periprocedural benefits in terms of outcomes in 383 patients with chronic stable angina or with NSTEMI. Indeed in this population there was lower incidence of postprocedural creatine kinase-myocardial band and troponin-I elevation greater than the upper limit of normal in the atorvastatin arm (13% vs. 24%, $p = 0.017$, and 37% vs. 49%, $p = 0.021$, respectively) and multivariable analysis identified atorvastatin reload as a predictor of decreased risk of 30-day incidence of major adverse cardiac events odds ratio: 0.50, 95% confidence interval: 0.20 to 0.80; $p = 0.039$), mainly in patients with acute coronary syndromes (82% relative risk reduction; $p = 0.027$) [32]. Likewise, the NAPLES II study underlines how 80 mg of atorvastatin the day prior to PCI prevent primary endpoints and specifically incidence of a periprocedural MI was 9.5% in the atorvastatin group and 15.8% in the control group (odds ratio: 0.56; 95% confidence interval: 0.35 to 0.89; $p = 0.014$) [33].

Moreover in a sub-study of PROVE IT-TIMI22, patients that receive high dose of atorvastatin versus lower dose have better outcomes after PCI. Kaplan–Meier curves of this study estimate of the rates of the primary end point at two years were 26.3 percent in the pravastatin group and 22.4 percent in the atorvastatin group, reflecting a 16 percent reduction in the hazard ratio in favour of atorvastatin ($P=0.005$; 95 % confidence interval, 5 to 26 %) [34].

Heart failure is another important condition where physicians can use statins with important benefits. They may inhibit or reverse myocardial remodelling, inhibit inflammation, improve endothelial function and restore anatomic nervous system balance.

A recent meta-analysis on eleven trials with 590 patients confirmed these data and demonstrated and improvement of cardiac function and clinical symptoms too. Pooled analysis showed that statin treatment was associated with a significant increase in left ventricular ejection fraction (WMD: 3.35%, 95% CI: 0.80 to 5.91%, $P = 0.01$). The beneficial effects of statin treatment were also demonstrated by the reduction of left ventricular end-diastolic diameter (WMD: -3.77 mm, 95% CI: -6.24 to -1.31 mm, $p = 0.003$), left ventricular end-systolic diameter (WMD: -3.57 mm, 95% CI: -6.37 to -0.76 mm, $p = 0.01$), B-type natriuretic peptide (WMD: -83.17 pg/mL, 95% CI: -121.29 to -45.05 pg/mL, $p < 0.0001$), and New York Heart Association functional class (WMD: -0.30, 95% CI: -0.37 to -0.23, $p < 0.00001$) [35]. Other works explain that these advantages occur also in severe heart failure and in patients with heart failure and metabolic syndrome in elderly patients [36-38]. Our group studied statins use in another field that is peripheral artery diseases [39-40]. In the management of this disease it is important start statins to exploit a triple effect: anti-inflammatory effect, anti-proliferation one and anti-thrombotic one. Considering mortality in these patients it's know that this is reduced with statins independent to CRP and D-Dimer levels and considering symptoms, they can reduce claudicatio intermittens, increasing meters that patients can walk without pain or discomfort [41]. The last application field for statin that we want to consider is aortic stenosis [42-45]. Different trials were conducted in this sense and in particular ASTRONOMER one demonstrated that statins didn't have any role in progression of stenosis or of diastolic dysfunction; so they aren't recommended in patients with aortic stenosis and without conventional indications for statins [46].

Adverse Effects and Interactions

The most important adverse effects of statins are myopathy and asymptomatic increase of hepatic transaminases.

In terms of percentage they are infrequent but they are common because statins are often used.

About hepatotoxicity, this occurs in 1% of case and it is dose dependent. Severe hepatotoxicity is rare but FDA reported 30 case of hepatotoxicity from 1987 to 2000. it is indicate to control transaminases levels after 3 months of use start and if normal it isn't necessary repeat them again. Sometimes this elevation is reversal but however statins are contraindicated in cholestasis and active liver diseases [47].

Myopathy is the second classical side effect but is the most important one. A common complaint is non specific muscle aches without associated increases in creatin-kinase without muscular pains. Severe myositis is rare and they are characterized by muscle aches, soreness, or weakness with associated elevated creatine kinase [48]. All of these can lead to rhabdomyolysis, myoglobinuria and acute renal necrosis. Myositis usually occurs in patients that use statins in combinations with other drugs and usually cyclosporine, fibrates, macrolide antibiotics and niacin.

About fatal rhabdomyolysis, FDA reports one case in a million of prescription among different statins but this is not for cerivastatin. Indeed rate of fatal rhabdomyolysis was 50 times higher for cerivastatin in monotherapy and for this reason it withdrawn from the market [49]. It is not clear the mechanism of myopathy but same data suggest an effect on mitochondrial respiratory pattern and a correlation with exercise as statins can exacerbate exercise induced skeletal muscle injury. However usually the mechanism at base of interaction is inhibition of cytochrome P450. [50-53].

To resume these considerations, these are conclusions of a big metanalysis reported in literature: "Eighteen trials including 71,108 persons, and 301,374 person-years of follow-up were represented in this analysis. There were 36,062 persons receiving a statin and 35,046 receiving a placebo. Statin therapy increased the risk of any adverse effect by 39% 9 (OR = 1.4; 95% CI, 1.09-1.80; p = 0.008; NNH ([number needed to harm] = 197) compared with placebo. Statins were associated with a 26% reduction in the risk of a clinical cardiovascular event (OR = 0.74; 95% CI, 0.69-0.80; p < 0.001; number needed to treat = 27). Treating 1000 patients with a statin would prevent 37 cardiovascular events, and 5 adverse effects would be observed. Serious events (creatine phosphokinase >10 times the upper limit of normal or rhabdomyolysis) are infrequent (NNH = 3400) and rhabdomyolysis, although serious, is rare (NNH = 7428). Atorvastatin was associated with the greatest risk of AEs and fluvastatin with the least risk. Simvastatin, pravastatin, and lovastatin had similar odds of AEs. Non urgent AEs such as myalgia and liver function elevations were responsible for approximately two thirds of AEs reported in trials." [54].

Despite these adverse effects, clinical benefit of statins is substantial so it is important to consider how to reduce possibility of side effects to exploit all statins power.

Statins and Cancer

Research today involves itself in study of correlation between statins and cancer and in particular different studies try to understand if statins can reduce cancer onset.

An important work on NEJM in 2005 demonstrated in 3968 patients a significant reduction of colorectal cancer risk after adjustment for other known risk factors. Indeed In analyses including 1953 patients with colorectal cancer and 2015 controls, the use of statins for at least five years was associated with a significantly reduced relative risk of colorectal cancer (odds ratio, 0.50; 95 percent confidence interval, 0.40 to 0.63). This association remained significant after adjustment for the use or nonuse of aspirin or other nonsteroidal anti-inflammatory drugs; the presence or absence of physical activity, hypercholesterolemia, and a family history of colorectal cancer; ethnic group; and level of vegetable consumption (odds ratio, 0.53; 95 percent confidence interval, 0.38 to 0.74) [55].

Another study find similar results for lung cancer: Of the 483,733 patients in this retrospective case-control study, 163,662 patients (33.8%) were receiving statins and 7,280 patients (1.5%) had a primary diagnosis of lung cancer. Statin use > 6 months was associated with a risk reduction of lung cancer of 55% (adjusted odds ratio, 0.45; 95% confidence interval, 0.42 to 0.48; $p < 0.01$). Furthermore, the protective effect of statin was seen across different age and racial groups and was irrespective of the presence of diabetes, smoking, or alcohol use [56].

Despite this, many of other studies didn't find a significant correlation like a on American Journal of Medicine published meta-analysis where estimated differences in absolute risk between statins treatment and placebo were as follows (negative risks indicate that treatment was safer than placebo): all nonfatal cancers, 0.0% (95% confidence interval : –0.8% to 0.8%); all fatal cancers, –0.1% (95% CI: –0.7% to 0.4%); all fatal and nonfatal cancers combined, –0.1% (95% CI: –1.0% to 0.7%); and all-cause mortality, –1.5% (95% CI: 2.8% to 0.2%) [57]. And more, another meta-analysis that was published in 2006 on JAMA shows in 6662 incident cancers and 2407 cancer deaths, that statins did not reduce the incidence of cancer (OR, 1.02; 95% CI, 0.97-1.07) or cancer deaths (OR, 1.01; 95% CI, 0.93-1.09) for any individual cancer type, and that this null effect on cancer incidence persisted when only hydrophilic, lipophilic, naturally derived, or synthetically derived statins were evaluated.

Conclusions of this study were: Statins have a neutral effect on cancer and cancer death risk in randomized controlled trials [58].

Naturally all of these results need to be confirmed or controvert a big blinded randomised trial that doesn't exist; so it is difficult say if there is a positive or negative or neutral correlation between statins and cancer and the debact is still open [59].

Conclusion

Evidence shows that statins can be used in all of described conditions but their management needs a watchful assessment of patient to choose the best drug and the best dosage. Goal of physician is attainment of guidelines cholesterol target that is different considering global cardiovascular risk of patient. New frontier in statins pharmacology is genetic background estimate to establish an appropriate therapy and so to avoid important described adverse effects.

Considering emerging role of statins in fields like oncology or aortic stenosis it is important to wait more data that can arrive only from big double blind randomized controlled trials.

References

[1] Stossel T.P., The Discovery of Statins. *Cell* 2008 Sep;134 (6):903-905.

[2] Yokoyama C., Wang X., Briggs M.R., Admon A., Wu J., Hua X., Goldstein J.L., Brown M.S., SREBP-1, a basic-helix–loop–helix-zipper protein that controls transcription of the low density receptor gene. 1993 *Cell* 75:185–197.

[3] Kim J.B., Spotts G.D., Halvorsen Y.D., Shih H.M., Ellenberger T., Towle H.C., Spiegelman B.M., Dual DNA binding specificity of ADD1/SREBP-1 controlled by a single amino acid in the basic helix–loop–helix domain. 1995 *Mol Cell Biol* 15:2582–2588.

[4] Horton J.D., Goldstein J.L., Brown MS., SREBPs: activators of the complete program of cholesterol and fatty acid synthesis in the liver. *J Clin Invest.* 2002 May;109(9):1125-31.

[5] Aguilar-Salinas CA, Barrett H, Schonfeld G. Metabolic modes of action of the statins in the hyperlipoproteinemias. Atherosclerosis. 1998 Dec;141(2):203-7.

[6] Ginsberg H.N., Effects of statins on triglyceride metabolism. *Am J Cardiol.* 1998 Feb 26;81(4A):32B-35B.

[7] Course J.R., Kastelein J., Isaacsohn J., et al. A large, 36 week study of the HDL-C raising effects and safety of Simvastatin versus atorvastatin. *Atherosclerosis* 2000; 151: 8–9.

[8] Hunninghake D.B., Stein E.A., Bays H.E., et al. Rosuvastatin improves the atherogenic and atheroprotective lipid profiles in patients with hypertriglyceridemia. *Coron Artery Dis.* 2004 Mar;15(2):115-23.

[9] Jones P., Kafonek S., Laurora I., Hunninghake D., Comparative dose efficacy study of atorvastatin versus simvastatin, pravastatin, lovastatin, and fluvastatin in patients with hypercholesterolemia (the CURVES study). *Am J Cardiol.* 1998 Mar 1;81(5):582-7.

[10] Littarru G.P., Langsjoen P., Coenzyme Q10 and statins: biochemical and clinical implications. *Mitochondrion.* 2007 Jun;7 Suppl:S168-74

[11] Liao J.K., Laufs U., Pleiotropic effects of statins. *Annu Rev Pharmacol Toxicol.* 2005;45:89-118.

[12] Albert M.A., Danielson E., Rifai N., et al, Effect of statin therapy on C-reactive protein levels: the pravastatin inflammation/CRP evaluation (PRINCE): a randomized trial and cohort study. *JAMA.* 2001 Jul 4;286(1):64-70.

[13] Koh K.K., Sakuma I., Quon M.J., Differential metabolic effects of distinct statins. *Atherosclerosis.* 2011 Mar;215(1):1-8.

[14] Heart Protection Study Collaborative Group. C-reactive protein concentration and the vascular benefits of statin therapy: an analysis of 20,536 patients in the Heart Protection Study. *Lancet.* 2011 Feb 5;377(9764):469-76.

[15] Liao J.K., Laufs U., Pleiotropic effects of statins. *Annu Rev Pharmacol Toxicol,* 2005;45:89-118.

[16] Wang P.S., Solomon D.H., Mogun H., Avorn J., HMG-CoA reductase inhibitors and the risk of hip fractures in elderly patients. *JAMA.* 2000 Jun 28;283(24):3211-6.

[17] Tang T.Y., Howarth S.P., Miller S.R., et al. The ATHEROMA (Atorvastatin Therapy: Effects on Reduction of Macrophage Activity) Study. Evaluation using ultrasmall

superparamagnetic iron oxide-enhanced magnetic resonance imaging in carotid disease. *J Am Coll Cardiol.* 2009 Jun 2;53(22):2039-50.

[18] Stancu C., Sima A., Statins: mechanism of action and effects. *J Cell Mol Med.* 2001 Oct-Dec;5(4):378-87.

[19] Chasman D.I., Posada D., Subrahmanyan L., et al. Pharmacogenetic study of statin therapy and cholesterol reduction. *JAMA*. 2004 Jun 16;291(23):2821-7.

[20] Fiegenbaum M., da Silveira F.R., Van der Sand C.R., et al. The role of common variants of ABCB1, CYP3A4, and CYP3A5 genes in lipid-lowering efficacy and safety of simvastatin treatment. *Clin Pharmacol Ther.* 2005 Nov;78(5):551-8.

[21] Scandinavian Simvastatin Survival Study Group. Randomised trial of cholesterol lowering in 4444 patients with coronary heart disease: the Scandinavian Simvastatin Survival Study (4S). *Lancet.* 1994 Nov 19;344(8934):1383-9.

[22] Sever P.S., Dahlöf B., Poulter N.R., et al. Prevention of coronary and stroke events with atorvastatin in hypertensive patients who have average or lower-than-average cholesterol concentrations, in the Anglo-Scandinavian Cardiac Outcomes Trial--Lipid Lowering Arm (ASCOT-LLA): a multicentre randomised controlled trial. *Lancet.* 2003 Apr 5;361(9364):1149-58.

[23] Van de Werf F., Bax J., Betriu A., et al. Management of acute myocardial infarction in patients presenting with persistent ST-segment elevation: the Task Force on the Management of ST-Segment Elevation Acute Myocardial Infarction of the European Society of Cardiology. *Eur Heart J.* 2008 Dec;29(23):2909-45.

[24] Hamm C.W., Bassand J.P., Agewall S., et al. ESC Guidelines for the management of acute coronary syndromes in patients presenting without persistent ST-segment elevation: The Task Force for the management of acute coronary syndromes (ACS) in patients presenting without persistent ST-segment elevation of the European Society of Cardiology (ESC). *Eur Heart J.* 2011 Dec;32(23):2999-3054.

[25] Lewis S.J., Lipid-lowering therapy: who can benefit? *Vasc Health Risk Manag.* 2011;7:525-34.

[26] McElduff P., Jaefarnezhad M., Durrington P.N., American, British and European recommendations for statins in the primary prevention of cardiovascular disease applied to British men studied prospectively. *Heart.* 2006 Sep;92(9):1213-8.

[27] Brugts J.J., Yetgin T., Hoeks S.E., et al. The benefits of statins in people without established cardiovascular disease but with cardiovascular risk factors: meta-analysis of randomised controlled trials. *BMJ.* 2009 Jun 30;338:b 2376.

[28] Taylor F., Ward K., Moore T.H., et al. Statins for the primary prevention of cardiovascular disease. *Cochrane Database Syst Rev.* 2011 Jan 19;(1):CD004816.

[29] Baigent C., Keech A., Kearney P.M., et al. Efficacy and safety of cholesterol-lowering treatment: prospective meta-analysis of data from 90,056 participants in 14 randomised trials of statins. *Lancet.* 2005 Oct 8;366(9493):1267-78.

[30] Albert M.A., Glynn R.J., Fonseca F.A., et al. Race, ethnicity, and the efficacy of rosuvastatin in primary prevention: the Justification for the Use of Statins in Prevention: an Intervention Trial Evaluating Rosuvastatin (JUPITER) trial. *Am Heart J.* 2011 Jul;162(1):106-14.e2.

[31] Kostapanos M.S., Elisaf M.S. JUPITER and satellites: Clinical implications of the JUPITER study and its secondary analyses. *World J Cardiol.* 2011 Jul 26;3(7):207-14.

[32] Di Sciascio G., Patti G., Pasceri V., et al. Efficacy of atorvastatin reload in patients on chronic statin therapy undergoing percutaneous coronary intervention: results of the ARMYDA-RECAPTURE (Atorvastatin for Reduction of Myocardial Damage During Angioplasty) Randomized Trial. *J Am Coll Cardiol.* 2009 Aug 4;54(6):558-65.

[33] Briguori C., Visconti G., Focaccio A,. et al. Novel approaches for preventing or limiting events (Naples) II trial: impact of a single high loading dose of atorvastatin on periprocedural myocardial infarction. *J Am Coll Cardiol.* 2009 Dec 1;54(23):2157-63.

[34] Rouleau J., Improved outcome after acute coronary syndromes with an intensive versus standard lipid-lowering regimen: results from the Pravastatin or Atorvastatin Evaluation and Infection Therapy-Thrombolysis in Myocardial Infarction 22 (PROVE IT-TIMI 22) trial. *Am J Med.* 2005 Dec;118 Suppl 12A:28-35.

[35] Zhang L., Zhang S., Jiang H., et al. Effects of statin treatment on cardiac function in patients with chronic heart failure: a meta-analysis of randomized controlled trials. *Clin Cardiol.* 2011 Feb;34(2):117-23.

[36] Fazio G., Amoroso G.R., Barbaro G., Novo G., Novo S., The role of statins in preventing the progression of congestive heart failure in patients with metabolic syndrome. *Curr Pharm Des*. 2008;14(25):2605-12.

[37] Zhang L., Zhang S., Jiang H., et al. Effects of statin treatment on cardiac function in patients with chronic heart failure: a meta-analysis of randomized controlled trials. *Clin Cardiol.* 2011 Feb;34(2):117-23.

[38] Horwich T.B., MacLellan W.R., Atorvastatin and statins in the treatment of heart failure. *Expert Opin Pharmacother*. 2007 Dec;8(17):3061-8.

[39] Aronow W.S., Office management of peripheral arterial disease. *Am J Med.* 2010 Sep;123(9):790-2.

[40] Vidula H., Tian L., Liu K., et al. Comparison of effects of statin use on mortality in patients with peripheral arterial disease with versus without elevated C-reactive protein and d-dimer levels. *Am J Cardiol.* 2010 May 1;105(9):1348-52.

[41] Coppola G., Novo S.. Statins and peripheral arterial disease: effects on claudicatio, disease progression, and prevention of cardiovascular events. Arch Med Res. 2007 Jul;38(5):479-88.

[42] Rossebø A.B., Pedersen T.R., Boman K., et al. Intensive lipid lowering with simvastatin and ezetimibe in aortic stenosis. *N Engl J Med.* 2008 Sep 25;359(13):1343-56.

[43] Cowell S.J., Newby D.E., Prescott R.J., et al. A randomized trial of intensive lipid-lowering therapy in calcific aortic stenosis. *N Engl J* . 2005 Jun 9;352(23):2389-97.

[44] Novo G., Fazio G., Visconti C., et al. Atherosclerosis, degenerative aortic stenosis and statins. *Curr Drug Targets*. 2011 Jan;12(1):115-21.

[45] Shavelle D.M., Takasu J., Budoff M.J., et al. HMG CoA reductase inhibitor (statin) and aortic valve calcium. *Lancet*. 2002 Mar 30;359(9312):1125-6.

[46] Chan K.L., Teo K., Dumesnil J.G., et al. Effect of Lipid lowering with rosuvastatin on progression of aortic stenosis: results of the aortic stenosis progression observation: measuring effects of rosuvastatin (ASTRONOMER) trial. *Circulation*. 2010 Jan 19;121(2):306-14.

[47] Cohen D.E., Anania F.A., Chalasani N.; National Lipid Association Statin Safety Task Force Liver Expert Panel. An assessment of statin safety by hepatologists. *Am J Cardiol.* 2006 Apr 17;97(8A):77C-81C.

[48] Thompson P.,D., Clarkson P., Karas R.H., Statin-associated myopathy. *JAMA*. 2003 Apr 2;289(13):1681-90.

[49] Graham D,J,, Staffa J,A,, Shatin D,, et al. Incidence of hospitalized rhabdomyolysis in patients treated with lipid-lowering drugs. *JAMA*. 2004 Dec 1;292(21):2585-90.

[50] Bellosta S., Paoletti R., Corsini A., Safety of statins: focus on clinical pharmacokinetics and drug interactions. *Circulation*. 2004 Jun 15;109(23 Suppl 1):III50-7.

[51] Bottorff M.B., Statin safety and drug interactions: clinical implications. *Am J Cardiol*. 2006 Apr 17;97(8A):27C-31C.

[52] McKenney J.M., Davidson M.H., Jacobson T.A., et al. Final conclusions and recommendations of the National Lipid Association Statin Safety Assessment Task Force. *Am J Cardiol*. 2006 Apr 17;97(8A):89C-94C.

[53] Armitage J. The safety of statins in clinical practice. *Lancet*. 2007 Nov 24;370(9601):1781-90.

[54] Silva M.A., Swanson A.C., Gandhi P.J., Tataronis GR. Statin-related adverse events: a meta-analysis. *Clin Ther*. 2006 Jan;28(1):26-35.

[55] Poynter J.N., Gruber S.B., Higgins P.D., et al. Statins and the risk of colorectal cancer. *N Engl J Med*. 2005 May 26;352(21):2184-92.

[56] Khurana V, Bejjanki H.R., Caldito G., Owens M.W. Statins reduce the risk of lung cancer in humans: a large case-control study of US veterans. *Chest*. 2007 May;131(5):1282-8.

[57] Bjerre L.M., LeLorier J. Do statins cause cancer? A meta-analysis of large randomized clinical trials. *Am J Med*. 2001 Jun 15;110(9):716-23.

[58] Dale K.M., Coleman C.I., Henyan N.N., Kluger J., White CM. Statins and cancer risk: a meta-analysis. *JAMA*. 2006 Jan 4;295(1):74-80.

[59] Marelli C, Gunnarsson C, Ross S,et al. Statins and risk of cancer: a retrospective cohort analysis of 45,857 matched pairs from an electronic medical records database of 11 million adult Americans. *J Am Coll Cardiol*. 2011 Jul 26;58(5):530-7.

In: Statins
Editors: Benedetta La Grua and Alessandro Molinelli ISBN: 978-1-62081-367-6

Chapter VII

Alzheimer's Disease Risk-Lowering Effect of Lipophilic Statins

Elisa Biondi*
Facoltà di Scienze Biologiche - Università di Torino
Torino, Italy

Abstract

Alzheimer's Disease (AD) is considered to be a multifactorial neurodegenerative disorder with a strong genetic component and the role of cholesterol in this pathology is attracting increasing attention. The association of genetic alterations of proteins involved in cholesterol production, distribution and removal from the central nervous system (CNS) and an higher risk of AD point an important link between this lipid and neurodegenerative disease.

Cholesterol has well-known neuroprotective effects, influences synaptic function and its disturbed homeostasis is involved in the pathogenesis of AD.

The use of pharmacological methods to reduce plasma cholesterol levels may have little effect on brain cholesterol if the drugs cannot cross the Blood-Brain-Barrier (BBB) but the most prescribed Statins for AD theraphies are lipophilic ones and long-term treatments could have adverse effects; in fact, a recent study shows an impaired synaptic vesicle release when neuronal cholesterol biosynthesis is inhibited with Lovastatin.

Probably Statins anti-atherosclerotic pleiotropic properties have influenced the outcome of many studies on AD patients because their anti-oxidant and anti-inflammatory effects improve oxygenation of the brain and they be responsible for the apparent reduction in AD risk.

Further studies are required, especially trials able to compare side effects on neuronal cholesterol of hydrophilic statins versus lipophilic ones and design of new drugs in neuropathology field must focus on the importance of brain lipidic pool, avoiding any alteration of it.

Keywords: Alzheimer's Disease, Statins, Cholesterol, Blood-Brain-Barrier

* E-mail: elisan@libero.it.

Alzheimer's Disease (AD) is a progressive and irreversible neuropathology with a diagnosis often missed or delayed because early symptoms resemble natural sign of ageing. Changes occurring in this disease are represented by extracellular senile plaques caused by Amyloid Beta protein (Abeta) accumulation, neurofibrillary tangles constituted by hyperphosphorylated Tau protein, synaptic alterations and inflammatory response. Amyloid peptide derives from the processing of the transmembrane Amyloid Precursor Protein (APP) and its production is a physiological event, necessary for several cellular functions, but changes in molecular composition of the membrane correlated with alteration in lipid concentration, could have an effect on APP cleavage creating a toxic accumulation of neuronal plaques.

Cholesterol is an essential component of the phospholipidic bilayer and for many years the importance of cholesterol in the Central Nervous System (CNS) hasn't been considered but a lot of studies suggest its beneficial role in the brain, one of the lipogenic human organs and the most richest in this lipid; cholesterol is crucial for the correct functioning of the CNS where is required for the formation of synapses, for the electrical transmission, and is the major component of the myelin sheath. Moreover, alteration of membrane cholesterol could affect APP cleavage, promoting Abeta toxic accumulation (amyloidosis) inside brain tissues.

Postmortem examinations of AD patients brains revealed that there is a reduction in the lipid bilayer width and low neuronal cholesterol concentration ; moreover, the association of genetic alteration of several proteins involved in the production and transport of cholesterol in the CNS and an increased risk of AD may point an important link between this sterol and neurodegenerative disease.

Brain cholesterol is independent from its serum oscillations and is originated from *de novo* synthesis by astrocytes, oligodendrocytes and in a small amount by neurons which use glial lipoprotein-derived cholesterol to maintain their extensive plasma membranes and synapses, and convert it to 24-hydroxycholesterol for excretion from the brain; for this reason the use of dietary or pharmacological methods to reduce circulating cholesterol levels and to increase HDL/LDL ratios may have little effect on its brain content.

Several clinical trials showed that patients with elevated serum cholesterol treated with blood cholesterol lowering drugs present a decreased incidence of AD and these evidence had led to the controversial hypothesis that high serum lipid levels results in Abeta protein accumulation in the brain and, for this reason, statins have been normally prescribed to AD patients.

Statins are pluripotent agents exhibiting multiple non-lipid lowering actions, like reducing oxidative stress, immunomodulatory , anti-inflammatory and anticoagulant effects blocking the production and the activity of reactive oxygen; their therapeutic use in hypercholesterolemia, dyslipidemias, metabolic syndrome and coronary heart disease is totally justify by current evidences but in neuropathologies like AD, conflicting messages coming from a great deal of reports and possible alterations in brain lipidic content caused by Blood-Brain-Barrier (BBB)-penetrating statins must focus the attention on the hyphotesis that these drugs could be not appropriate therapeutic tools for this kind of disease.

Studies on rodents showed that the treatment of the animals with Lovastatin, a lipophilic statin able to cross the BBB, causes amyloid production and senile plaques deposition.: a treatment over a period of 23 days caused an altered membrane function in young and middle-age mice and before complete destruction of the neuritic network a decrease in dendritic outgrowth, attenuated axonal branching and depolymerization of microtubules associated with hyperphosphorylation of tau protein were observed [1].

Clinical studies examinig statin treatments have not produced consistent data: in patients with mild to moderate AD, Atorvastatin (another lipophilic statin) can reduce cholesterol levels and improve cognitive impairment and subjects with advanced AD do not receive any benefit from the drug [2,3,4]. Several results showed an involvement of cholesterol in the production and/or degradation of the Abeta peptide: in particular, in this sense, much effort has been paid in determine the implication of cholesterol-rich lipid rafts in Abeta metabolism, being this membrane domains well known to play a central role in membrane-occurring signalling events.

Mailman *et al.* [5] demonstrated how inhibition of neuronal cholesterol biosynthesis with Lovastatin leads impaired synaptic vesicle release : after treatment of primary hippocampal neurons with low level of Lovastatin for one week neither lipoproteins nor geranylgeraniol fully counteracted the drug-induced decrease of vesicle exocytosis, even when cholesterol depletion was prevented. They also tried to restore neuronal cholesterol synthesis with Mevalonate but this treatment prevented vesicle alterations without fully normalizing neuronal lipid content. A lot of findings suggest that statins affected not only the formation of new synapses, but also synapse maturation or remodeling [6].

For this reason the use of statins in older subjects with neurological disorders should be revised and exhaustive trials comparing the effects of lipophilic versus hydrophilic ones must be done. High throughput screenings on statins must be done using in vitro BBB model: this kind of procedure substantially reduces the use of experimental animals, facilitates the process of obtaining a functional in vitro BBB system, can gives predictions about whether a compounds' interaction with the BBB is likely to compromise its functionality and results were similar to the standard co-cultured system.

Other kind of compounds, like Probucol, a non-statin cholesterol-loweing drug with anti-inflammatory and antioxidant properties, can low levels of Abeta peptide avoiding possible statins side effects (liver damage, neuropathy, rhabdomyolysis, memory loss), but commercial power of this product is uncomparable to statins' one and no sufficient clinical trials were actually performed.

Santos *et al.* [7] showed for the first time *in vivo* how Probucol is able to counteract the cognitive/biochemical impairments induced by intracerebroventricular (i.c.v) injection of aggregated Abeta peptides in an experimental model of AD, but the correct mechanism related to the beneficial effects of Probucol cannot be completely explained only based on these results. More recently, Pallebage-Gamarallage *et al.* [8] found that Probucol also suppresses enterocytic accumulation of Abeta peptide induced by saturated fat and cholesterol feeding.

The field of lipid lowering drugs is full of controversies that must be cleared up and non-statin drugs could be promising molecules for further pharmacological studies on the search for therapeutic strategies to treat and/or prevent Alzheimer's Disease. The importance of cholesterol in the CNS has been underestimated for many years and therapeutical approach for neuropathology must take new directions, designing new molecules able to restore histological and chemical alterations caused by AD,even if the pass the BBB and act directly inside the brain.

References

[1] Eckert GP; Kirsch C; Mueller WE. Differential effects of Lovastatin treatment on brain cholesterol levels in normal and apoE-deficient mice. *NeuroReport*, 2001, 12, 883-887.

[2] Sparks DL; Lopez J; Connor D; Sabbagh M; Seward J; Browne P. A position paper: based on observational data indicating an increased rate of altered blood chemistry requiring withdrawal from the Alzheimer's Disease Cholesterol Lowering Treatment Trial. *J. Mol. Neurosci.*, 2003, 20, 407-410.

[3] Sparks DL; Sabbagh MN; Connor DJ *et al.* Atorvastatin for the treatment of mild to moderate Alzheimer's Disease: preliminary results. *Arch. Neurol.*, 2005, 62,753-757.

[4] Sparks DL; Sabbagh MN; Connor DJ *et al.* Atorvastatin therapy lowers circulating cholesterol but not free radical activity in advance of identifiable clinical benefit in the treatment of mild-to-moderate AD. *Curr. Alzheimer Res.*, 2005, 2, 343-353.

[5] Mailman T; Hariharan M; Karten B. Inhibition of neuronal cholesterol biosynthesis with Lovastatin leads to impaired synaptic vesicle release even in the presence of lipoproteins or geranylgeraniol. *J Neur*, accepted article, doi: 10.1111/j.1471-4159.2011.07474.x.

[6] Bruel-Jungerman E; Davis S; Laroche S. Brain plasticity mechanisms and memory: A party of four. *Neuroscientist*, 2007, 13, 492-505.

[7] Santos DB; Peres KC; Ribeiro R *et al.* Probucol, a lipid-lowering drug, prevents cognitive and hippocampal synaptic impairments induced by amyloid beta peptide in mice. *Exp Neurol.*, 2012, accepted article, doi: 10.1016/j.expneurol.2011.11.036.

[8] Pallebage-Gamarallage MM; Galloway S; Takechi R; Dhaliwal S; Mamo JC. Probucol suppresses enterocytic accumulation of amyloid-beta induced by saturated fat and cholesterol feeding. *Lipids*, 2012, 47(1), 27-34.

Index

B

C

D

E

F

G

H

I

J

K

N

Q

R

S

T

U

V

W

X

Y